Oral and Maxillofacial Pain

Editor

STEVEN J. SCRIVANI

ORAL AND MAXILLOFACIAL SURGERY CLINICS OF NORTH AMERICA

www.oralmaxsurgery.theclinics.com

Consulting Editor
RICHARD H. HAUG

August 2016 • Volume 28 • Number 3

ELSEVIER

1600 John F. Kennedy Boulevard • Suite 1800 • Philadelphia, Pennsylvania, 19103-2899

http://www.oralmaxsurgery.theclinics.com

ORAL AND MAXILLOFACIAL SURGERY CLINICS OF NORTH AMERICA Volume 28, Number 3
August 2016 ISSN 1042-3699, ISBN-13: 978-0-323-45981-5

Editor: John Vassallo; j.vassallo@elsevier.com
Developmental Editor: Colleen Viola

Oral and Maxillofacial Surgery Clinics of North America (ISSN 1042-3699) is published quarterly by Elsevier Inc., 360 Park Avenue South, New York, NY 10010-1710. Months of issue are February, May, August, and November. Business and Editorial Offices: 1600 John F. Kennedy Blvd., Suite 1800, Philadelphia, PA 19103-2899. Periodicals postage paid at New York, NY and additional mailing offices. Subscription prices are $385.00 per year for US individuals, $628.00 per year for US institutions, $100.00 per year for US students and residents, $455.00 per year for Canadian individuals, $753.00 per year for Canadian institutions, $520.00 per year for international individuals, $753.00 per year for international institutions and $235.00 per year for Canadian and foreign students/residents. To receive student/resident rate, orders must be accompanied by name or affiliated institution, date of term, and the *signature* of program/residency coordinator on institution letterhead. Orders will be billed at individual rate until proof of status is received. Foreign air speed delivery is included in all *Clinics* subscription prices. All prices are subject to change without notice. **POSTMASTER:** Send address changes to *Oral and Maxillofacial Surgery Clinics of North America,* Elsevier Periodicals **Customer Service, 11830 Westline Industrial Drive, St. Louis, MO 63146. Tel: 1-800-654-2452 (U.S. and Canada); 314-447-8871 (outside U.S. and Canada). Fax: 314-447-8029. E-mail: journals customerservice-usa@elsevier.com (for print support); journalsonlinesupport-usa@elsevier.com (for online support).**

Reprints. For copies of 100 or more, of articles in this publication, please contact the Commercial Reprints Department, Elsevier Inc., 360 Park Avenue South, New York, NY 10010-1710. Tel.: 212-633-3874; Fax: 212-633-3820; Email: reprints@elsevier.com.

Oral and Maxillofacial Surgery Clinics of North America is covered in *MEDLINE/PubMed (Index Medicus), Science Citation Index Expanded (SciSearch®), Journal Citation Reports/Science Edition,* and *Current Contents®/Clinical Medicine.*

Contributors

CONSULTING EDITOR

RICHARD H. HAUG, DDS
Professor and Chief, Oral Maxillofacial Surgery,
Carolinas Medical Center, Charlotte, North
Carolina

EDITOR

STEVEN J. SCRIVANI, DDS, DMSc
Director, Orofacial Pain Residency Training
Program, Chief, Division of Oral and
Maxillofacial Pain, Department of Oral and
Maxillofacial Surgery, Massachusetts General
Hospital, Boston, Massachusetts

AUTHORS

JEREMY J. ABBOTT, DDS
West Coast Ear, Nose and Throat Medical
Group, Thousand Oaks, California

JORDAN BACKSTROM, MDiv, PsyD
Boston Pain Care Center, Waltham,
Massachusetts

ZAHID H. BAJWA, MD
Director, Clinical Research, Boston Pain Care;
Director, Boston Headache Institute; Lecturer,
Tufts University School of Medicine, Waltham,
Massachusetts

JENNIFER BROWNSTEIN, MA
Department of Diagnostic Sciences,
Craniofacial Pain and Headache Center, Tufts
University School of Dental Medicine;
Department of Anesthesia, Critical Care and
Pain Medicine, Massachusetts General
Hospital, Harvard Medical School, Boston,
Massachusetts

GLENN T. CLARK, DDS, MS
Professor and Program Director; Orofacial Pain
Graduate Residency Program; Director of
Orofacial Pain and Oral Medicine Center,
Herman Ostrow School of Dentistry of USC,
Los Angeles, California

SHUCHI DHADWAL, DMD
Department of Diagnostic Sciences, Craniofacial
Pain and Headache Center, Tufts University
School of Dental Medicine, Boston,
Massachusetts

DAVID DiBENNEDETTO, MD, DABPM
Department of Diagnostic Sciences, Boston
Pain Care, Tufts University School of Dental
Medicine, Boston, Massachusetts

RAYMOND DIONNE, DDS, PhD
Research Professor, Department of
Pharmacology, Brody School of Medicine,
East Carolina University, Schools of Medicine
and Dental Medicine, Greenville, North
Carolina

MARY HIL EDENS, DDS
Resident, Oral Medicine Residency
Program, Department of Oral Medicine,
Carolinas Healthcare System, Charlotte,
North Carolina

ELIAV ELI, DMD, PhD
Professor; Director, Eastman Institute for Oral
Health, University of Rochester Medical
Center, Rochester, New York

MATTHEW FINKELMAN, PhD
Department of Biostatistics and Experimental Design, Tufts University School of Dental Medicine, Boston, Massachusetts

JAMES FRICTON, DDS, MS
Senior Researcher, HealthPartners Institute for Education and Research, Professor Emeritus, University of Minnesota School of Dentistry, Edina, Minnesota

DONALD GOODMAN, PhD
Lecturer; Director of Psychological Services, Graduate Orofacial Pain Program, UCLA School of Dentistry, Los Angeles, California

STEVEN B. GRAFF-RADFORD, DDS
The Pain Center; Director, The Program for Headache and Orofacial Pain, Cedars-Sinai Medical Center; Adjunct Professor, UCLA School of Dentistry, Los Angeles, California

MIRIAM GRUSHKA, MSc, DDS, PhD
Certified Specialist, Oral Medicine, Diplomate, American Board of Oral Medicine, Diplomate, American Board of Orofacial Pain, Active Staff, William Osler Health Centre, Toronto, Ontario, Canada

HOWARD A. ISRAEL, DDS
Professor of Clinical Surgery, Division of Oral amd Maxillofacial Surgery, Weill-Cornell Medical College, Cornell University, New York, New York

YASSER KHALED, BDS, MDSc, MMSc
Resident, Oral Medicine Residency Program, Department of Oral Medicine, Carolinas Healthcare System, Charlotte, North Carolina

SHEHRYAR N. KHAWAJA, BDS, MS
Resident, Orofacial Pain Training Program, Department of Oral and Maxillofacial Surgery, Massachusetts General Hospital, Boston, Massachusetts

GARY D. KLASSER, DMD
Certificate Orofacial Pain, Associate Professor, Department of Diagnostic Sciences, Louisiana State University Health Sciences Center, School of Dentistry, New Orleans, Louisiana

JONATHAN K. KLEEN, MD, PhD
UCSF Department of Neurology, University of California San Francisco Medical Center, San Francisco, California

RONALD J. KULICH, PhD
Department of Diagnostic Sciences, Craniofacial Pain and Headache Center, Tufts University School of Dental Medicine; Department of Anesthesia, Critical Care and Pain Medicine, Massachusetts General Hospital, Harvard Medical School, Boston, Massachusetts

MORRIS LEVIN, MD
UCSF Headache Center, UCSF Department of Neurology, University of California San Francisco Medical Center, San Francisco, California

ROBERT L. MERRILL, DDS, MS
Clinical Professor; Director, Graduate Orofacial Pain Program, UCLA School of Dentistry, Los Angeles, California

JOEL J. NAPEÑAS, DDS, FDSRCS(Ed)
Director, Oral Medicine Residency Program, Department of Oral Medicine, Carolinas Healthcare System, Charlotte, North Carolina

MARIELA PADILLA, DDS, MEd
Assistant Professor; Assistant Director of Distance Education, Herman Ostrow School of Dentistry of USC, Los Angeles, California

BENOLIEL RAFAEL, BDS (Hons)
Professor, Department of Diagnostic Sciences; Associate Dean for Research; Director, Center for Orofacial Pain and Temporomandibular Disorders; Rutgers School of Dental Medicine, Rutgers, The State University of New Jersey, Newark, New Jersey

SARAVANAN RAM, DDS, MS
Associate Professor and Program Director; Oral Medicine Graduate Residency Program, Herman Ostrow School of Dentistry of USC, Los Angeles, California

STEVEN J. SCRIVANI, DDS, DMSc
Director, Orofacial Pain Residency Training
Program, Chief, Division of Oral and
Maxillofacial Pain, Department of Oral
and Maxillofacial Surgery, Massachusetts
General Hospital, Boston,
Massachusetts

SARAH S. SMITH, ANP-BC, GNP-BC
Nurse Practitioner, Boston Pain Care,
Boston Headache Institute, Waltham,
Massachusetts

TEICH SORIN, DMD, MBA
Associate Professor; Associate Dean of Clinical
Operations, Department of Comprehensive
Care, CWRU School of Dental Medicine,
Cleveland, Ohio

EGILIUS L.H. SPIERINGS, MD, PhD
Clinical Professor of Neurology and Craniofacial
Pain, Tufts University Schools of Medicine and
Dental Medicine, Boston, Massachusetts

NAN SU, BSc, MBBS
Toronto, Ontario, Canada

Contents

Pain in the orofacial region is a common presenting symptom. The majority of symptoms are related to dental disease, and the cause can readily be established, the problem dealt with, and the pain eliminated. However, pain may persist and defy attempts at treatment. Intractable oral or facial pain can be diagnostically challenging. To make a definitive diagnosis and initiate proper treatment, a rigorous protocol for evaluation includes a thorough history and an appropriate comprehensive clinical examination and diagnostic testing, including chief complaint, history of present illness, medical history, physical examination, diagnostic studies, including imaging, and psychosocial evaluation.

Patients with chronic orofacial pain disorders have significant psychological distress that plays an important role in modulating and maintaining their pain. For many patients, doing procedures or giving them medications does not relieve their pain. This article discusses the role of cognitive behavioral therapy and other related types of therapy, including mindfulness practices in modulating their pain disorders and helping patients to understand and participate in exercises and practices that will downregulate their pain and add to their toolbox of things they can do to gain relief.

This article describes a model of opiate risk stratification with a special focus on dentistry and oral surgery. A brief overview covers the scope of the US opioid abuse and misuse epidemic and the role of the dentist in mitigating the problems of diversion and misuse of controlled substances. The expanding role of dentistry is summarized. An assessment outlines gathering critical risk information, screening questionnaires, access to state prescription monitoring programs, and communication with cotreating providers. Special populations are discussed. Barriers and possible solutions for effective implementation of these strategies are summarized.

Those experiencing intraoral pain associated with dental and oral diseases are likely to pursue treatment from medical and dental providers. The causes for intraoral pain include odontogenic, periodontal, oral mucosal, or contiguous hard and soft tissue structures to the oral cavity. Providers should be vigilant when diagnosing these, as they should be among the first in their differential diagnoses to be ruled out. This review provides brief overviews of frequently encountered oral/dental diseases that cause intraoral pain, originating from the teeth, the surrounding mucosa and gingivae, tongue, bone, and salivary glands and their causes, features, diagnosis, and management strategies.

More than 100 million adults in the United States have chronic pain conditions, costing more than $500 billion annually in medical care and lost productivity. They are the most common reason for seeking health care, for disability and addiction, and the highest driver of health care costs. Myofascial pain is the most common condition causing chronic pain and can be diagnosed through identifying clinical characteristics and muscle palpation. Management is focused on integrating patient training in changing lifestyle risk factors with evidence-based treatment. Understanding the cause, diagnosis, and management of myopain conditions will help prevent the impact of chronic pain.

Internal derangement is caused by loss of the structure and function of the intra-articular tissues, leading to a failure in the biomechanics of the temporomandibular joint. This tissue failure is usually caused by joint overload, leading to an inflammatory/degenerative arthropathy of the temporomandibular joint. The intra-articular changes associated with internal derangement of the temporomandibular joint can also be caused by a systemic arthropathy or a localized atypical arthropathy involving the temporomandibular joint. Clinicians must be diligent in establishing the correct diagnosis and cause of the internal derangement, which ultimately leads to the appropriate management of patients with these disorders.

Temporomandibular disorders (TMD) and primary headaches can be perpetual and debilitating musculoskeletal and neurological disorders. The presence of both can affect up to one-sixth of the population at any one time. Initially, TMDs were thought to be predominantly musculoskeletal disorders, and migraine was thought to be solely a cerebrovascular disorder. The further understanding of their pathophysiology has helped to clarify their clinical presentation. This article focuses on the role of the trigeminal system in associating TMD and migraine. By discussing recent descriptions of prevalence, diagnosis, and treatment of headache and TMD, we will further elucidate this relationship.

Advances in diagnostic modalities have improved the understanding of the pathophysiology of neuropathic pain involving head and face. Recent updates in nomenclature of cranial neuralgias and facial pain have rationalized accurate diagnosis.

Clear diagnosis and localization of pain generators are paramount, leading to better use of medical and targeted surgical treatments.

Peripheral nerve blocks are an increasingly viable treatment option for selected groups of headache patients, particularly those with intractable headache or facial pain. Greater occipital nerve block, the most widely used local anesthetic procedure in headache conditions, is particularly effective, safe, and easy to perform in the office. Adverse effects are few and infrequent. These procedures can result in rapid relief of pain and allodynia, and effects last for several weeks or months. Use of nerve block procedures and potentially onabotulinum toxin therapy should be expanded for patients with intractable headache disorders who may benefit, although more studies are needed for efficacy and clinical safety.

ORAL AND MAXILLOFACIAL SURGERY CLINICS OF NORTH AMERICA

THE CLINICS ARE NOW AVAILABLE ONLINE!
Access your subscription at:
www.theclinics.com

Preface
Oral and Maxillofacial Pain

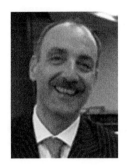

Steven J. Scrivani, DDS, DMSc
Editor

Painful conditions in the oral and maxillofacial region are common. Due to the complex anatomy of this region of the body with specialized structures and physiology, evaluation, diagnosis, and management can be difficult. Making an accurate diagnosis and providing diagnosis-specific, evidence-based therapy are essential to successful patient care.

The articles in this issue explore the differential diagnosis of painful conditions in the oral and maxillofacial region. Specific pain disorders are presented by a panel of experts in the field who review common and uncommon conditions and potentially dangerous conditions that present with pain. Current diagnostic classifications and guidelines for treatment are highlighted.

Steven J. Scrivani, DDS, DMSc
Division of Oral and Maxillofacial Pain
Department of Oral and Maxillofacial Surgery
Massachusetts General Hospital
Warren 1201
55 Fruit Street
Boston, MA 02114, USA

E-mail address:
sscrivani1@partners.org

Oral Maxillofacial Surg Clin N Am 28 (2016) xiii
http://dx.doi.org/10.1016/j.coms.2016.06.013
1042-3699/16/$ – see front matter © 2016 Published by Elsevier Inc.

Classification and Differential Diagnosis of Oral and Maxillofacial Pain

Steven J. Scrivani, DDS, DMSc[a],*,
Egilius L.H. Spierings, MD, PhD[b]

KEYWORDS

- Orofacial pain • Maxillofacial pain • Craniofacial pain • Classification • Differential diagnosis
- Diagnostic evaluation • Physical examination • Diagnostic imaging

KEY POINTS

- Most orofacial pain is related to dental disease and the cause can be readily established, the problem dealt with expeditiously, and the pain eliminated.
- The formal medical evaluation includes the chief complaint, history of present illness, medical history, physical examination, diagnostic studies, including imaging, and psychosocial evaluation.
- The physical examination consists of a muscle examination, temporomandibular joint examination, intraoral examination, neurologic examination, and vascular examination.
- Diagnostic studies include blood tests, diagnostic injections, biopsies of suspicious lesions, radiographs, computed tomography, soft tissue MRI, technetium bone scan, salivary gland scintigraphy, and ultrasonography.

INTRODUCTION

Orofacial pain syndromes are common in clinical practice and tend to be unique in their presentation owing to the complex anatomy and specialized sensory innervation of the face, head, and neck. Although nociceptive transmission in the trigeminal and spinal systems is similar, the 2 systems have important differences. The 3 trigeminal cutaneous divisions are completely separate in a rostrocaudal pattern with topographical representation in the brainstem. They are also bilaterally distinct and separate. Additionally, however, there is a circumferential, cutaneous, perioral organization that is also topographically organized in the brainstem adjacent to the rostrocaudal organization in a complex somatotopic fashion.[1–3]

In the perioral region, the trigeminal divisions contain afferent fibers that subserve the dermatomes, which include the lips, teeth, gingiva, anterior two-thirds of the tongue, upper pharynx, uvula, and soft palate. In addition to this cutaneous distribution, the trigeminal nerve contains afferent fibers that provide sensory innervation to a variety of deep structures in the face, including the muscles of mastication and facial expression, the nasal and oral mucosa, the corneae, tongue, tooth pulp, temporomandibular joints, dura mater, intracranial vessels, external auditory meati, and ears (partially, and with cranial nerves [CN] VII, IX, and X).

The trigeminal system carries somatosensory information from these cutaneous and deep structures as well as from specialized organs that have principally nociceptive innervation. Most nociceptive afferent fibers relay through the trigeminal brainstem complex, with oral and perioral structures represented more rostrally than the peripheral sites on the face.[1–4]

[a] Division of Oral and Maxillofacial Pain, Department of Oral and Maxillofacial Surgery, Warren 1201, Massachusetts General Hospital, 15 Parkman Street, Suite 230, Boston, MA 02114, USA; [b] Tufts University Schools of Medicine and Dental Medicine, Boston, MA 02111, USA
* Corresponding author.
E-mail address: sscrivani1@partners.org

Oral Maxillofacial Surg Clin N Am 28 (2016) 233–246
http://dx.doi.org/10.1016/j.coms.2016.04.003
1042-3699/16/$ – see front matter © 2016 Elsevier Inc. All rights reserved.

In addition, nociceptive afferents from other CN and the upper cervical spinal segments (C2–C4) also are relayed through the trigeminal brainstem complex.[5,6] In the subnucleus caudalis, cells relaying nociceptive signals (nociceptive-specific cells and wide dynamic range cells) are localized primarily to analogous regions of laminae I and V in the spinal cord.[5,7] Deep afferent fibers also converge on cells that receive cutaneous nociceptive input, providing a substrate for referred pain in the face, head, and neck through the trigeminal system.[5,6] This anatomic and physiologic construct has very important implications with regard to pain patterns in the face, head, and neck region and the source or generator of the pain disorder. Structures in the facial region and the cervical region can alternatively be involved in the production of pain in these respective areas and make the differential diagnosis confusing and sometimes elusive (**Figs. 1** and **2**).[5,6,8] Finally, the trigeminal nociceptive relay cells are modulated strongly by central pathways (descending opioidergic, noradrenergic, and serotonergic) that may dynamically modulate nociception under a variety of environmental situations and behavioral states.[1,4–6]

Although the trigeminal dermatomes do not overlap generally with those supplied by the adjacent cervical spinal nerves and other CN, they overlap extensively in the spinal afferent system. Because the peripheral sensory nerves overlap so little with the trigeminal system, nerve lesions may result in more pronounced central somatosensory changes than those evoked by similar lesions in spinal nerves. These changes may partly underlie trigeminal neuropathic pain disorders and may also influence the development of chronic orofacial pain.[9]

As with other chronic pain conditions, psychosocial factors explain much of the variance in the outcome of persistent orofacial pain disorders (see article by Kulich RJ, et al: A Model for Opioid Risk Stratification: Assessing the Psychosocial Components of Orofacial Pain, in this issue). Affective and anxiety symptoms, especially emotional trauma, have been implicated in precipitating and maintaining chronic orofacial pain.[10] Marked somatic overconcern or somatization disorder can also compromise treatment in these disorders. Similarly, chronic disability behavior further compromises the patient's status. Validated self-report orofacial pain scales also address psychosocial issues, and their use within multidisciplinary facial pain facilities is common.[11–13]

DIAGNOSTIC EVALUATION

Pain in the orofacial region is a common presenting symptom in clinical practice. The majority of symptoms are related to dental disease and, in most cases, the cause can be established readily, the problem dealt with expeditiously, and the pain eliminated. However, in many patients, pain may persist and defy attempts at treatment. Intractable oral or facial pain can be challenging diagnostically, given the many potential causes of pain, the anatomic complexity of the region, and the psychosocial importance of the mouth and face. To formulate a differential diagnosis and ultimately make a definitive diagnosis to initiate proper

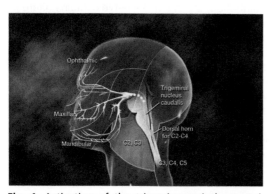

Fig. 1. Activation of the trigeminocervical network (TNC) may result in referred pain that could be perceived anywhere along the TNC. The TNC, which includes the 3 branches of the trigeminal nerve (the ophthalmic branch [V1], the maxillary branch [V2], and the mandibular branch [V3]) as well as the sensory nerves for the posterior head and neck (C2, C3, C4, C5) feed into the TNC. Activation of the TNC may result in referred pain to various locations along the TNC. Pain may be perceived on one or both sides of the head, the eyes or sinuses, and the posterior head and neck.

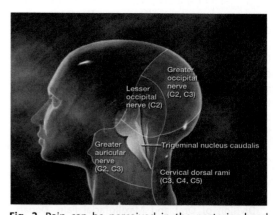

Fig. 2. Pain can be perceived in the posterior head and neck regions. Because activation of the trigeminocervical network can result in referred migraine pain to all regions supplied by the upper cervical nerves (C2, C3, C4, C5), patients may present with posterior head and neck pain.

treatment, a rigorous protocol for evaluating these patients includes a thorough history and an appropriate comprehensive clinical examination and diagnostic testing. This formal diagnostic medical evaluation contains the following components: chief complaint, history of present complaint, medical history, physical examination, diagnostic imaging, and psychosocial evaluation.

Chief Complaint

The patient's description of the pain may provide clues as to its cause. Primary neuralgias are frequently described as sharp and lancinating; neuropathic pain disorders may have a burning, searing quality; vascular headaches can be throbbing; and muscle pain is often described as a deep and dull ache. However, many of these descriptions overlap. Corroborating information from relatives and friends may be needed to build a general picture of the pain as it affects the patient. Each pain complaint should be listed by severity. Additional associated complaints should be sought, because they may provide helpful information.

History of Present Complaint

The intensity of the pain needs to be measured against the patient's own experience of pain, need for medication, and effect on lifestyle. For example, does the pain interfere with work, sleep, talking, eating, or social activities? How severe is it on a 0 to 10 numerical pain rating scale? Does it fluctuate over time? The origin of the pain should be determined by asking the patient to indicate the site of the pain or the site of maximum pain intensity. Its anatomic distribution should be traced accurately in terms of local anatomy.

The patient should be encouraged to remember the events surrounding the onset of the pain, even if it was several years ago. Any other instance of similar pain should be ascertained, even though the patient may not associate these with the present problem. The time relations of the pain should be clarified in terms of duration and frequency of attacks, as well as possible remissions.

Aggravating factors should be determined. Is the pain aggravated by the ingestion of specific foods or beverages, chewing, by lying down, during times of stress, talking, brushing the teeth, shaving, applying make-up, or by other identifiable factors? If so, do any of these factors evoke a short, shocklike pain or a continuous, lingering pain? In addition, relieving factors (eg, lying down, sleep, heat, cold, medications, surgery, and other treatments) are important clues. Finally, the presence or absence of associated factors (eg,

redness or swelling of the face, flushing, tearing, nasal congestion, eyelid ptosis, facial numbness, or facial weakness) needs to be ascertained. Any history of a CN abnormality needs to be noted and investigated further.

The key to the diagnosis is commonly in the cluster of symptoms reported by the patient and then the signs of a problem found on the physical examination. The clinical pattern of many pain disorders can be typical and almost pathognomonic for certain conditions; therefore, pattern recognition in the history is critical.

Medical History

A careful medical history should be taken. A thorough review of organ system disease should be performed, including surgical history, hospitalizations, habit history, psychosocial history, illegal drug use or abuse, allergies, current medical treatments, and current medications. Especially note any trauma to the face, mouth, or head. Identify current and past medications, relevant family history, and the use of over-the-counter medications, supplements, and alternative or complementary therapies. Identify any jaw habits, such as clenching, grinding, posturing the jaw, or gum chewing, including occupational or vocational habits (eg, playing a wind instrument, scuba diving, and so on). A comprehensive psychosocial history is imperative for all patients with a chronic pain disorder as well as establishment of the details of any pending or planned disability claims or litigation.

Physical Examination

The purpose of the physical examination is to discover any possible anatomic or physiologic basis for the pain; therefore, it is important to proceed systematically. Patients with orofacial pain should undergo a complete face, head, and neck examination, oral cavity examination, and neurologic examination; they should be examined directed by a presumed diagnosis. The examination should include inspection, palpation, percussion, and auscultation. Findings of swellings, masses, lesions, and discolorations should be noted. The submandibular region and anterior and lateral neck should be examined for any lymphadenopathy or other kinds of masses. Hyperesthesia, hypoesthesia, anesthesia, paresthesia, dysesthesia, and allodynia should also be noted as well as tenderness and pain in any area.

Muscle examination
The muscles of mastication as well as those of the face, neck, shoulders, and upper back (the suprascapular and pectoral girdle) are common causes

of face, head, and neck pain, so the neck, shoulder, and masticatory muscles should be thoroughly assessed. The size of the muscles can be assessed visually (eg, temporal hollowing, masseteric hypertrophy). The muscles should be palpated, tender and trigger points noted (with a twitch response and referral pattern of pain) and head/neck posture should be assessed. A more thorough evaluation of the masticatory muscles includes evaluating mandibular function and measuring the maximum opening and lateral and protrusive excursions. Tremors, deviations, and fasciculation should be noted as well.

Temporomandibular joint examination
Palpate the lateral pole of the mandibular condyle for tenderness and/or swelling with the mouth open and closed. With mandibular movements, the condylar movement should be evaluated for symmetry and ease. The condyles should also be assessed for pain on movement, shifting of the mandible with movement, and any intermittent locking pattern. Course and fine crepitations should be noted and joint noises auscultated. Clicks and pops and their position in the opening or closing cycle of the joints should be observed. Determining whether the sounds are eliminated or not by changing the maxillomandibular height relation or by posturing the jaw forward will determine their functional importance.

Intraoral examination
Note how the maxillary and mandibular teeth interdigitate when the mouth is closed (dental occlusion), as well as the state of the dentition, evidence of dental decay, gingival health, and oral hygiene. Look for evidence of wear on teeth, excessive toothbrush abrasion, or erosion of teeth. The health of the oropharyngeal mucosa should be recorded, as well as the color and moistness of the mucosa. Inspect and palpate for any swellings, masses, lesions, or areas of discoloration. The parotid and submandibular glands should be inspected and palpated for any masses or areas of tenderness and can be milked to evaluate the quality and quantity of saliva expressed. The tongue, tongue base, lateral pharyngeal walls, tonsillar pillars, tonsillar fossa, and soft palate should be centered midline and move freely and symmetrically. The tongue and palate can be inspected and palpated for lesions, masses, tenderness, and discolorations. Excessive draping of the soft palate, as seen in sleep apnea, should be noted and a Mallampatti classification recorded.

Neurologic examination
The most important part of the neurologic evaluation is the examination of the CNs V (trigeminal) and VII (facial) and the upper cervical nerve roots (C2–C4). The 3 divisions of the trigeminal nerve, that is, ophthalmic (first), maxillary (second), and mandibular (third), through their peripheral mucocutaneous branches, supply the majority of sensation to the face, head, and mouth (and all associated structures). Examine the skin distribution of all 3 divisions, as well as the intraoral distribution of the second and third divisions. Sensory testing with directional sense, sharp (pain) touch, light touch, hot and cold, pressure, 2-point discrimination, and sensory perception with "von Frey hairs" (Semmes-Weinstein microfilaments) may help with the diagnosis. Taste may need to be tested in certain situations. Pain to pressure over the bony foramina (supraorbital, infraorbital, and mental) may indicate trigeminal involvement. Corneal and gag reflexes should be assessed. The size and strength of the masticatory muscles reflect the motor division of CN V. Facial nerve function can be assessed by asking the patient to whistle, purse the lips, smile, close the eyes, and frown. Tongue movements and posture should be evaluated and taste can also be assessed.

CN I can be grossly evaluated with specific, definable noxious or nonnoxious smells.

CN II should be evaluated for visual acuity and visual fields, and CN II and III can be assessed by examining pupil size, direct and consensual pupillary light reflexes, and evidence of an afferent pupillary defect. Funduscopic examination can be performed as needed. CN III, IV, and VI can be evaluated with eye movements in the 6 cardinal fields of gaze to assess extraocular muscle function.

CN VIII can be evaluated with gross hearing perception and, additionally, bone conduction versus air conduction can be assessed with the Weber and Rinne tests. CN IX and X can be evaluated with sensory perception in the posterior tongue, soft palate elevation with phonation, and by the gag reflex. CN XI is evaluated with shoulder shrug and head rotation to commands and against resistance. CN XII is evaluated with straight tongue protrusion and side-to-side movements.

Upper cervical nerve sensation can be accessed on the posterior scalp for C2 (greater occipital nerve at the back of the head and the lesser occipital nerve behind the ear) and at the angle of the jaw and upper neck for C3 and C4. Pressure over the midsuperior nuchal line directly can affect the greater occipital nerve and may reproduce headache or cause shocklike radiating pain. The upper cervical nerves can also be assessed for any sensory alteration in the distribution of the greater auricular, transverse cervical, and supraclavicular branches.

Vascular examination

The carotid arteries should be palpated individually and assessed for pulse rate, full and bounding quality, and auscultated for bruits. The superficial temporal arteries should be inspected and palpated for prominence, tortuosity, pulsations, nodules, and tenderness or pain. Auscultation for bruits can also be performed over the eyes.

Diagnostic Imaging

Panoramic and periapical dental radiographs are inexpensive, readily available, do not expose patients to excessive radiation, and offer detailed information about the teeth and jaws. Other plain radiographs may occasionally be helpful. Computed tomography can provide more detailed images of the bony structures of the maxillofacial skeleton, including nose and sinuses, temporomandibular joints, and skull base. Three-dimensional imaging can be helpful in some instances. MRI is best for evaluating the soft tissues and can be used for assessing the deep oropharyngeal and nasopharyngeal anatomy and the internal anatomy of the temporomandibular joints. In addition, the brain can be evaluated with MRI with and without intravenous gadolinium contrast. MRI studies can also help to determine if there is any intracranial structural pathology or vascular abnormality (MR angiography/MR venography) or alteration in intraparenchymal brain or cerebrospinal-fluid system.

Bone scan with technetium-99m will highlight areas of increased metabolic activity within the bone and can help to identify infection, tumor, or degenerative changes in the temporomandibular joints. Scintigraphy can also be used to evaluate salivary gland function along with contrast injection sialography and computerized sialography. Ultrasonography can be used to evaluate the major salivary glands, carotid arteries, and masses in the neck, particularly in the thyroid gland. Formal contrast injection angiography is rarely warranted.

Other Diagnostic Studies

Routine blood studies may need to be assessed in certain situations. Hematology, blood chemistry, coagulation studies, microbiological studies, and inflammatory and immunologic studies may all contribute important information in cases where these seem warranted by history or physical examination. Diagnostic injections (local anesthetic, corticosteroid) of nerve branches (nerve blocks), muscles (trigger point injections), or joints may be of some value. Biopsy of any suspicious mass or lesion (fine needle aspiration, core needle, or incisional/excisional) is often deemed appropriate. Therapeutic procedures (injection, pharmacologic, surgical) can also be part of the diagnostic process in some cases and be very helpful.

Psychosocial Evaluation

An important part of the evaluation of the patient with a pain disorder, particularly chronic pain, is a thorough psychosocial evaluation. There are standardized questionnaires that have been well-validated in evaluating pain patients. Additionally, specific questions and a review of systems specifically geared toward the psychosocial component of the pain disorder patient can be used without much difficulty (**Boxes 1** and **2**).

Summary

The goal of the diagnostic evaluation of the patient with a pain problem is to establish a definitive diagnosis and provide the most appropriate and evidence-based treatment approaches for the alleviation of the pain, suffering, and associated medical conditions. To this end, formulating a comprehensive differential diagnosis to rule out ominous and potentially life-threatening conditions

---

Box 1
Psychological disorders and chronic pain – why?

1. High prevalence of psychological comorbidities among patients with chronic pain.

2. Presence of chronic pain may cause emotional distress and exacerbate premorbid psychological disorders.

3. Emotional problems may increase perceived pain intensity and disability, and perpetuate dysfunction.

4. Unrecognized and untreated psychological distress may interfere with successful treatment of chronic pain.

Adapted from Flor H, Turk DC. Chronic pain: an integrated biobehavioral approach. Seattle (WA): IASP Press; 2011.

Box 2
Psychological conditions associated with chronic pain

- Mood disorders
- Anxiety disorders
- Somatic symptoms disorders
- Personality disorders
- Other conditions

is mandatory. Once this has been accomplished, the differential diagnostic list can be treated as a problem list that then needs potential further evaluations, consultations, and diagnostic studies. Stratifying this list into categories based on the common diagnostic classifications for face, head, and neck pain disorders can help to focus the clinician toward eliminating potentially incorrect diagnoses. The following section and other articles in this issue focus on this classification and common oral and maxillofacial pain conditions.

CLASSIFICATION

The common descriptive terms and diagnostic categories for orofacial pain complaints and clinical diagnoses are frequently misleading. To avoid confusion, clinicians should be familiar with the International Headache Society's Diagnostic Classification for Headache (Head, Face, and Neck Pain) Disorders, the "International Classification of Headache Disorders III (Beta Version)" (**Boxes 3–6**).[14] Clinicians need to be able to distinguish among painful conditions that arise from

Box 3
International Headache Society's International Classification of Headache Disorders III (ICHD III-Beta)

14 Categories

- Primary headaches: 1 to 4
- Secondary headaches: 5 to 12
- Painful cranial neuropathies, other facial pains and other headaches: 13 to 14
- Appendix

From Headache Classification Committee of the International Headache Society (IHS). The international classification of headache disorders, 3rd edition (beta version). Cephalalgia 2013;33:636–42; with permission.

Box 4
International Classification of Headache Disorders primary headache categories

1. Migraine
   a. Without aura
   b. With aura
2. Tension-type headache
3. Trigeminal autonomic cephalalgias
4. Other primary headaches

From Headache Classification Committee of the International Headache Society (IHS). The international classification of headache disorders, 3rd edition (beta version). Cephalalgia 2013;33:636–42; with permission.

structural pathology of the oral and facial structures and those related to temporomandibular joint disorders, myofascial pain disorders, headache syndromes, and cranial neuralgias. In addition, there is a more focused and specific classification of head, face, and neck pain disorders by the American Academy of Orofacial Pain; "Orofacial Pain: Guidelines for Assessment, Diagnosis and Treatment" (**Boxes 7–9**).[15]

Box 5
International Classification of Headache Disorders secondary headache categories

1. Attributed to trauma or injury to the head and/or neck
2. Attributed to cranial or cervical vascular disorder
3. Attributed to nonvascular intracranial disorder
4. Attributed to a substance or its withdrawal
5. Attributed to infection
6. Attributed to disorder of homeostasis
7. Headache or facial pain attributed to disorder of cranium, neck, eyes, ears, nose, sinuses, teeth, mouth, or other facial or cranial structures
8. Attributed to psychiatric disorder

From Headache Classification Committee of the International Headache Society (IHS). The International classification of headache disorders, 3rd edition (beta version). Cephalalgia 2013;33:636–42; with permission.

Box 6
International Classification of Headache Disorders painful cranial neuropathies and other facial pains

1. Trigeminal neuralgia
   a. Classical trigeminal neuralgia
      i. Classical trigeminal neuralgia, purely paroxysmal
      ii. Classical trigeminal neuralgia with concomitant persistent facial pain
   b. Painful trigeminal neuropathy
      i. Painful trigeminal neuropathy attributed to acute herpes zoster
      ii. Postherpetic trigeminal neuropathy
      iii. Painful posttraumatic trigeminal neuropathy
      iv. Painful trigeminal neuropathy attributed to multiple sclerosis plaque
      v. Painful trigeminal neuropathy attributed to space-occupying lesion
      vi. Painful trigeminal neuropathy attributed to other disorder
2. Glossopharyngeal neuralgia
3. Nervus intermedius (facial nerve) neuralgia
4. Occipital neuralgia
5. Optic neuritis
6. Headache attributed to ischemic ocular motor nerve palsy
7. Tolosa-Hunt syndrome
8. Paratrigeminal oculosympathetic (Raeder's) syndrome
9. Recurrent painful ophthalmoplegic neuropathy
10. Burning mouth syndrome
11. Persistent idiopathic facial pain
12. Central neuropathic pain
    a. Central neuropathic pain attributed to multiple sclerosis
    b. Central poststroke pain

From Headache Classification Committee of the International Headache Society (IHS). The International classification of headache disorders, 3rd edition (beta version). Cephalalgia 2013;33:629–808; with permission.

Box 7
Guidelines from orofacial pain: guidelines for assessment, diagnosis, and treatment

- Introduction to orofacial pain
- General assessment of the orofacial pain patient
- Diagnostic classification of orofacial Pain
- Vascular and nonvascular intracranial disorders
- Primary headache disorders
- Episodic and continuous neuropathic pain
- Intraoral pain disorders
- Temporomandibular disorders
- Cervicogenic mechanisms of orofacial pain and headaches
- Extracranial causes of orofacial pain and headaches
- Sleep and orofacial pain
- Axis II biobehavioral considerations

From De Leeuw R, Klasser GD, editors. Orofacial pain: guidelines for assessment, diagnosis and management. American Academy of Orofacial Pain. 5th edition. Quintessence Books; 2013.

Box 8
Temporomandibular joint articular disorders

1. Congenital or developmental
   a. Aplasia
   b. Hypoplasia
   c. Hyperplasia
2. Joint Pain
   a. Arthralgia
   b. Arthritis
3. Joint disorders
   a. Disc–condyle complex disorders
   b. Other hypomobility disorders – adhesions, ankylosis
   c. Hypermobility disorders – subluxation, dislocation
4. Joint diseases
   a. Degenerative joint diseases – osteoarthritis/arthrosis
   b. Condylysis – idiopathic condylar resorption
   c. Osteonecrosis
   d. Systemic arthritides – Rheumatoid arthritis (RA), ankylosing spondylitis (AS), Rieter's, etc
   e. Neoplasm
   f. Synovial chondromatosis
5. Fractures

---

history. Looking carefully at the patient's history of the pain problem, along with the physical examination findings, diagnostic studies, and past evaluations and interventions, and including epidemiologic considerations, the clinician can better make a determination of the pain diagnosis and then better facilitate further evaluations and treatments.

Given the clinical presentation, there are pain conditions that are relatively common and need to be considered first. Some are more ominous and potentially life-threatening and these need to be considered as well. Keys to making the correct diagnosis are generally related to the history of the pain disorder, a cluster of positive symptoms and/or signs and recognition of a pattern of a particular pain disorder.

Painful disorders of the oral cavity (see article by Fricton J: Myofascial Pain: Mechanisms to Management, in this issue) are related generally to structures in the mouth or associated structures in the maxillofacial complex. The odontogenic structures are a common cause of pain and can be diagnosed easily with history, physical examination, and imaging or other local testing (**Box 10, Table 1**). Painful disorders of the oral mucous membranes very often present with lesions of some sort that are definable and can be biopsied and studied microscopically (**Box 11**). Disorders of the salivary glands often present with swelling and possibly localized pathology or constitutional signs of generalized illness and can also be evaluated with diagnostic testing, particularly, imaging modalities (computed tomography, MRI, scintigraphy, sialography) or fine needle aspiration biopsy (**Box 12**). Disease of the paranasal sinuses can present with "sinusitis-like" symptoms or that of

---

With the large number of pain conditions affecting the face, head, and neck region, clinicians need to organize and prioritize their differential diagnosis based on the patient's

---

Box 9
Masticatory muscle disorders

1. Muscle pain limited to the orofacial region
   a. Myalgia
   b. Tendonitis
   c. Myositis
   d. Spasm
2. Myofibrotic contracture
3. Hypertrophy
4. Neoplasms
5. Movement disorders – dyskinesia/dystonia
6. Masticatory muscle pain owing to systemic/central disorders

---

Box 10
Features of odontogenic pain

- Presence of etiologic factors for an odontogenic origin of pain
- Unilateral pain
- Localized pain (diagnosis specific)
- Pain qualities (sharp, dull, aching, throbbing)
- Sensitivity to temperature
- Sensitivity to pressure, palpation, percussion
- Pain reduction by local anesthetic injection?

From Scrivani SJ, Mehta MR, Keith DA, et al. Facial pain. In: Fishman SM, Ballantyne JC, Rathmell JP, eds. Bonica's Management of Pain. Philadelphia: Wolters Kluwer, 2009; with permission.

Table 1
Odontogenic pain

Diagnosis	Pulpitis	Periodontal	Cracked Tooth	Dentinal
Diagnostic features	Spontaneous and/or evoked deep/diffuse pain in compromised dental pulp. Pain may be sharp, throbbing, or dull.	Localized deep continuous pain in compromised periodontium (eg, gingiva, periodontal ligament) exacerbated by biting or chewing.	Spontaneous or evoke brief sharp pain in a tooth with history of trauma or restorative work (eg, crown, root canal).	Brief, sharp pain evoked by different kinds of stimulus to the dentin (eg, hot or cold drinks).
Diagnostic evaluation	Look for deep caries and recent or extensive dental work. Pain provoked/exacerbated by percussion, thermal or electric stimulation of affected tooth. Dental radiographs helpful (periapical).	Tooth percussion over compromised periodontium provokes pain. Look for inflammation or abscess (eg, periodontitis, apical dental radiographs helpful (bitewings, periapical).	Presence of tooth fracture may be detectable by radiograph. Percussion should elicit pain. Dental radiographs are helpful (periapical taken from different angles).	Exposed dentin or cementum owing to recession of periodontium. Possible erosion of dentinal structure. Cold stimulation reproduce pain.
Treatment	Medication: nonsteroidal anti-inflammatory drugs, nonopiate analgesics. Dentistry: remove carious lesion, tooth restoration, endodontic treatment or tooth extraction.	Medication: nonsteroidal anti-inflammatory drugs, nonopiate analgesics, antibiotics, mouth washes. Dentistry: drainage and debridement of periodontal pocket, scaling and root planning, periodontal surgery, endodontic treatment or tooth extraction.	Medication: nonsteroidal anti-inflammatory drugs, nonopiate analgesics. Dentistry: depends on level of the tooth fracture restoration; treatment; or extraction of the tooth.	Medication: mouthwash (fluoride), desensitizing toothpaste. Dentistry: fluoride or potassium salts, tooth restoration, endodontic treatment. Patient education, diet, tooth brushing force and frequency, proper tooth paste.

From Scrivani SJ, Mehta MR, Keith DA, et al. Facial pain. In: Fishman SM, Ballantyne JC, Rathmell JP, eds. Bonica's Management of Pain. Philadelphia: Wolters Kluwer, 2009; with permission.

Box 11
Common painful mucosal conditions

Infections
- Herpetic stomatitis
- Varicella zoster
- Candidiasis
- Acute necrotizing gingivostomatitis

Immune/autoimmune
- Allergic reactions (toothpaste, mouthwashes, topical medications)
- Erosive lichen planus
- Benign mucous membrane pemphigoid
- Aphthous stomatitis and aphthous lesions
- Erythema multiform
- Graft-versus-host disease

Traumatic and iatrogenic injuries
- Factitial, accidental (burns: chemical, solar, thermal)
- Self-destructive (rituals, obsessive behaviors)
- Iatrogenic (chemotherapy, radiation)

Neoplasia
- Squamous cell carcinoma
- Mucoepidermoid carcinoma
- Adenocystic carcinoma
- Brain tumors

Neurologic
- Burning mouth syndrome and glossodynia
- Neuralgias
- Postviral neuralgias
- Posttraumatic neuropathies
- Dyskinesias and dystonias

Nutritional and Metabolic
- Vitamin deficiencies (B_{12}, folate)
- Mineral deficiencies (iron)
- Diabetic neuropathy
- Malabsorption syndromes

Miscellaneous
- Xerostomia, secondary to intrinsic or extrinsic conditions
- Referred pain from esophageal or oropharyngeal malignancy
- Mucositis secondary to esophageal reflux
- Angioedema

Box 12
Salivary gland disease

- Inflammatory
- Noninflammatory
- Infectious
- Obstructive
- Immunologic (Sjogren's syndrome)
- Tumors
- Others (red herrings)

an upper respiratory tract infection but with pain being a primary and persistent complaint after common medical therapy is used. Pain from anatomic pathology, in particular benign and malignant tumors, often presents with unilateral complaints or with an atypical pain presentation or "pattern." Chronic facial pain and headache is not typically owing to sinus disease or other common upper respiratory tract disease. Pain in or around the ear or the eye can be owing to a number of different causes and needs to be carefully evaluated with additional studies and medical and surgical consultations (**Boxes 13–16, Table 2**). A differential diagnosis for this can potentially be one of the trigeminal autonomic

Box 13
Red flags for a patient with eye pain

- New visual acuity defect, color vision defect, or visual field loss
- Relative afferent pupillary defect
- Extraocular muscle abnormality, ocular misalignment, or diplopia
- Proptosis
- Lid retraction or ptosis
- Conjunctival chemosis, injection, or redness
- Corneal opacity
- Hyphema or hypopyon
- Iris irregularity
- Nonreactive pupil
- Fundus abnormality
- Recent ocular surgery (<3 months)
- Recent ocular trauma

Box 14
Pain in or around the eye: "quite eye" and normal examination

- Cluster headache and cluster–tic syndrome
- Paroxysmal hemicrania
- Short-lasting, unilateral, neuralgiform headache attacks with conjunctival injection and tearing (SUNCT)/short-lasting unilateral neuralgiform headache attacks with cranial autonomic symptoms (SUNA) syndrome
- Migraine and tension-type headache
- Ice-pick headache/ice cream headache/Valsalva headache
- Trigeminal neuralgia
- Sinus disease (acute)
- Teeth, jaws (temporomandibular disorder)
- Carotid disease
- Temporal arteritis
- Eye pain, headache and lung cancer

---

cephalalgias, ophthalmologic disorders, otologic disorders, trigeminal neuralgia, or other trigeminal neuropathic disorders and temporomandibular disorders. Additionally, local malignant disease and metastatic disease can also present in this way.

Temporomandibular disorders, although a common diagnosis, consists of a large variety of often confusing subtypes of problems. The term temporomandibular disorder is also nonspecific and, hence, confusing. It is a poorly construed "classification" for a multitude of problems and should avoid being used as a definitive diagnosis of any oral or maxillofacial pain problem. With accurate history, detailed physical examination, diagnostic testing, and appropriate imaging, if needed, a more specific and accurate diagnosis can be made. Specific disorders of the temporomandibular joint articular apparatus (see article by Israel HA, et al: Internal Derangement of the Tempromandibular Joint: New Perpsectives on an Old Problem, in this issue) and structures and the masticatory and/or cervical musculoskeletal complex (see article by Graff-Radford SB, Abbott JJ: Temporomandibular Disorders and Headache, in this issue) need to be diagnosed to afford the correct treatment (see **Boxes 8 and 9**).

Box 15
Pain in or around the eye - "Quite Eye" and ophthalmologic findings

- Ocular processes
  - Glaucoma, corneal disease, uveitis, scleritis, intraocular tumors, ocular ischemia, hemorrhage
- Processes affecting the optic nerve
  - Optic neuritis, ischemic, compressive or infiltrative optic neuropathy
- Orbital processes
  - Tumor, infection, inflammatory, vascular, posttraumatic
- Cavernous sinus/retroorbital processes
  - Aneurysm, tumor, thrombosis, infection, inflammatory, C-C fistula, posttraumatic
- Intracranial processes
  - Tumor, pseudotumor cerebri, infection, inflammatory, vascular, ICP changes

---

Box 16
Headache and facial pain syndromes with predominant ophthalmologic findings

- Carotid artery disease
- Orbital inflammatory pseudotumor
- Increased intracranial pressure (pseudotumor cerebri)
- Intracranial hemorrhage and stroke
- Intracranial arteriovenous malformation
- Tolosa-Hunt syndrome
- Raeder's paratrigeminal syndrome
- Gradenigo's syndrome
- Postherpetic neuralgia

Cranial neuralgias (see article by Bajwa ZH: Cranial Neuralgias, in this issue) present almost exclusively as episodic, unilateral, sharp, severe, lancinating pain (**Table 3**). They are more common in an older population or after some definable trigeminal injury or disorder. Neuropathic facial pain disorders (see article by Rafael B, et al: Painful Traumatic Trigeminal Neuropathy, in this issue) can be more episodic or continuous and have a different pattern of the pain and may be related to systemic disease, infection, or trauma (nerve injury), even routine dental surgical procedures (including local anesthetic injection), or ill-defined trauma. Their presentation is often

complex with other associated cranial neuropathy findings and/or autonomic epiphenomena and may be analogous to chronic regional pain syndrome. Burning mouth/tongue syndrome (see article by Klasser GD, et al: Burning Mouth Syndrome, in this issue) is certainly a well-defined and localized, very interesting enigma of a problem. Although it can be owing to localized or systemic diseases, it is more often than not a disorder of undefined etiology, but generally thought of as a neuropathic pain disorder or localized painful trigeminal neuropathy. It seems to have very specific characterizations and patient presentation.

Headache disorders (see article by Clark GT, et al: Medication Treatment Efficacy and Chronic Orofacial Pain, in this issue) are a very broad group of pain problems that often overlap with face and neck pain disorders. There may be a bidirectional association for many of the primary headache disorders (particularly migraine and tension-type headache) and some of the more common oral and maxillofacial pain problems (temporomandibular disorders). The trigeminal autonomic cephalalgias can often present with face and head pain, particularly in the area of the temple, eye, and periorbital region and maxilla. The large group of secondary headache disorders needs to be carefully eliminated, since many have potentially ominous and even life-threatening causes (**Box 17**). Movement disorders of the oral and maxillofacial complex (see article by Clark G, Ram S: Orofacial Movement Disorders, in this issue), although often not having pain as a primary complaint, can cause associated problems that can be painful and troublesome in many others ways.

Treatment for all of these complex pain disorders in the face, head, and neck is predicated on a correct diagnosis. Once that is made, a variety of therapeutic options are available to try to best treat these problems and ultimately eliminate pain and suffering. The treatments can and are often interprofessional in nature, combining pharmacologic, surgical, physical medicine and rehabilitation, biobehavioral and psychological therapies, injection therapy, and many others. A holistic and patient-centered approach to these pain disorders is paramount. The clinician must be able to evaluate, diagnose, and then treat all of the complex associated conditions that often go along with a pain disorder.

One of the essential qualities of the clinician is interest in humanity, for the secret in the care of the patient is in the caring for the patient.
                            —*Francis Weld Peabody*

Table 2
Ear and throat pain

Ear	Throat
Ext/middle ear	Carotid dissection
Temporomandibular disorder (joint or muscle)	Laryngeal nerve
	Myogenous
	Parotid gland
Ramsey-Hunt syndrome	Temporomandibular disorder (muscle)
Parotid gland	Submandibular gland
Myogenous	Lymphadenopathy
Carotid dissection	

Less common	
Geniculate nerve	Glossopharyngeal nerve
Glossopharyngeal nerve	Eagle syndrome
Eagle syndrome	Ernst syndrome
Ernst syndrome	Carotidynia
Carotidynia	

Table 3
Trigeminal neuropathic pain disorders

Diagnosis	Trigeminal Neuralgia	Deafferentation Pain	Acute and Postherpetic Neuralgia	Burning Mouth Syndrome
Diagnostic features	Brief severe lancinating pain evoked by mechanical stimulation of trigger zone (pain-free between attacks). Usually unilateral, affects the V2/V3 areas (rarely V1). Possible pain remission periods (for months or years)	Spontaneous or evoked pain with prolonged after-sensation after tactile stimulation. Trigger zone owing to surgery (tooth extraction) or trauma. Positive and negative descriptors (eg, burning, nagging, boring).	Pain associated with herpetic lesions, usually in the V1 dermatoma. Spontaneous pain (burning and tingling), but may present as dull and aching. Occasional lancinating evoked pain.	Constant burning pain of the mucous membranes of the tongue, mouth. Hard or soft palate or lips. Usually affects women age >50 y.
Diagnostic evaluation	MRI for evidence of tumor or vasocompression of the trigeminal tract or root (cerebropontine angle). Rule-out MS, especially in young adults.	Etiologic factors such as trauma or surgery in the painful area. Order MRI if the area is intact to rule-out peripheral or central lesions.	Small cutaneous vesicles (AHN) or scarring (PHN), usually affecting V1. Loss of normal skin color. Corneal ulceration can occur. Sensory changes in affected area (eg, hyperesthesia, dysesteshia).	Rule-out salivary gland dysfunction (xerostomia) or tumor, Sjögren syndrome, candidiasis, geographic or fissured tongue, and chemical or mechanical irritations. Nutrition and menopause.
Treatment	Medication: anticonvulsants (eg, carbamazepine, gabapentin); antidepressants (eg, amitriptyline, nortriptyline, desipramine); nonopiate analgesics, BTX. Combination of baclofen and anticonvulsants can produce good results. Surgery: microvascular decompression of trigeminal root, ablative surgeries (eg, rhizotomy, gamma knife).	Medication: anticonvulsants (eg, carbamazepine, gabapentin); antidepressants; nonopiate analgesics; topical agents (eg, lidocaine 5% patches). Surgery: ablative surgeries (eg, rhizotomy, gamma knife).	Medication: acyclovir (acute phase) anticonvulsants, antidepressants; nonopiate analgesics; topical agents (eg, lidocaine 5% patches). Surgery: ablative surgeries (eg, rhizotomy, gamma knife).	Medication: anticonvulsants, benzodiazepines, antidepressants; nonopiate analgesics; topical agents (eg, lidocaine, mouth washes). Cognitive-behavior: biofeedback, relaxation, coping skills.

Abbreviations: AHN, adenomatous hyperplastic nodule; BTX, benzene, toluene, xylene; PHN, postherpetic neuralgia.

Box 17
"Red Flags" in the headache history

- Headache accompanied by unconsciousness
- First-worst headache (appearing suddenly)
- Headache accompanied with neurologic abnormalities during and/or after the headache
- Headache associated with fever or stiff neck
- Headache developing after 50 years of age
- A change in characteristic response to previous treatments of headache
- Headache associated with alterations in behavior and personality
- Headache initiated by Valsalva maneuver

REFERENCES

1. Maciewicz R, Mason P, Strassman A, et al. Organization of the trigeminal nociceptive pathways. Semin Neurol 1988;8:255–64.
2. Sato F, Akhter F, Haque T, et al. Projections from the insular cortex to pain-receptive trigeminal caudal subnucleus (medullary dorsal horn) and other lower brainstem areas in rats. Neuroscience 2013;233:9–27.
3. Haque T, Akhter F, Kato T, et al. Somatotopic direct projections from orofacial areas of secondary somatosensory cortex to trigeminal sensory nuclear complex in rats. Neuroscience 2012;219:214–33.
4. Mason P, Strassman A, Maciewicz R. Is the jaw-opening reflex a valid model of pain? Brain Res 1985;357:137–46.
5. Le Doaré K, Akerman S, Holland PR, et al. Occipital afferent activation of second order neurons in the trigeminocervical complex in rat. Neurosci Lett 2006; 403:73–7.
6. Bartsch T, Goadsby PJ. The trigeminocervical complex and migraine: current concepts and synthesis. Curr Pain Headache Rep 2003;7:371–6.
7. Mørch CD, Hu JW, Arendt-Nielsen L, et al. Convergence of cutaneous, musculoskeletal, dural and visceral afferents onto nociceptive neurons in the first cervical dorsal horn. Eur J Neurosci 2007;26:142–54.
8. Bartsch T, Goadsby PJ. Increased responses in trigeminocervical nociceptive neurons to cervical input after stimulation of the dura mater. Brain 2003;126:1801–13.
9. Bennett GJ. Neuropathic pain in the orofacial region: clinical and research challenges. J Orofacial Pain 2004;18:281–6.
10. De Leeuw R, Bertoli E, Schmidt JE, et al. Prevalence of traumatic stressors in patients with temporomandibular disorders. J Oral Maxillofac Surg 2005;63:42–50.
11. Kafas P, Leeson R. Assessment of pain in temporomandibular disorders: the bio-psychosocial complexity. J Oral Maxillofac Surg 2006;35:145–9.
12. Levitt SR, McKinney MW. Validating the TMJ scale in a national sample of 10,000 patients: demographic and epidemiologic characteristics. J Orofac Pain 1994;8:25–35.
13. Schiffman E, Orbach R, Truelove E, et al. Diagnostic criteria for temporomandibular disorders (DC/TMD) for clinical and research applications: recommendations of the international RDC/TMD consortium network and orofacial pain special interest group. J Oral Facial Pain Headache 2014;28:6–27.
14. Headache Classification Committee of the International Headache Society (IHS). The international classification of headache disorders, 3rd edition (beta version). Cephalalgia 2013;33:629–808.
15. De Leeuw R, Klasser GD, editors. Orofacial pain: guidelines for assessment, diagnosis and management. American Academy of orofacial pain. 5th edition. Chicago, IL: Quintessence Books; 2013.

Chronic Orofacial Pain and Behavioral Medicine

Robert L. Merrill, DDS, MS*, Donald Goodman, PhD

KEYWORDS

- Chronic pain • Somatic arousal • Somatic quieting • Cognitive-behavioral therapy • Mindfulness

KEY POINTS

- Most patients with orofacial pain have chronic pain disorders that are heavily impacted by psychological issues that require recognition and management if patients are to recover.
- Patients with orofacial pain are somatically aroused, and treatment of their pain should include techniques that can provide somatic quieting.
- Focused breathing mindfulness has been shown to be very effective in causing somatic quieting.

INTRODUCTION

Patients with chronic orofacial pain (OFP) present in various types of pain clinics with a variability of complex problems that have a significant impact on their pain and impose roadblocks to the clinician who is trying to help patients. The clinician needs to identify and address these roadblocks if he or she is to effectively treat patients. Furthermore, whether the clinicians realize it or not, they may become part of patients' problems by avoiding or ignoring these roadblocks; they may be reinforcing the factors that cause the pain to be persistent. One of the primary roadblocks to managing patients' chronic pain is *somatic arousal*. This phenomenon is commonly observed in patients with chronic pain, and failure to address it leads to frustration and failure for both patients and the clinician. In this article, the authors discuss somatic arousal and review strategies that will directly address it.

The International Association for the Study of Pain[1,2] defines pain as "an unpleasant sensory and emotional experience associated with actual or potential tissue damage, or described in terms of such damage." This definition recognizes the association between the sensory and emotional aspects of pain. Chronic pain has been recognized as pain that persists past the normal time of healing, often described as persisting for more than 3 months. With the advent of functional MRI studies that allow for real-time brain imaging in experimental conditions, we can see what areas of the brain are activated by acute and chronic pain; those areas include lobes in the limbic system, consistent with the definition of pain as not only a sensory but also an emotional experience. This new ability now allows us to observe what is happening in the brain in real-time in response to different treatment modalities, including psychological interventions.

Over several decades of evaluating patients with chronic pain with various behavioral or personality inventories, the most frequently observed personality trait observed in patients with chronic pain was somatic overfocus. Patients who suffer from chronic pain are highly sensitive to their body symptoms and begin to focus on their symptoms with heightened awareness, in part, because of their frustration that doctors have not been able to give a definitive diagnosis or apply effective treatment. This circumstance leads to constant worry or anxiety that the pain is symptomatic of some potentially devastating problem, such as cancer, that is not being found. The wise clinician will recognize this problem during the initial visit and start to use somatic quieting exercises to

Graduate Orofacial Pain Program, UCLA School of Dentistry, Los Angeles, CA, USA
* Corresponding author.
E-mail address: rmerrill@ucla.edu

Oral Maxillofacial Surg Clin N Am 28 (2016) 247–260
http://dx.doi.org/10.1016/j.coms.2016.03.007
1042-3699/16/$ – see front matter © 2016 Elsevier Inc. All rights reserved.

help refocus and restructure the cognitions. Often, the clinician, becoming aware of the psychological impact on the patients' pain, will make a referral to a psychologist without realizing that the physical medicine program itself, used as part of the treatment administered by the clinician, can begin to address many of the behavioral aspects of the patients' chronic pain and start the process of somatic quieting.

The most pervasive problem seen in the OFP population is muscle pain. Although the spectrum of OFP problems involves neuropathic pain, headaches, and musculoskeletal pain, patients with nonmusculoskeletal pain conditions often have head and neck muscle pain in addition to the other types of pain conditions. Physical medicine protocols are given to these patients in addition to directly addressing the nonmusculoskeletal pain with disorder-appropriate procedures and medicines. The physical medicine modalities given to patients with chronic OFP include recommending a soft diet, use of moist heat and ice, and muscle specific stretches. Although it is obvious that the stretching part of the physical medicine program is addressing the muscle component of their pain, there are other techniques that can be given to patients to enhance the physical medicine protocols. These other modalities of the physical medicine program include focused breathing, time outs from the current stress, focused relaxation, and mindfulness practices. These aspects of the physical medicine program are important for all categories of chronic OFP disorders and should be incorporated into the overall management program that is taught to patients, not only to address the painful muscles but also for neuropathic pain and headache because the procedures use techniques that aid in somatic quieting.

This article focuses on the psychological aspects of chronic pain, whether it is musculoskeletal, neuropathic, or neurovascular, and discusses the aforementioned techniques that are used effectively to mediate patients' pain through using behavioral interventions involving somatic quieting.

OROFACIAL PAIN DISORDERS AND SOMATIC FOCUS

Patients with chronic OFP usually present with complex pain and abnormal sensation disorders in the orofacial region. The average general dentist or graduate from a dental specialty has little or no training or experience in dealing with these disorders. Most dental school training focuses on managing acute pain conditions, which does not prepare the student to recognize, diagnose, and treat the chronic pain disorders, including temporomandibular disorders (TMDs). This circumstance is particularly problematic because failure to recognize OFP disorders and using acute dental pain management techniques can push suffering patients down the pathway to frustration, distress, and somatization. The 3 main subtopics of OFP are neuropathic pain, neurovascular pain, and musculoskeletal pain. Each of these general disorders can be associated with comorbid somatization. Within the rubric of neuropathic pain, the International Headache Society (IHS) has classified neuropathies of the head and neck as "painful cranial neuropathies and other facial pains." Within this category, the system lists classic trigeminal neuralgia and painful trigeminal neuropathy as the neuropathic disorders of the trigeminal nerve. However, going further into the breakdown of this category of pain are burning mouth syndrome (BMS), persistent idiopathic facial pain, and central neuropathic pain. BMS has been particularly frustrating to diagnose and treat and has long been shackled with the assessment that patients are somatizing. The pathophysiology of BMS is still unknown, and the most effective treatment to date is use of clonazepam specifically but not the other benzodiazepine-type drugs. Most of the patients with BMS are postmenopausal women who are depressed and are an easy target for attributing the disorder to somatization. The hallmark of BMS is bilateral burning pain in the anterior mouth or tongue, including the lips. Topical or local anesthetic does not block the pain, and it probably represents a centralized pain disorder. These patients do become somatically aroused because no one is giving them a diagnosis or effective treatment, and fear of a serious life-threatening condition is always present.[3]

Persistent idiopathic facial pain has replaced the previous IHS classification of atypical facial pain in an attempt to disentangle these facial pain disorders from the psychological burden of somatization. Nevertheless, this remains a poorly defined category of pain and probably represents several different facial pain syndromes that could be categorized under neuropathic pain disorders but continue to be unclearly or inaccurately described.[4–6] Solberg and Graff-Radford[6] have reported on a group of these patients who were eventually diagnosed with centralized neuropathic pain that responded to stellate ganglion blockade.

An additional category of disorder often seen in the dental office is occlusal dysesthesia. This disorder is created by the unsuspecting dentist who has attempted to treat a complaint of *my bite is off*, by readjusting the occlusion after patients suffered a trauma to the jaw or had recent dental work done. Readjusting the bite over and over reinforces patients' obsessive checking of the bite and demanding that the bite be adjusted again. Patients become somatically overfocused, and subsequent bite adjustments only aggravate the problem.[2]

All of these facial pain disorders, including occlusal dysesthesia, are characterized by somatic arousal. Because none of these problems respond predictably to topical or systemic medications, using mindfulness breathing and relaxation techniques with cognitive-behavioral therapy (CBT) and physical medicine protocols may be the most effective treatment that can be offered to achieve somatic quieting or at least taught to be practiced along with medications.

HISTORICAL REVIEW OF COGNITIVE-BEHAVIORAL THERAPY AND THE THIRD-WAVE DEVELOPMENTS
Psychotherapy (Wave 1)

Before the 1970s, the primary approach to treating depression, anxiety, and other psychological problems was through using psychotherapy and psychoanalytic techniques. Although antidepressants were available, medications were often regarded as emergency or short-term measures that could interfere with psychotherapy or psychoanalysis because the medications lowered patients' drive to go through with the traditional psychotherapeutic processes. However, these modalities of treatment were very slow and expensive.

The Biopsychosocial Model of Health

In the 1970s, George Engel, a psychiatrist, developed a medical health concept that explained the interplay between patients' biological, social, and psychological factors. This concept became known as the biopsychosocial model that is the basis for CBT (**Fig. 1**).[7,8]

This model became very important for treating patients with chronic pain because the developing chronicity of their pain impacted on the 3 aspects of the biopsychosocial model. The importance of this model is woven into physical medicine treatment protocols that can be used with patients with chronic pain to speed the healing response to their pain. Note that the psychological circle includes cognitions, behaviors, and emotions, which is the basis of CBT. However, each of the circles becomes a focus of psychotherapy and change.

Although the treating OFP specialist is not a psychologist, it should become apparent that the factors noted in the biopsychosocial model need to be addressed by the pain specialist to optimize treatment outcomes and bring about beneficial change. In essence, the OFP specialist becomes a proxy for the CBT psychologist in the realm of treating the patients' pain disorder in the clinic.

Cognitive-Behavioral Therapy (Wave 2)

The advent of CBT caused a paradigm shift away from the psychoanalytic approaches and is considered a second wave of psychotherapy that was based on identifying cognitive, behavioral, and emotional aspects of the patients problems,

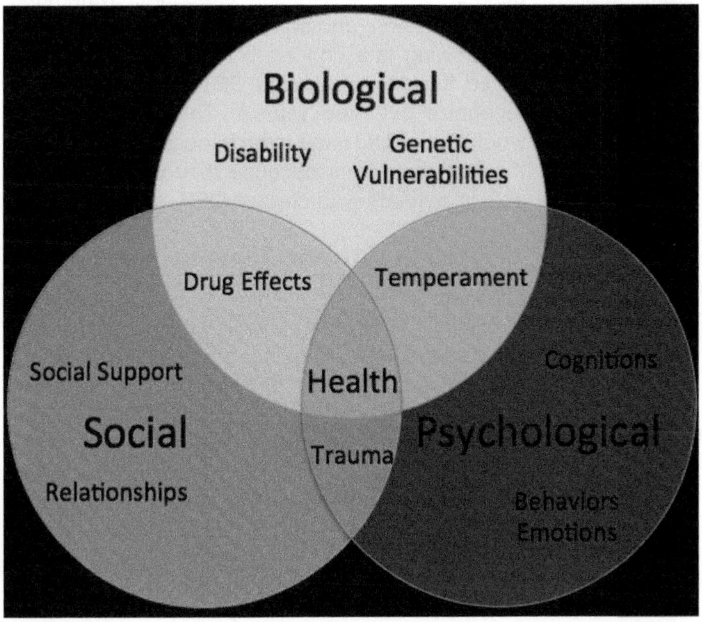

Fig. 1. The biopsychosocial model of health. This model, developed by George Engel, seeks to explain the complex interaction between the 3 main variables that impact an individual's health. Within each of the main variables are secondary variables that modify the primary variable or its relationship with the overlapping primary variables. The net result of these overlapping variables impacts our health. (*Adapted from* Engel G. The predictive value of psychological variables for disease and death. Ann Intern Med 1976;85(6):673–4; with permission).

bringing about change more quickly and cost-effectively.

Third-Wave Therapies

Subsequently a third-wave behavioral therapy has been developed that is used in addition to CBT to help solidify the changes made with CBT only or to address other types of problems that do not respond as well to CBT, such as borderline personality disorder.[9] Acceptance and commitment therapy (ACT) teaches patients to accept and embrace unwanted thoughts and events.[10] Suffering is caused by avoidance, rumination, and fear. The so-called mindfulness techniques help to bring the individuals' thoughts to the present moment and to accept and embrace them. Patients who have chronic pain conditions have uncontrolled and wondering thought processes that continue to focus on their pain, creating somatic arousal and suffering that exacerbate their pain. ACT helps to relieve the suffering aspect of their reaction to the pain and consequently decreases the pain itself. Mindfulness-based cognitive therapy (MBCT) became the next development in CBT by including mindfulness practices into the CBT process. The net result of mindfulness inclusion was strengthening the changes brought about by CBT and reducing relapse.

COGNITIVE-BEHAVIORAL THERAPY

One of the great composers of our time, Igor Stravinsky, once stated that the hardest thing about composing was knowing what not to compose. This article describes and explains the ins and outs of CBT in a concise and understandable way. Additionally there will be a description of mindfulness-based cognitive behavioral therapy and mindfulness-based stress reduction (MBSR).

As stated earlier, CBT has come to be thought of as the second wave of psychotherapy following the first wave of psychoanalytic and psychodynamic. Although codified by Albert Ellis in the 1950s and later Aaron T. Beck in the early 1960s, CBT was formulated before by many others, including Alfred Adler, Meichenbaum, and even the Stoic philosophers of the past, such as Marcus Aurelius and Epictetus who stated: "Men are disturbed not by things but by the views which they take of them."

CBT is thought of as an umbrella term for therapies that help the individual change their thoughts and behaviors through empowered choice. Therapies under this umbrella include rational emotive therapy (RET), cognitive therapy (CT), dialectal behavioral therapy, schema therapy, biofeedback, hypnotherapy, relaxation,

visualization, meditation, heart rate variability, breathing, yoga, and so forth. Ellis, a behaviorist, worked on a method of therapy (RET) that focused on how events lead to thoughts, behaviors, and emotions. Beck worked on his method of therapy (CT) stating that thoughts, feelings, and behaviors are all connected and they can be confronted in a healthy way in order to reduce dysfunction and negativity.

Combining CT and RET, Beck and Ellis formed CBT creating a collaborative style of therapy whereby the therapists and patients work together toward a common goal. In this developing paradigm, patients now play an integral part in their curative process. The therapist now assigns homework for patients to engage in between sessions. In this new paradigm, psychotherapy focuses on symptom relief. The stereotypical need to go back into the patients' past, determining how and whether patients were nurtured well or not is secondary. Now, the therapists and patients look for evidence to support or dispute the automatic thoughts and behaviors. For patients with OFP, some of these automatic thoughts might be as follows: I am having this jaw pain and it is never going away; I had my tooth pulled last week and it is still killing me; It must be something the dentist did. These thoughts add to the problems of somatic arousal.

With CBT one tool we might use would be to ask patients to keep a thought record to first recognize the automatic negative thoughts and then look for evidence as to whether they can substantiate the thought. Other tools include journaling, thought records, pleasant activity scheduling, behavioral experiments, imagery-based exposure, systematic desensitization, and so forth.

Following is a concise list of some of the distorted thinking styles that CBT has been able to recognize over the years.[11] The OFP specialist would be well advised to be acquainted with these thought processes because they will be identifiable in patients with chronic OFP.

15 Styles of Distorted Thinking

Filtering
You take the negative details and magnify them, while filtering out all positive aspects of a situation. A single detail may be picked out, and the whole event becomes colored by this detail. When you pull negative things out of context, isolated from all the good experiences around you, you make them larger and more awful than they really are.

Polarized thinking
The hallmark of this distortion is an insistence on dichotomous choices. Things are black or white,

good or bad. You tend to perceive everything at the extremes, with very little room for a middle ground. The greatest danger in polarized thinking is its impact on how you judge yourself. For example, you have to be perfect or you are a failure.

Overgeneralization

You come to a general conclusion based on a single incident or a piece of evidence. If something bad happens once, you expect it to happen over and over again. *Always* and *never* are cues that this style of thinking is being used. This distortion can lead to a restricted life, as you avoid future failures based on the single incident or event.

Mind reading

Without their saying so, you know what people are feeling and why they act the way they do. In particular, you are able to divine how people are feeling toward you. Mind reading depends on a process called projection. You imagine that people feel the same way you do and react to things the same way you do. Therefore, you do not watch or listen carefully enough to notice that they are actually different. Mind readers jump to conclusions that are true for them, without checking whether they are true for the other person.

Catastrophizing

You expect disaster. You notice or hear about a problem and start *what ifs*: What if that happens to me? What if tragedy strikes? There are no limits to a really fertile catastrophic imagination. An underlying catalyst for this style of thinking is that you do not trust in yourself and your capacity to adapt to change.

Personalization

Personalization is the tendency to relate everything around you to yourself. For example, thinking that everything people do or say is some kind of reaction to you. You also compare yourself with others, trying to determine who's smarter, better looking, and so forth. The underlying assumption is that your worth is in question. You are, therefore, continually forced to test your value as a person by measuring yourself against others. If you come out better, you get a moment's relief. If you come up short, you feel diminished. The basic thinking error is that you interpret each experience, each conversation, each look as a clue to your worth and value.

Control fallacies

There are 2 ways you can distort your sense of power and control. If you feel externally controlled, you see yourself as helpless, a victim of fate. The fallacy of internal control has you responsible for the pain and happiness of everyone around you. Feeling externally controlled keeps you stuck. You do not think you can really affect the basic shape of your life, let alone make any difference in the world. The truth of the matter is that we are constantly making decisions and that every decision affects our lives. On the other hand, the fallacy of internal control leaves you exhausted as you attempt to fill the needs of everyone around you and feel responsible in doing so (and guilty when you cannot).

Fallacy of fairness

You feel resentful because you think you know what is fair, but other people will not agree with you. Fairness is so conveniently defined, so temptingly self-serving, that each person gets locked into his or her own point of view. It is tempting to make assumptions about how things would change if people were only fair or really valued you. But the other person hardly ever sees it that way, and you end up causing yourself a lot of pain and an ever-growing resentment.

Blaming

You hold other people responsible for your pain or take the other tack and blame yourself for every problem. Blaming often involves making someone else responsible for choices and decisions that are actually our own responsibility. In blame systems, you deny your right (and responsibility) to assert your needs, say no, or go elsewhere for what you want.

Shoulds

You have a list of ironclad rules about how you and other people should act. People who break the rules anger you, and you feel guilty if you violate the rules. The rules are right and indisputable; as a result, you are often in the position of judging and finding fault (in yourself and in others). Cue words indicating the presence of this distortion are *should*, *ought*, and *must*.

Emotional reasoning

You think that what you feel must be true—automatically. If you *feel* stupid or boring, then you must *be* stupid and boring. If you feel guilty, then you must have done something wrong. The problem with emotional reasoning is that our emotions interact and correlate with our thinking process. Therefore, if you have distorted thoughts and beliefs, your emotions will reflect these distortions.

Fallacy of change

You expect that other people will change to suit you if you just pressure or cajole them enough.

You need to change people because your hopes for happiness seem to depend entirely on them. The truth is the only person you can really control or have much hope of changing is yourself. The underlying assumption of this thinking style is that your happiness depends on the actions of others. Your happiness actually depends on the thousands of large and small choices you make in your life.

Global labeling
You generalize one or 2 qualities (in yourself or others) into a negative global judgment. Global labeling ignores all contrary evidence, creating a view of the world that can be stereotyped and one dimensional. Labeling yourself can have a negative and insidious impact on your self-esteem, although labeling others can lead to snap judgments, relationship problems, and prejudice.

Being right
You feel continually on trial to prove that your opinions and actions are correct. Being wrong is unthinkable, and you will go to any length to demonstrate your rightness. Having to be right often makes you hard of hearing. You are not interested in the possible veracity of a differing opinion, only in defending your own. Being right becomes more important than an honest and caring relationship.

Heaven's reward fallacy
You expect all your sacrifice and self-denial to pay off, as if there were someone keeping score. You feel bitter when the reward does not come as expected. The problem is that, although you are always doing the right thing, if your heart really is not in it, you are physically and emotionally depleting yourself.

List of Tools and Specific Descriptions

Cognitive rehearsal
In this technique, patients are asked to recall a problematic situation of the past.[11] The therapists and patients work together to find a solution to the problem or a way in which the difficult situation, if occurs in the future, may be sorted out.

Validity testing
It is one of the CBT techniques in which the therapist tests the validity of beliefs or thoughts of patients. Initially, patients are allowed to defend their viewpoint by means of objective evidence. The faulty nature or invalidity of the beliefs of patients is exposed if they are unable to produce any kind of objective evidence.

Writing in a journal
It is the practice of maintaining a diary to keep an account of the situations that arise in day-to-day life. The thoughts that are associated with these situations and the behavior exhibited in response to them are also mentioned in the diary. The therapist, along with the patients, reviews the diary/journal and finds out the maladaptive thought pattern and how they actually affect the behavior of an individual.

Guided discovery
The objective/purpose behind using this technique is to help patients and enable them to understand their cognitive distortions.

Modeling
It is one of the CBT techniques in which the therapists performs role-playing exercises that are aimed at responding in an appropriate way to overcome difficult situations. Patients make use of the therapist's behavior as a model in order to solve the problems they comes across.

Homework
The homework is actually a set of assignments given by therapists to patients. The patients may have to take notes while a session is being conducted, review the audiotapes of a particular session, or have to read articles/books that are related to the therapy.

Aversive conditioning
Among the different CBT techniques used by therapists, the aversive conditioning technique makes use of dissuasion for lessening the appeal of a maladaptive behavior. Patients are exposed to an unpleasant stimulus while being engaged in a particular behavior or thought for which they have to be treated. Thus, the unpleasant stimulus gets associated with such thoughts/behaviors and then the patients exhibit an aversive behavior towards them.

Systematic positive reinforcement
The systematic positive reinforcement is one of the CBT techniques in which certain (positive) behaviors of a person are rewarded with a positive reinforcement. A reward system is established for the reinforcement of certain positive behaviors. Just like positive reinforcement helps in encouraging a particular behavior, withholding the reinforcement deliberately is useful in eradicating a maladaptive behavior.

What CBT attempts to do is work to eliminate the distorted thoughts through the methods listed previously. As stated earlier, chronic pain, although bio-physiological in nature, cannot be separated from the psychological. Chronic pain has to be evaluated both as an emotion and a perception; we cannot separate the emotions, feelings, and thoughts from the physical expressions of the human being. We are and, it is hoped, never will be robots. Our thoughts, feelings, and emotions play a major role in how we interpret our discomfort. But, if our pain is a perception and emotion, it can be changed and we can choose how to feel it and how to change it.

Empowered choice is the goal. Freeing patients from their automatic negative thoughts is the aim. The great irony is that so much of what we either suffer from or enjoy is really ultimately in our heads.

Patients with classic OFP are somatically over-focused; tend to exaggerate their discomfort; are highly involved in rumination, negative thinking, catastrophizing, and blaming; and are probably depressed and anxious. All of these behaviors exaggerate somatic arousal.

The physical medicine program involving stretching, posture, and breathing exercises stimulates somatic quieting. In order to implement somatic quieting processes, we teach among, other techniques, the power of diaphragmatic breathing, which in turn elicits a profound relaxation response in addition to a reduction in anxiety and subsequent reduction in automatic negative thinking and rumination.

CBT as a second-wave therapy has a deep history of research on its effectiveness in treating chronic pain.[12] For a review of relevant studies on CBT and chronic pain, see Akerblom and colleagues.[13]

THE NEUROSCIENCE OF MINDFULNESS BEHAVIOR
Patients with Temporomandibular Disorders and Somatic Arousal

TMDs involve not only peripheral mechanisms of nociception, inflammation, and modulation but also involve central pain processes. These processes included increased temporal summation, central modulation and spread, central sensitization, motor dysfunction, cognitive dysfunction, maladaptive brain plasticity affecting learning and motivation, and learned helplessness.[14,15] Ploghaus and colleagues[16] have shown that thinking about pain increases the sensation of pain. Thinking about pain activates brain areas that are activated during actual pain. In addition, they have found that distraction relieves pain.[16] Ploghaus and colleagues[16] have shown that the pain experience activates the anterior and caudal cingulate cortex, the midinsular cortex, and the

anterior cerebellum, whereas the anticipation of pain activates the medial frontal cortex, the anterior insula, and the posterior cerebellum. Decreasing motor activity as a protection against aggravating pain becomes pathologic and actually increases nociceptive activity, altering the trigeminal nerve microstructure.[17,18] Boudreau and colleagues[19] found that nociception inhibits motor cortex (M1) activity and that task training activity was inhibited by pain, that is, the animal cannot learn new motor tasks in the presence of pain. In addition, the inhibition of motor activity leads to disuse atrophy of the orofacial region of M1. As altered motor function becomes pathologic, it leads to heightened pain.

Hollins and colleagues[20] described increases in hypervigilance and somatic overfocus in patients with TMDs, which is analogous to somatic arousal. The area of the ventrolateral prefrontal cortex was the focus area. The frontal pole is involved in complex executive function and requires extensive resources to evaluate and execute. Chronic pain depletes these resources and distracts from the patients' ability to give attention to other executive tasks.[21]

Pain has been shown to interrupt thought processes and becomes the primary focus of thinking. Van Damme and colleagues[22,23] have shown that when pain intrudes into cognition, it is difficult to disengage cognitive focus from the pain.[22,23] These changes in cognitive focus are associated with grey matter changes in the brain and white matter changes in the cingulate cortex and the insular cortex.[24,25]

Default Mode Network and Chronic Pain

Killingsworth and Gilbert[26] reported that mind-wandering activity represented about 50% of our waking life and was associated with lower levels of happiness. The mind-wandering activity represented ongoing surveying of concerns of the individual. For patients with pain, this would represent focused concern regarding their pain and worry about the meaning or implication of the pain, for example, is it cancer, and so forth. Raichle[27] described a network of brain areas that are associated with self-referencing activity. This activity has been described as selfing, and the brain areas active during this process were described as the default mode network (DMN). The 2 primary parts of the DMN are the posterior cingulate cortex (PCC) and the medial prefrontal cortex (mPFC).[27]

Brewer reported that experienced meditators demonstrated decreased DMN activation during meditation. He found that the areas that were activated during meditation were coincidental with the areas of the DMN that were active during the mind-wandering or selfing activity.

Buckner and colleagues reported that the involved brain areas included mPFC, PCC, inferior parietal lobe (IPL), medial temporal lobe (MTL), and the lateral temporal cortex (LTC) (Buckner and colleagues, 2008) (**Fig. 2**).

Somatic Arousal and Patients with Chronic Pain

Traditionally, the minnesota multiphasic personality inventory (MMPI) and other psychological instruments, such as the symptom checklist-90-revised (SCL-90-R), have been used to evaluate patients with chronic pain to determine the various psychological variable that may be impacting their pain and present roadblocks to effective treatment. Patients who are somatically overfocused generally show elevations of the first 3 clinical scales on the MMPI. Those scales are measuring hypochondriasis, depression, and hysteria. Other scales representing anxiety, distrust, or social isolation may also be elevated; but the first 3 scales tend to be the driving force in chronic pain (**Fig. 3**).

Somatic arousal or somatic overfocus represents a form of selfing in which are distressed and spend excessive amounts of time ruminating and worrying about their pain, consequently making it more difficult to treat without using strategies to help patients disengage from the somatically arousing thoughts. Somatic quieting provides one of the most effective ways of bringing about this disengagement. The physical medicine protocol incorporates stretching and breathing exercises that provide the time and change of focus for somatic quieting.

MINDFULNESS-BASED COGNITIVE THERAPY

MBCT is another of the third-wave therapies that grew out of MBSR. Explaining what MBCT requires that we first define mindfulness. In doing so, we need to look at the writings of Thich Nhat Hanh and Jon Kabat-Zinn. Both leading proponents of mindfulness taught the importance of being in the moment. Thich Nhat Hanh taught to wash dishes and only focus on the washing of the dishes. Jon Kabat-Zinn showed that the present-day coveted skills of multitasking are in reality antithetical to mindfulness and being in the moment. In fact research has shown degradation in areas of the brain when subjects are engaged in multitasking.[28,29]

Why is it so difficult to be to be in the moment? What is it about our brains that causes us to either ruminate about the past or stress about tomorrow. The main purpose of the brain is to protect the individual. By asking questions about past events and past consequences, the brain is then obligated, especially if there have been traumatic events in the past, to avoid allowing those events from happening again in the future. We have seen that this function of the brain going into the past to protect the individual from possible future challenges increases anxiety. Furthermore, depression in and of itself occurs when the individual's thinking is stuck in the past; anxiety occurs when the individual's thoughts are constantly worrying about tomorrow.

By learning to live in the moment, without judging the thoughts, without criticizing the self, one can quickly lower anxiety and relieve depression as well as lower other distorted thinking styles. In fact, mindfulness teaches a type of

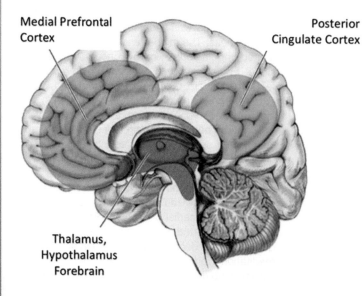

Medial Prefrontal Cortex

Posterior Cingulate Cortex

Thalamus, Hypothalamus Forebrain

Fig. 2. Areas of the default mode network. This diagram shows the primary areas of the default mode network that are active during periods of mind-wandering or selfing. These areas have been found to be active in patients with chronic pain. Patients with chronic pain tend to ruminate (selfing) over their pain. The psychological implications of this are somatic overfocus or somatic arousal.

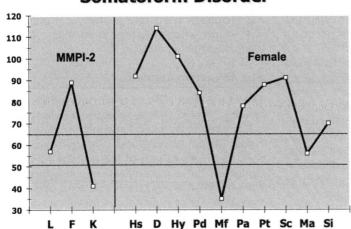

Somatoform Disorder

MMPI-2   Female

L F K   Hs D Hy Pd Mf Pa Pt Sc Ma Si

Fig. 3. Representative MMPI scale of a patient with chronic pain. The MMPI shows very significant elevations of several clinical scales. The triad of chronic pain is seen in elevated Hs, D, and Hy scales. This represents somatic overconcern. This triad does not suggest that the patient is fabricating his or her pain (psychosomatic pain) but does suggest that the patient is hyperfocused on his or her pain. The elevation of the F scale in the 3 validity scales also indicates that the patient is acting out, resentful, and trying to look bad.

thinking and meditation that allows for acceptance and being in the moment. When acceptance occurs and negative thoughts are recognized but not focused on, the negative thoughts come into awareness and are then allowed to just leave.

MBCT is now thought of as part of the third wave of psychotherapy and differs from second-wave CBT. MBCT helps to bring about a more powerful and long-lasting change in patients with fewer relapses. Mindfulness is now being used in conjunction with many traditional types of therapy for several reasons.

CBT, RET, dialectical behavioral therapy (DBT), and psychodynamic and psychoanalytic therapies have all been very effective. One of the problems that occurs with these therapies is the development of patient boredom with the techniques. The therapists have noted that the process of "looking for evidence," might inadvertently increase anxiety down the road. High levels of anxiety serve to increase pain, perpetuate illness and cause somatic arousal (SNS activation—Fight, Flight or Freeze). The third wave of psychotherapy has as its aim activation of the parasympathetic nervous system (PNS activation—Rest and Digest). By so doing, the brain and body release chemicals that clearly shut down the sympathetic nervous system (SNS) and its resultant adrenaline, norepinephrine and cortisol consequences. By activating the PNS the patient is brought out of the battle-hypervigilant mode and out of the DMN (Default Mode Network) to the relaxed, clear-thinking, healing mode.

Extensive research has shown that meditation, mindfulness, acceptance and breathing all combine to activate the parasympathetic faster and more easily without dependence on medications or other ancillary aids.

The addition of mindfulness to CT, DBT, or CBT is like adding a pinch of salt to a recipe: it brings out the flavor and makes it more desirable and more effective.

Referring back to the aforementioned somatically overfocused patients, how would we expect them to respond to CT that included mindfulness? What would the treatment plan like?

Instead of doing thought records whereby we would ask patients to record all negative thoughts and then look for evidence to support those thoughts, we might now ask patients to accept the thoughts without judgment and just let them pass by (acceptance).

THE MINDFULNESS-BASED PHYSICAL MEDICINE PROGRAM-SOMATIC QUIETING

TMD and OFP disorders are associated with increased temporal summation, pain facilitation, and expanding of the receptive field, motor dysfunction, cognitive dysfunction, maladaptive brain plasticity, and learned helplessness. All of these factors converge into the state of somatic arousal.

Patients who have OFP disorders will benefit from using a mindfulness-based physical medicine program during the day to provide episodes of somatic quieting. The exercises should be given not only to the patients with musculoskeletal pain but also patients with neurovascular and neuropathic pain because patients who are seen in OFP clinics with the last two pain disorders usually have gone from doctor to doctor without benefit of correct diagnosis or appropriate treatment. This circumstance results in creating a state of hypervigilance or somatic arousal in patients that needs to be downregulated with somatic quieting. The mindfulness-based physical medicine program reduces the hypervigilance and should be initiated on the first visit and reviewed on each succeeding office visit (**Box 1**).

One of the key factors in creating somatic arousal in patients is stress. The two stress-related systems are the sympathetic-adrenal medullary system, involving release of epinephrine/norepinephrine (catecholamines), and the hypothalamic-pituitary-adrenal axis that stimulates release of cortisol. These two systems bring about significant somatic alerting. Benson and colleagues[30] coined the term "relaxation response" to describe the effect of focused attention and guided imagery on decreasing the stress response. They reported that using these techniques decreased blood

pressure, blood sugar, cortisol, and the catecholamines (ie, somatic arousal) as well as enhanced the endorphin and γ-aminobutyric acid systems, the neurochemical substrate of somatic quieting, sleep, and pain modulation.[31,32]

The Relaxation Response

One of the most effective treatment modalities for treating chronic OFP is utilization of stretching/posture exercises that incorporate breathing exercises. Deep breathing and exhaling have been used for years as part of the physical medicine protocols, but a more effective routine incorporates the mindfulness breathing into the stretching exercises. These exercises are beneficial not only for patients with musculoskeletal pain but also patients with headache and neuropathic pain. Patients are taught the stretching exercises that require bringing the awareness to the immediacy of the stretch itself and also bringing the thoughts to the breathing that is done at the same time. These exercises help bring about somatic quieting.

Benson and colleagues[30–32] showed that the effectiveness of the relaxation response using a progressive relaxation procedure helped keep the thought processes focused on the present and current moment (**Box 2**).

As can be appreciated in **Box 2**, there are several tools that can bring about the relaxation response, for example, focused concentration, physical medicine protocols, focused stomach breathing, and progressive relaxation. The relaxation response is quieting the somatic overfocus. These tools cause the cognitive focus to change from the pain to relaxation and breathing process.

Mindfulness-Based Physical Medicine Protocol

The mindfulness-based physical medicine protocol begins by eliminating possible provoking factors related to the OFP complaint. For musculoskeletal pain involving the masticatory muscles, this involves putting patients on a soft diet and eliminating any oral/jaw habits that may involve masticatory muscle activity. This protocol also applies to cervical muscle pain. In addition, patients are instructed to use moist heat and ice for 10 minutes 2 times per day. During the time with moist heat, patients are to do focused breathing.

The second step is to correct both jaw and cervical posture. Patients are taught how to do a jaw posture exercise by placing the tip of the tongue on the palate behind the teeth, bringing attention to the feel of the tongue touching the palate and slowly inhaling through the nose and exhaling,

---

Box 1
Physical medicine program

Patients are given the following:

- Treatment plan
- Treatment contract
- Pain diary
- Somatic quieting protocols
  - N-position stretch
  - N-position rest: practice the focused breathing from this position
  - Chin tuck/shoulder stretch
  - Instructions for moist heat and ice
  - Focused breathing
  - The relaxation response instructions plus handout
  - Walk 10 minutes per day in sun.
- Review sleep problems.
- Stabilize pain medication and/or give nonsteroidal antiinflammatory drugs or other pain medications as needed. All medications should be taken time contingently, *not* as needed for PAIN.
- Make referral for physical therapy if needed.
- Make referral for behavioral medicine if needed.

After the assessment, patients are given a diagnosis and treatment plan. Included in the treatment plan are some physical medicine protocols that are designed to bring about somatic quieting. These protocols involve stretching exercises, instruction for use of moist heat and ice over the tender muscles, as well as instructions for focused breathing. These instructions are accompanied with printed instructions and an explanation of the relaxation response.

Box 2
Benson's steps for inducing the relaxation response

1. Sit quietly in a comfortable position.

2. Close your eyes.

3. Deeply relax all your muscles, beginning at your feet and progressing up to your face. Keep them relaxed. (Relax your tongue and thoughts will cease.)

4. Breathe through your nose. Become aware of your breathing. As you breathe out, say the word *one*[a] silently to yourself. For example, breathe in and then out and say *one*,[a] in and out, and repeat *one*.[a] Breathe easily and naturally.

5. Continue for 10 to 20 minutes. You may open your eyes to check the time, but do not use an alarm. When you finish, sit quietly for several minutes, at first with your eyes closed and later with your eyes opened. Do not stand up for a few minutes.

6. Do not worry about whether you are successful in achieving a deep level of relaxation. Maintain a passive attitude and permit relaxation to occur at its own pace. When distracting thoughts occur, try to ignore them by not dwelling on them and return to repeating *one*.[a]

7. With practice, the response should come with little effort. Practice the technique once or twice daily but not within 2 hours after any meal, because the digestive processes seem to interfere with the elicitation of the relaxation response.

[a] Choose any soothing, mellifluous-sounding word, preferably with no meaning or association, in order to avoid stimulation of unnecessary thoughts.
Data from Refs.[30–32]

---

bringing attention to the sensation of air going through the nose and the sensation of the jaw muscles becoming relaxed and the jaw feeling heavy and relaxed. This tongue position should be maintained throughout the day with the focus on the relaxed sensation and bringing the attention to the breathing.

The next step involves having patients open the jaw as far as they can without removing the tongue from the palate. Patients are instructed to hold this stretched position and continue the focus on the breathing for 6 seconds. The jaw is then relaxed; patients then inhale through the nose and a then subsequently exhale, and then this jaw stretch procedure is repeated. This exercise should also be taught to patients with neuropathic pain and chronic headache because this is an active part of somatic quieting. This exercise is to be repeated every 2 hours throughout the waking day.

A neck muscle stretch is also taught on this first visit. This exercise involves taking a breath and holding it, and then gently pulling the head forward moving the chin to the chest with a hand and exhaling at the same time. The head position is adjusted to move the head back over the shoulders first and then to do the stretch from this position. It should be repeated 6 times in a row with the focus being on the breathing. This stretching exercise is to be done 6 times during the day with focus on the relaxation and breathing. Patients are to use the hand to gently stretch and bring the chin to the chest, holding that position and focusing on the breathing. In addition, it should also be taught to patients with neuropathic pain and with chronic headache because this is an active part of somatic quieting. Patients are instructed to repeat the exercises every 2 hours throughout the waking day.

On the first visit after the initial examination and instruction period of physical medicine and focused breathing, patients are asked to demonstrate the exercises given on that first visit. This time is for correcting stretches and breathing exercises that are being done incorrectly. Patients are then given instructions for 3 neck exercises that are to be done in addition to the jaw posture and stretching and the neck stretching. These 3 neck exercises are as follows.

Cervical rotation
Rotate the head to look over the shoulder. An inhale is initially done; the head is rotated to look over the shoulder; a slow exhale is done, and then the head is brought back to center. This stretching exercise with the breathing is repeated 6 times in a row on one side and then repeated on the other side.

Nose to armpit stretch
The hand is placed on the crown of the head and the neck is gently stretched, pulling the nose toward the armpit on the side of the hand. Patients are instructed to inhale, hold, and release the air through the nose as the head is guided down. This stretching exercise with the breathing is

repeated 6 times in a row on one side then repeated on the other side.

Ear to shoulder stretch

From the position of the head centered over the shoulders, one hand is brought to the crown of the head and the head/neck is stretched by bringing the ear to the shoulder by the hand. Patients are instructed to inhale, hold, and release the air through the nose as the head is guided down to the side. This stretching exercise with the breathing is repeated 6 times in a row on one side then repeated on the other side.

Each succeeding visit is used first to check on the patients' compliance and technique of stretching the jaw and neck muscles. The third follow-up visit is used to teach a spray-and-stretch technique if patients have persistent muscle tightness.

All of these protocols, posture correction, stretching, breathing, and spray-and-stretch technique increase patients' ability to take control and modify their pain. Previous to visiting the OFP specialist, most patients have had unfortunate and unsuccessful visits with dentists and/or physicians who were not able to diagnose or treat their pain. Their sense of loss of control and hopelessness has been confirmed by each of these failures. Giving them tools they can use to manage their pain is one of the most beneficial and effective things we can do in the realm of chronic orofacial pain.

MINDFULNESS-BASED STRESS REDUCTION

In 1979, Jon Kabat-Zinn was teaching MBSR using 2 meditation practices, breathing medication and mountain meditation, and yoga. These practices were introduced into many different health care settings and have become the most widely studied techniques for stress reduction. MBSR is a third-wave addition to CBT and helps to build concentration, present focus, acceptance, and somatic quieting. In 2004, Grossman and colleagues[33] published a meta-analysis of 20 high-quality MBSR studies that covered a wide spectrum of patients, including individuals with cancer, chronic pain, cardiovascular disease, depression, and anxiety. They found a moderate to strong effect size beneficial response to MBSR for reducing stress in the various disorders studied. The MBSR uses the focused breathing exercises to bring attention back from the mind-wandering to the present moment.

So again, Mindfulness is the aware, balanced acceptance of the present experience. It isn't more complicated than that. It is opening to or receiving the present moment, pleasant or unpleasant, just as it is, without either clinging to it or rejecting it.

—Sylvia Boorstein

MBSR is a program designed initially to assist people with chronic pain and other issues developed by Jon Kabat-Zinn at the University of Massachusetts Medical Center. It uses a combination of mindfulness meditation, body awareness, and yoga to help people become more mindful.

Generally, MBSR has been used as a group program that focuses on teaching mindfulness awareness. The program is an 8-week workshop taught by certified trainers that entails weekly group meetings, homework, and instruction in 3 formal techniques: mindfulness meditation, body scanning, and simple yoga postures. According to Kabat-Zinn, the basis of MBSR is mindfulness, which he defined as "moment-to-moment, nonjudgmental awareness."

To quote Kabat-Zinn in 2011: "I bent over backward to structure it (MBSR) and find ways to speak about it that avoided as much as possible the risk of it being seen as Buddhist, 'New Age,' 'Eastern Mysticism' or just plain 'flaky.' To my mind this was a constant and serious risk that would have undermined our attempts to present it as a common-sensical, evidence-based, and ordinary, and ultimately a legitimate element of mainstream medical care."[34,35]

The goal is to focus patients on the experience of the moment as it passes and then help patients to allow that moment to leave and the next to move into place. ACT therapy, previously mentioned—a nice acronym for acceptance, choice, and taking action—then becomes the therapy du jour. Acceptance implies the ability to let go of questions, judgments, blaming, and criticism. Living in the moment would preclude the ability to ruminate on questions and judgments. Choice is the place where all patients, whether in psychotherapy or medical treatment, have to arrive. All patients have to realize that they have, for the most part, the choice to think positively or negatively and the choice to move forward or stay in the past. The idea of taking action puts patients back in the driver's seat, responsible for their own process of healing and cure as well as for their own discomfort.

MBSR teaches how to be in the moment through mindfulness training and dovetails with ACT. The idea of stress reduction is interesting. For almost 30 years, the word *stress* had not been a part of the psychologist's lexicon. Somehow it came back in the early 2000s, possibly due to an increased awareness of the significance of stress on disease or possibly due to a realization that medication was not the long-term answer to wellness. Regardless, we now understand that stress and anxiety, depression, feelings, thoughts, and emotions are major components to health and well-being. We also now know that rather than fighting against negative behaviors, be they thoughts, actions, or feelings, and trying with all our might to win the battle, it is more efficacious to accept, breathe, meditate, love, and care for oneself and then to let go.

Referring back to the patients with OFP, the authors would incorporate into their treatment relaxation exercises, breathing exercises, mindfulness meditation, and possibly some mild yogic exercises. This treatment would generate somatic quieting, decrease anxiety, and ultimately decrease chronic pain. To be sure, this is a process. Probably the most challenging aspect of introducing and maintaining CBT, MBCT, or MBSR treatment is overcoming the expectation on the part of patients to receive immediate and complete relief. The age of immediate satisfaction and gratification has taken its toll on us all. It has also precluded us as clinicians and patients from taking responsibility for the work that is required to overcome our emotional and physical challenges. Of course, medication has its role; but time has shown us that its effects do not, for the most part, lead to a cure. We have seen that once patients with chronic pain discontinue the medication, whether pain medication or antidepressant, the pain can return with a vengeance.

Somatic quieting is a step-by-step process whereby patients and the clinician work collaboratively to decrease baselines levels of rumination or somatic focus. If patients present with chronic pain between 8 and 10, our first goal is to reduce it to a 6 to 8 or a 7 to 9 and let it stabilize there for a period of time. Then we can continue to lower that baseline in the same way. The process requires patience, faith, hope, and work. It is advisable for the clinician to develop rapport and trust with patients in order to help move them through the process.

The approach with CBT, MBCT, or MBSR is effective, although it takes time. It is an important and integral part of pain management, and results are seen relatively quickly. The patients who have chronic neuropathic pain that is not responding to medication management need to be working with a behavioral medicine doctor who has expertise in CBT and the third-wave techniques. Additionally, the OFP specialist should be able to guide patients in the physical medicine protocols that include focused breathing practices to help achieve somatic quieting.

REFERENCES

1. IASP. Classification of chronic pain. Seattle (WA): IASP Press; 1994.
2. Reeves JL 2nd, Merrill RL. Diagnostic and treatment challenges in occlusal dysesthesia. J Calif Dent Assoc 2007;35(3):198–207.
3. Patton LL, Siegel MA, Benoliel R, et al. Management of burning mouth syndrome: systematic review and management recommendations. Oral Surg Oral Med Oral Pathol Oral Radiol Endod 2007; 103(Suppl):S39.e1–13.
4. Graff-Radford SB, Solberg WK. Is atypical odontalgia a psychological problem? Oral Surg Oral Med Oral Pathol 1993;75(5):579–82.
5. Graff-Radford SB, Solberg WK. Atypical odontalgia. J Craniomandib Disord 1992;6(4):260–5.
6. Graff-Radford SB, Solberg WK. Atypical odontalgia. CDA J 1986;14(12):27–32.
7. Engel G. The predictive value of psychological variables for disease and death. Ann Intern Med 1976; 85(6):673–4.
8. Engel G. The clinical application of the biopsychosocial model. Am J Psychiatry 1980;137(7): 535–44.
9. Vowles KE. Editorial overview: third wave behavior therapies. Curr Opin Psychol 2015;2:v–vii.
10. Scott W, McCracken LM. Psychological flexibility, acceptance and committment therapy, and chronic pain. Curr Opin Psychol 2015;2:91–6.
11. McKay M, Davis MP, Fanning P. Thoughts & feelings: the art of cognitive stress intervention. Oakland (CA): New Harbinger Publications; 1981.
12. Keefe FJ. Cognitive behavioral therapy for managing pain. Clin Psychol 1996;49(3):4–5.
13. Akerblom S, Perrin S, Fischer MR, et al. The mediating role of acceptance in multidisciplinary cognitive-behavioral therapy for chronic pin. J Pain 2015;16(7):606–15.
14. Goldberg MB, Mock D, Ichise M, et al. Neuropsychologic deficits and clinical features of posttraumatic temporomandibular disorders. J Orofac Pain 1996;10(2):126–40.
15. Goldberg RT, Maciewicz RJ. Prediction of pain rehabilitation outcomes by motivation measures. Disabil Rehabil 1994;16(1):21–5.
16. Ploghaus A, Tracey I, Gati JS, et al. Dissociating pain from its anticipation in the human brain. Science 1999;284(5422):1979–81.
17. Hodges PW, Tucker K. Moving differently in pain: a new theory to explain the adaptation to pain. Pain 2011;152(3 Suppl):S90–8.
18. Teutsch S, Herken W, Bingel U, et al. Changes in brain gray matter due to repetitive painful stimulation. Neuroimage 2008;42(2):845–9.
19. Boudreau S, Romaniello A, Wang K, et al. The effects of intra-oral pain on motor cortex

neuroplasticity associated with short-term novel tongue-protrusion training in humans. Pain 2007; 132(1–2):169–78.

20. Hollins M, Harper D, Gallagher S, et al. Perceived intensity and unpleasantness of cutaneous and auditory stimuli: an evaluation of the generalized hypervigilance hypothesis. Pain 2009;141(3):215–21.

21. Koechlin E. Frontal pole function: what is specifically human? Trends Cogn Sci 2011;15(6):241–3.

22. Van Damme S, Crombez G, Eccleston C. Disengagement from pain: the role of catastrophic thinking about pain. Pain 2004;107(1–2):70–6.

23. Van Damme S, Crombez G, Eccleston C. The anticipation of pain modulates spatial attention: evidence for pain-specificity in high-pain catastrophizers. Pain 2004;111(3):392–9.

24. Moayedi M, Weissman-Fogel I, Salomons TV, et al. White matter brain and trigeminal nerve abnormalities in temporomandibular disorder. Pain 2012; 153(7):1467–77.

25. Moayedi M, Weissman-Fogel I, Salomons TV, et al. Abnormal gray matter aging in chronic pain patients. Brain Res 2012;1456:82–93.

26. Killingsworth MA, Gilbert DT. A wandering mind is an unhappy mind. Science 2010;330(6006):932.

27. Raichle ME. The brain's default mode network. Annu Rev Neurosci 2015;38:433–47.

28. Rosen C. The myth of multitasking. New Atlantis 2008;20:105–10.

29. Levitin DJ. The Organized Mind: Thinking straight in the age of information overload. New York: Dutton; 2014. p. 16.

30. Benson H, Beary JF, Carol MP. The relaxation response. Psychiatry 1974;37(1):37–46.

31. Benson H. The relaxation response: history, physiological basis and clinical usefulness. Acta Med Scand Suppl 1982;660:231–7.

32. Benson H. The relaxation response: therapeutic effect. Science 1997;278(5344):1694–5.

33. Grossman P, Niemann L, Schmidt S, et al. Mindfulness-based stress reduction and health benefits. A meta-analysis. J Psychosom Res 2004;57(1):35–43.

34. Wllliams JMG, Kabat-Zinn J. Mindfulness: diverse perspectives on its meaning, origins, and multiple applications at the intersection of science and dharma. Contemp Buddhism 2011;12:1–18.

35. Williams JMG, Kabat-Zinn J, editors. Mindfulness: diverse perspectives on its meaning, origins and applications. London; New York: Routledge; 2013.

A Model for Opioid Risk Stratification
Assessing the Psychosocial Components of Orofacial Pain

Ronald J. Kulich, PhD[a,b,1,*], Jordan Backstrom, MDiv, PsyD[c,2],
Jennifer Brownstein, MA[a,b,1,*], Matthew Finkelman, PhD[d,*],
Shuchi Dhadwal, DMD[a,3,*],
David DiBennedetto, MD, DABPM[e,2]

KEYWORDS

• Opioid • Risk-management • Dentistry • Substance abuse • Interprofessional

KEY POINTS

• Deaths related to opioid abuse continue to be a national epidemic, with diversion and nonmedical use of prescription medications often occurring as a result of prescriptions written for acute pain by dentistry.
• Dentists are assuming increased responsibilities in the public health arena and now play an important role in the judicious monitoring of the dispensing of controlled substances.
• Dentists also now are in a position to use formal screening strategies for the patient at risk for substance abuse, an important role in risk mitigation.
• After assessing risk, the dentist's responsibilities include counselling the patient, referral, and close collaboration with cotreating physician colleagues.

In the last 20 years, there is evidence of increasing deaths due to overdose because controlled substances are more widely available.[1] Dentistry has been particularly affected by the national crisis in opioid abuse. Dentistry, largely as a result of analgesic prescriptions for surgical procedures, had been identified as the second highest opioid prescriber group. There has been an overall drop in opioid prescribing by dentists, largely due to a combination of continuing educational efforts and emphasis from the general media on the apparent risks.[2] An especially important tool in mitigating this risk is the psychosocial assessment. Nonetheless, evidence of more judicious screening for the high-risk patient and counseling or referral for substance abuse care remains lacking.

Disclosure Statement: All authors have nothing to disclose.
[a] Department of Diagnostic Sciences, Craniofacial Pain and Headache Center, Tufts School of Dental Medicine, Boston, MA, USA; [b] Department of Anesthesia, Critical Care and Pain Medicine, Massachusetts General Hospital, Harvard Medical School, Boston, MA, USA; [c] Boston Pain Care Center, Waltham, MA, USA; [d] Department of Biostatistics and Experimental Design, Tufts University School of Dental Medicine, 1 Kneeland Street, 7th Floor, Boston, MA 02129, USA; [e] Department of Diagnostic Sciences, Boston Pain Care, Tufts School of Dental Medicine, Boston, MA, USA
[1] Present address: 15 Parkman St, Boston, MA 02114.
[2] Present address: 85 First Avenue, Waltham, MA 02451.
[3] Present address: 1 Kneeland Street, 7th Floor, Boston, MA 02129.
* Corresponding authors. 1 Kneeland Street, 6th Floor, Boston, MA 02129.
E-mail address: rkulich@mgh.harvard.edu

Oral Maxillofacial Surg Clin N Am 28 (2016) 261–273
http://dx.doi.org/10.1016/j.coms.2016.03.006
1042-3699/16/$ – see front matter © 2016 Elsevier Inc. All rights reserved.

As interdisciplinary clinics and research programs become more common, the practice of implementing a psychosocial assessment as part of a comprehensive care plan has become the standard of care. This change has developed in parallel with the general recognition that patients presenting with orofacial pain experience higher levels of psychological distress and have more psychiatric comorbidities than other dental patient populations.[3,4] Patients with temporomandibular disorders often endorse depressed mood, anxiety, and posttraumatic stress disorder at rates significantly higher than controls.[5] Indeed, the literature has developed sufficiently now to demonstrate a clear etiologic link between psychological factors and problems of the masticatory muscles, the temporomandibular joint, and associated physiologic structures.[6] Specifically, the psychological factors of personality traits, stress reactivity, somatic focus, and the tendency toward catastrophizing, have an exacerbating influence on myofascial pain and increase the risk of chronic painful temporomandibular disorders.[6] Yet, even as the presence and expectation of psychosocial assessment in the orofacial pain setting becomes more ubiquitous, the dual function, both as a diagnostic instrument in holistic patient care and as a tool for risk assessment, remains confused, particularly in the context of opioid prescribing.

Traditionally, the central components of the assessment have included[7]

- Patient rapport building
- Acquisition of medical and psychiatric history with identification of recent medical changes and life stressors
- Exploration of the patient's lifestyle such as diet, exercise, and social support
- Current level of function
- Any relevant legal issues
- A mental status examination with suicide risk assessment and exploration of any substance use disorder.

Although all these areas remain central to the provision of a quality psychosocial assessment, the assessment rubric must be flexible and organized under the conceptual primacy of opiate risk if these medications could potentially be part of the orofacial pain patient's overall treatment plan. This article describes a way forward, emphasizing both quality patient care and a method of risk-mitigation for the dentists and pain specialists who provide that care.

The scope of the opioid problem dates to the mid-1990s, when adequate treatment of acute and chronic pain was identified as an international public health concern. Multiple international health care agencies identified access to pain care as part of the problem, with debate in the United States continuing as to whether there has been any clear progression.[8,9] It is argued that there needs to be a balance between risk mitigation and access to effective analgesic use for the patient with pain.[10] The widely disseminated Institute of Medicine report, *Relieving Pain in America*, highlights issues of access with its first principle, "Effective pain management is a moral imperative, a professional responsibility, and the duty of people in the healing professions."[11(pp3)] Despite this attention, concern about opioid abuse, diversion, and the increasing number of opioid-related deaths persist.

Diversion of prescription medications has also been recognized as a growing problem. For example, individuals with substance abuse issues often obtained their medication from family members and friends. In a survey of dental patients, Ashrafioun and colleagues[12] (2014) found that approximately 5% to 10% of patients reported that in the past 30 days they sometimes or rarely took someone else's medications. Although diversion may seem to involve relatively few patients within a dental practice, the high volume of patients seen in dentistry underscores the magnitude of the problem. By 2010, 81.6% of individuals ages 12 years and older who used opioids illicitly were obtaining them from a friend or relative, with 54.2% obtaining it without a monetary fee. By 2011, 52 million people in the United States ages 12 years and older used prescription drugs, nonmedically, 1 or more times in their lifetime. Of these individuals, more than 6% were found to be using prescription drugs illicitly within the prior month.[13]

As opioid-related deaths increased concurrent with an increase in sales, the pharmaceutical industry and prescribers were considered largely responsible. Among the most common drugs implicated in deaths were the short-acting analgesics, including hydrocodone and oxycodone, with methadone being a particular risk when prescribed for pain. Dentists were writing prescriptions for 1 to 1.5 billion doses of immediate opioids per year, only exceeded by primary care physicians and internists.[14,15] Deaths were also attributed to polypharmacy, with benzodiazepines significantly adding to the risk. Drug overdose became the leading cause of death, exceeding motor vehicle accidents in many states.[16]

Dentistry began to respond to the public health crisis. Levy and colleagues[17] (2015) found that the largest drop in percentage of prescribing from 2007 to 2012 was from emergency medicine

(−9%) and dentistry (−6%). Meanwhile, other researchers, such as Rasubala and colleagues[2] (2015), suggested a more precipitous drop in opioid prescriptions in dentistry by as much as 70%. This decrease in opioid prescribing by dentistry may have resulted in fewer drugs being available on the street; however, patients already abusing opioids now seem to be shifting to cheaper alternatives to address their addiction (eg, heroin). Hence, deaths continue at high levels despite the changes in clinician prescribing practices.[18,19]

As encouraged by Denisco and colleagues[20] (2011), dentists and other health care providers may have been writing prescriptions for fewer pills or have simply declined to write any opioids for patients who seemed to be at risk. Other practitioners completely modified their practice, with typical comments in continuing education conferences such as: we just do not write for opioids in our practice anymore, it is not worth the hassle, and I cannot be bothered checking the prescription monitoring program all the time. As a consequence of dentists prescribing fewer pills or none at all, acute pain care may be compromised. Additionally, this trend may perpetuate missed opportunities to assess and refer the high-risk patients for substance use treatment.

Despite a decrease in prescribing opiates, substance use risk assessment does seem be viewed as important by many dentists, with three-fourths of dentists reporting that they ask their patients about substance abuse. Nonetheless, dentists remain ambivalent, with two-thirds of the same population feeling that such screening is not necessarily compatible with their professional role.[21] Dental societies and governmental organizations are seeking to challenge this attitude with a host of educational programs and published guidelines that underscore the increasing role of dentistry in risk assessment, emphasizing the profession's role in the public health arena.

The dentist's responsibilities are expanding, a development that is especially the case when the clinician encounters at-risk populations with complex medical or psychiatric comorbidities.[20,22,23] Substance misuse and abuse assessment, counseling the patient, referral, and interprofessional collaboration now seem to be increasingly within the dentist's professional role. The American Dental Association recently readdressed the issue with educational efforts such as The Practical Guide to Substance Abuse Disorders (2015),[23] providing another template for underscoring the importance of comprehensive risk assessment. Educational efforts may eventually have an impact. Parish and colleagues[21] (2015) found that prior experience and knowledge about substance misuse were the strongest predictors of whether the clinician queried the patient on this substance abuse and accepted this type of screening as part of their role in patient care.

SUBSTANCE USE DISORDERS

The definition of addiction has evolved, with the most recent Diagnostic and Statistical Manual of Mental Disorders, 5th edition, moving toward the term substance use disorders.[24,25] Problems with the older definition included confusion concerning terms such as physical dependence, with an effort to clarify and strengthen the criteria while avoiding cultural biases. The new definition classifies substance use disorders according to criteria that include impaired control, substance overuse, social impairment, and risky use. The criteria also provide for a designation of mild, moderate, or severe substance use. Definitions of terms typically considered in the assessment of substance use disorders remain the same and are of particular importance in treating the at-risk patient. For example, tolerance is still defined as "a state of adaptation in which exposure to the drug induces changes that result in a diminution of one or more of the drug's effects over time," whereas physical dependence is "the state of adaptation this is manifested by a drug class specific withdrawal syndrome that can be produced by abrupt cessation, rapid dose reduction, decreasing blood level of the drug, and/or administration of an antagonist."[26(pp2)]

The diagnostic criteria also address specific characteristics of the particular drug being abused. In the case of opioid use disorder, these include "a strong desire for opioids, inability to control or reduce use, continued use despite interference with major obligations or social functioning, use of larger amounts over time, development of tolerance, spending a great deal of time to obtain and use opioids, and withdrawal symptoms that occur after stopping or reducing use (eg, negative mood, nausea or vomiting, muscle aches, diarrhea, fever, and insomnia)."[18,19]

Special considerations also have arisen with respect to dental patients taking opioids, particularly with use over an extended period of time and at high doses. One of many unforeseen consequences has included an increase in pain, an outcome seen years early in patients managed in methadone maintenance programs. Building on the early work of Ballantyne and Mao[27] (2003), opioid-induced hyperalgesia has been defined by nociceptive sensitization caused by exposure to opioids. The response has been considered paradoxic, wherein the patient responds to painful stimuli with heightened sensitivity and loss of opioid efficacy. Further increases in opioid dosing may result in transient improvement in the patient's pain, although pain ultimately increases in time, independent of nociception.[28] Although relevant in the setting of chronic pain management, the phenomenon also takes on importance in the context of the acute pain patient who arrives at the dental practice already on high doses of opioids. It also is important to underscore that opioid-induced hyperalgesia not only is seen with opioid-related substance use disorders but also with chronic cancer and some noncancer conditions in which chronic opioid therapy is used.

In addition to opioids, some at-risk patients may present positive for a range of substances, including illicit drugs such as cocaine, as well as prescription medications being used illicitly such as benzodiazepines, stimulants, various sedatives, and/or alcohol.[29] Other prescription drugs, including barbiturates, antiseizure agents, and various other psychotropic drugs, may be misused, further complicating care. The number of legal and illicit substances of abuse remains large and the options continue to grow for those who actively abuse substances. Although alcohol abuse has been widely studied and has been shown to be predictive of a poor outcome with many dental and medical conditions, tobacco smoking (nicotine) also has been shown to be 1 of the better predictors of a problematic course with opioid therapy.[30]

Substance-use disorders remain a public health problem with 24 million Americans suffering from some type of substance abuse and only 10% may be receiving treatment.[21,24] Given the incidence in the general population, as many as 15% of patients who present to any dental or medical practice may be at risk. Failing to recognize and conduct judicious screening places the patient in a vulnerable position and may predict medico-legal risks for the clinician.

A MODEL FOR RISK ASSESSMENT AND PATIENT MANAGEMENT

Notwithstanding this expanding role for dentistry in the area of substance use screening, it is both unrealistic and inappropriate to expect the practicing oral surgeon or primary care dentist to assume the role of a mental health practitioner or primary care physician. For the dentist, assessment of substance use risk must be brief and cost-effective. If possible, the assessment should be tailored to the specific practice of dentistry, and the predictive validity and reliability of any assessment protocol should be well established for the general dental population. The fields of primary care and pain medicine have made advances in the development of risk screening tools, as well as templates for counseling the at-risk patient. Dentistry can adapt and use these tools, although the special needs of dentistry require consideration.

Within the context of a dental practice, screening for substance abuse and related risk factors requires brief, directed questioning, as well as access to other sources of patient information. Substance use risk items can be integrated into a dental office-screening questionnaire, although a checklist is typically insufficient in the absence of the necessary interactive query between the clinician and patient. Other professionals in the office can greatly assist. For example, dental hygienists can also play cost-effective roles in the clinical assessment, as they do in other critical components of the patient's care. The National Institute on Drug Abuse offers a brief assessment tailored to primary physician practices yet relevant for general dentistry.[18]

Notwithstanding the importance of specific risk questionnaires, a thorough history-taking remains the first step in assessment. Although many patients may be reluctant to disclose current or past misuse of substance, it is frequently the clinician's reticence to engage in this interactive query that remains the primary barrier. In some cases, patients with a substance use history also may fear obtaining inadequate pain relief for a dental procedure because they are perceived as being high-risk, a fear that may not be unfounded. These barriers can be overcome and part of that process involves a dialogue with the patient while integrating other patient information into the interview. Prescription monitoring program results, detail from previous medical and dental records, and cross-communication with other health care providers provides data for fruitful discussion with the patient.

Box 1 provides an inventory of the risk factors for a likely problematic course with opioid therapy, as well as risks for substance misuse. No single risk is definitively predictive, and the relative contribution of each factor may vary within the individual. For example, a patient may have a significant early history of substance abuse, although he or she has been abstinent from drugs for many years, has established positive relationships with his or her health care providers, has worked reliably, and has readily shared sensitive information about his care. In contrast, a patient may deny most risk factors or provide inconsistent history of medication use after worrisome results from the prescription monitoring program. Although clinical judgment remains crucial, there are tools to substantially improve the assessment process.

Medical risk indicators can be as important as psychosocial risk factors. Although history of bipolar disorder or post-traumatic stress disorder indicates possible risk with opioid therapy, there are other medical factors potentially predictive of a problematic course. A history of kidney disease, pancreatitis, chronic pulmonary disease, history of heart failure, and diagnosis of pain conditions such as peripheral neuropathy are predictors of risk for substance abuse as well as risk for overdose.[31] Zedler and colleagues[31] (2015) provide a

brief screen in **Table 1** for overdose or risk of respiratory depression and each item is weighted for quick scoring. Oral consequences of substance use also can occur with common drugs of abuse. For example, movement disorders such as buccolingual dyskinesia can occur with cocaine abuse. Many other illicit drugs have various oral manifestations. Prolonged opioid abuse can be evidenced with multiple decayed or missing teeth, or poor nutrition, with the underlying cause being chronically poor hygiene for some patients. Nonetheless, with the recent increase in opioid misuse and abuse, a patient may have few observable risk factors and appear quite healthy.

Although a basic review of the patient's mental status and other behavioral observations are important, patients on stable high doses of opioids tend to show minimal cognitive impairment in contrast to individuals using a range of other illicit drugs or alcohol. Infections or cellulites may be present in the area where the drug has been injected, and observation of specific risk factors such as track marks should be noted in the record and addressed within an overall risk assessment and communication with the patient.

Prescription Monitoring Programs

The addition of the prescription monitoring program seems to positively affect more than 70% of prescribing physicians by reducing inappropriate prescribing.[2,32] Conversely, the prescription monitoring program also may facilitate appropriate prescribing for patients requiring necessary pain control. Irvine and colleagues[32] (2014) found that almost all users reported discussing problematic prescription monitoring program data with the patient, with 54% making substance abuse or mental health referrals. Given the promising data with medical providers, the American Dental Association has encouraged use of the prescription monitoring program for several years, with some states now mandating its use by dentists. Practical barriers are being removed to provide ease-of-use in dental settings. Most states now permit practice assistants or delegates to assist with accessing the electronic data. Other states permit batch queries so all patient prescription monitoring program results can be accessed at the beginning of a day. Barriers still exist because some prescription monitoring program systems remain difficult to use and many states experience slowed access because of delays in the reporting by pharmacies. Cross-state communication also remains poor and most states do not require use of the prescription monitoring program, resulting in gaps in reporting for some high-risk groups. For example,

Table 1
Determine score for Risk Index for Overdose or Serious Opioid-induced Respiratory Depression (RIOSORD)[a]

Question	Points for Yes Response
In the past 6 mo, has the patient had a healthcare visit (outpatient, inpatient or ED) involving any of the following health conditions?[b]	
Opioid dependence?[c]	15
Chronic hepatitis or cirrhosis?	9
Bipolar disorder or schizophrenia?	7
Chronic pulmonary disease (eg, emphysema, chronic bronchitis, asthma, pneumoconiosis, asbestosis)?	5
Chronic kidney disease with clinically significant renal impairment?	5
An active traumatic injury, excluding burns (eg, fracture, dislocation, contusion, laceration, wound)?	4
Sleep apnea?	3
Does the patient consume:	
An extended-release or long-acting (ER/LA) formulation of any prescription opioid?[d] (eg, OxyContin, Oramorph-SR, methadone, fentanyl patch)	9
Methadone? (Methadone is a long-acting opioid so also check "ER/LA formulation" [9 points])	9
Oxycodone? (If it has an ER/LA formulation [eg, OxyContin] also check "ER/LA formulation" [9 points])	3
A prescription antidepressant? (eg, fluoxetine, citaJopram, venlafaxine, amitriptyline)	7
A prescription benzodiazepine? (eg, diazepam, alprazolam)	4
Is the patient's current maximum prescribed opioid dose[e]:	
≥100 mg morphine equivalents per day?	16
50–<100 mg morphine equivalents per day?	9
20–<50 mg morphine equivalents per day?	5
In the past 6 mo, has the patient:	
Had one or more emergency department (ED) visits?	11
Been hospitalized for one or more days?	8
Total point score (maximum 115)	

[a] This risk is intended for completion by a health care professional.
[b] The condition does not have to be the *primary* reason for the visit but should be entered in the chart or EHR as *one* of the reasons or diagnoses for the visit.
[c] The International Classification of Disease (9th and 10th Revisions) codes the diagnosis of substance "addiction" as substance "dependence."
[d] A patient consuming one or more opioids with an ER/LA formulation receives 9 additional points regardless of the number of different ER/LA products consumed.
[e] Include *all* prescription opioids consumed on a daily basis.
From Zedler B, Xie L, Wang L, et al. Development of a risk index for serious prescription opioid-induced respiratory depression or overdose in Veteran's Health Administration patients. Pain Med 2015;16(8):1574; with permission.

methadone maintenance clinics are not required to report due to federal regulations and access to the Veterans Administration Hospital System varies by state. Despite these barriers, use of state program prescription monitoring programs has proven valuable in identifying the high-risk patient and providing a clinical opportunity to counsel and refer. Psychiatry, dentistry, and surgery remain among the least likely professions to use of the prescription monitoring program, although ongoing efforts, such as required use, are being taken to address this issue.[32]

Medical or Dental Records and Cross-Communication with Treating Providers and Others

A copy of medical records from a primary care physician typically provides a trove of valuable information when considering controlled substances for the complex patient. Few dentists request this information because it adds additional time for patient care and might be perceived as irrelevant. If the primary physician is the major prescriber of controlled substances, insight into the patient's history may be well-documented in their record, including commentary on any worrisome issues about medication misuse or relevant medical and psychiatric comorbidities not mentioned by the patient. Especially in cases in which the patient is being maintained on chronic opioids, records may reveal results from urine toxicology or other risk assessments not commonly conducted by the dentist. A brief record review can be cost-effective if undertaken in the presence of the patient. This approach provides a forum for a frank discussion about any inconsistencies. Some practices also require complex patients to arrive with a copy of primary care records dating from the last year, a process that also engages the patient in the assessment and treatment planning process. Failure to permit direct communication with other clinicians should always be considered a risk factor or flag, thus it is reasonable to make continuing care contingent on that communication.

Documented telephone conversations or secure email correspondence with the provider is another valuable avenue for cross-communication. In the high-risk patient, a telephone conversation with the physician in the patient's presence may also engage the patient in the process and facilitate adherence. Although federal privacy guidelines do not require a formal signed release for communication among treating health care providers (Health Insurance Portability and Accountability Act [HIPPA]), full disclosure to the patient is always preferred to maintain trust and rapport.[33]

Traditionally, clinicians have preferred to avoid sharing worrisome information with the patient. This reticence may be the result of discomfort on the part of the clinician and reluctance to precipitate a confrontation. Irvine and colleagues[32] (2014) reported frequent denial and anger when patients were confronted with inconsistent prescription monitoring program results, although having this patient-clinician dialogue remains an important component of risk mitigation.[34] Clinician hesitation to share information is nothing new, and has been reinforced by a centuries-old paternalistic view of the patient-clinician relationship. In 1891, Oliver Wendell Holmes, the noted physician and anatomist, concluded that, "your patient has no more right to all the truth you know than he has to all the medicine in your saddlebag ... he should only get just so much as is good for him."[35(pp388)] Although there may be some truth

to this statement, it clearly is always beneficial for the patient and clinician to share information on substance use risk.

Family members provide another critical source for assessing risk and maximizing adherence. During a treatment planning meeting, it can be important to include significant others because they often have first-hand knowledge of the patient's risk factors, may readily disclose their concerns, and may provide support throughout their partner's treatment. Alternatively, the dentist may discover that a family member is strongly encouraging inappropriate opioid use or acting as unexpected consumer of diverted opioids.

Finally, patients may not be candid about their risk factors for many reasons and a smaller number may engage in illegal drug seeking or other aberrant behaviors. For example, altering prescriptions is a crime that may place others at risk. In such cases, the clinician should contact law enforcement authorities without fear of repercussion. Involvement by the police also does not necessarily predict poor patient outcome. When the severity of behavior reaches this level for substance abusing patients, the criminal justice system seems to have a positive impact when long-term treatment programs are mandated.[36]

Risk-Screening Questionnaires for Opioid Therapy

In the last 10 years, several brief risk screening questionnaires have been developed, although most of them have been studied with patients who were being considered or are currently maintained on chronic opioid therapy by their physician.[37] Validity, reliability, and/or normative data for dental populations are lacking. Some of the most well-known questionnaires used in medicine include the Screener and Opioid Assessment for Patients with Pain (SOAPP) and its revised version (SOAPP-R). These self-report questionnaires seek to predict aberrant medication-related behavior among patients who have chronic pain and are being considered for opioid therapy.[38–40] One difference between the questionnaires is that the original SOAPP was conceptually derived, whereas the SOAPP-R was empirically derived.[39] Additionally, the SOAPP-R was designed to be less transparent to respondents in terms of its scoring and, therefore, less prone to overt deception.[39] The original validation study of the SOAPP-R suggested that this screener has adequate reliability, sensitivity, and specificity.[39] A cross-validation study indicated a degree of shrinkage in the statistical parameters of the SOAPP-R but concluded that it is a reliable and valid tool.[40]

Another self-report screener that has gained prominence in the field is the Current Opioid Misuse Measure (COMM).[41] Unlike the SOAPP and SOAPP-R, the COMM is not designed to predict future aberrant medication-related behaviors. Instead, it assists providers in monitoring such behaviors among chronic pain patients who are currently on long-term opioid therapy. Both the original validation study and a cross-validation study found the COMM to have satisfactory reliability and predictive validity.[41,42] The Opioid Risk Tool (ORT) is another brief, validated screening tool for the prediction of aberrant behaviors among opioid-treated patients that may have greater utility in the dental setting.[43] Specific questionnaires addressing risk for opioid prescribing in the dental population are still lacking although efforts are underway to modify questionnaires to better address this need. Despite this barrier, dentists should still pursue a multimodal approach to risk assessment and avoid overreliance on any single measure.

Although there is significant evidence that the aforementioned questionnaires are valuable tools, any screening instrument has limitations that should be considered before their use. Providers should bear in mind that these brief questionnaires are intended as a complement to other risk assessment practices, rather than as a substitute for clinical judgment.[40,44] Another practical consideration is that efficiency is often critical in health care delivery; therefore, a questionnaire should not contain more items than are necessary for its purpose.[45] At 24 and 17 items, respectively, the SOAPP-R and COMM are not unduly lengthy; nevertheless, shorter instruments may be preferred in some contexts such as a general dental practice. A 5-item version of the SOAPP has been studied as well.[46]

For questionnaires administered via computer, it also may be possible to track the answers of respondents and stop the assessment once enough information has been obtained, thus potentially reducing respondent burden.[44,47]

There also are outstanding brief questionnaires that address overall substance use risk, with likely value for use in a dental setting. The National Institute of Drug Abuse (NIDA) Quick Screen is available online and can be easily adapted to computer-based patient records (**Fig. 1**).[18] Although initially developed for adolescents, it has seen widespread use across populations with reasonable reliability and validity in adult populations but more work needs to be done. Parish and colleagues[21] (2015) have addressed its use in a dental population, and its brevity and ease of scoring may allow for easy use in a dental practice. Although an at-risk score does not necessarily define the patient as being a substance abuser, patients can be counseled on risk factors, cross-communication can occur with other providers, and the patient can be counselled and referred for further substance use assessment and treatment.[48]

Counseling the Patient

NIDA provides a template for addressing dental patients who seem to be high-risk per the Quick Screen results, suggesting that the interaction be structured around the 5 As of Intervention: ask, advise, assess, assist, arrange. These provide a useful framework for screening and feedback for the patient.[49]

Ask

Follow-up on the office-administered NIDA Quick Screen. The assessment ends if there are no at-

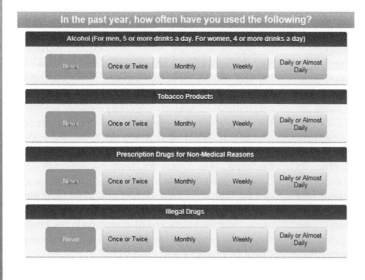

Fig. 1. National Institute on Drug Abuse quick screen. (*From* The NIDA quick screen. [Internet]. Available at: http://www.drugabuse.gov/publications/resource-guide-screening-drug-use-in-general-medical-settings/nida-quick-screen. Accessed December 7, 2015.)

risk responses to the items, other risk factors are absent (eg, problematic prescription monitoring program results), and the patient's responses are consistent with other measures.

Advise

The clinician should provide clear, direct advice to the patient as clinically indicated. The patient should be approached in a nonconfrontational and nonjudgmental manner, reinforcing that the assessment is administered to all patients, and the results provide an opportunity to improve patient care. For example, the clinician may state, "Your screening and the other information we have suggests that you may be having a problem with managing your medications (or using alcohol). I wanted us to see if we can come up with a plan so we find the most effective medications for your treatment."

Assess

Discuss and further assess the patient's current use of medication or other substances, and make an assessment with respect to readiness to change behavior, such as discontinuing drinking or improving adherence with an opioid regimen. The clinician may ask, "Given what we've talked about, what are your feelings about getting this assistance and following-up with the recommendation to meet with a [counselor, primary care physician, pain specialist]?"

Assist

This step involves assisting the patient in making a change. Collaboration in contacting the consulting clinician is discussed. It also is sometimes helpful for the clinician and patient to jointly formulate a brief, written treatment pain listing the action items and enter this into the progress note. In some cases, the patient can be asked to make the telephone call within the time of the dental visit to maximize adherence or to provide a follow-up call to the dental office to confirm the contact was made. Patients who resist the communication and are not interested in completing a change plan should be encouraged to consider an interim goal, such as returning home to discuss the recommendations with a family member or proactively cutting back on substances such as alcohol before the next visit.

Arrange

Because the screening does not provide a diagnosis of substance use disorder, there often is a need to refer the high-risk patient for a full assessment. Ideally, the dentist should have resources available for collaboration and referral. If a clear resource is not available for counseling or substance use assessment, consider using the Substance Abuse and Mental Health Services Administration (SAMHSA) treatment locator (http://findtreatment.samhsa.gov/).[50] Direct communication with the patient's primary care also is recommended, as well as documentation of the recommendations and the patient's response.

Although the above approach may result in valuable assessment data and successful referral, the process should not be a static, single-session event; it should be ongoing throughout the patient's care. The following dialogue illustrates an interaction with a patient who presents worrisome results from a prescription-monitoring program check after several weeks of care.

Clinician: I see that you've seen another doctor for hydrocodone since I saw you last, and your primary doctor is writing you methadone for pain. Some of this care wasn't clearly reflected in your medical history. We want to help you get the best care, so I'd like you to help us understand the inconsistencies.

Patient: What do you mean inconsistent? I didn't list everything because that medication is for my back pain. The other dentist sent me here to get this tooth taken care of and that's it. Along with my back, this problem is terrible, I don't sleep, I'm miserable…"

Clinician: I understand the problem, but I'm trying to work with you for the best care plan. Because you may need certain medications for pain after surgery, I would like to first speak to your primary care physician so we can best coordinate your care. There are also alternative medications for your pain care that might be more effective. It sounds like it's been difficult to deal with this, and I'm sure it's been stressful. We also may be able to help by offering you a referral to get through this difficult time. Are you seeing a counselor or therapist?

Patient: I see someone but that's my business. At this point I just need to get this pain taken care of and this tooth fixed.

Follow-up would include the clear request to speak with the patient's primary care physician and/or mental health provider, even if communication had already occurred in the past. New issues may develop in time with the patient. It also may be an erroneous assumption that the patient's current opioid provider is familiar with the recent stressful events. Any refusal to permit cross-communication among providers can be grounds for discharge because patients with severe substance use disorders also may engage in elaborate efforts to acquire drugs. The determined substance-abusing patient is typically more skillful in his or her efforts to acquire more drugs than the clinician is in detecting the abuse. Requiring substance abuse evaluation and insisting on clinician cross-communication are the best avenues for successful care in this situation.

SPECIAL AT-RISK POPULATIONS
The Patient Currently on Opioids and the Patient Abusing Substances

The patient currently on a stable chronic opioid regimen presents some challenges for the clinician considering a surgical approach. The first step involves a conversation with the physician managing the patient on chronic opioids. Ideally, the dentist would provide a short-term pain management treatment plan that addressed the needs for acute pain care during and after oral surgery. Issues such as intraoperative pain management, the impact of the patient's currently prescribed opioid medications on the planned anesthetic, the potential need for additional opioid and adjuvant medications to address acute postoperative pain, and the identification of risk factors that adversely affect surgical recovery and complicate pain management efforts must be considered before undertaking a surgical procedure. It is critical that the clinician consult with a patient's prescribing physician for guidance in developing a rational plan for intraoperative and postoperative pain management when contemplating a surgical procedure for patients on high-dose opioid treatment (daily dose ≥90 mg in morphine equivalents) or on low-dose opioid treatment with significant comorbid medical conditions such as chronic obstructive pulmonary disease or sleep apnea.

Surgical delay to allow sufficient time for consultation and proper case planning is often prudent when a procedure is elective and issues such as active substance abuse, opioid-induced hyperalgesia, or complex medical/psychiatric issues are of concern. Comorbid psychiatric issues that adversely affect both postoperative pain management and surgical outcomes such as severe depression, somatization, anxiety, and catastrophization disorders require preoperative investigation. For example, a prospective study by Granot and Ferber[51] demonstrated a correlation between catastrophization and anxiety with increased postoperative pain scores; whereas a meta-analytical study by Theunissen

and colleagues[52] showed a statistically significant correlation between catastrophization, anxiety and the development of chronic postsurgical pain.

Preoperative consultation with behavioral health professionals experienced in treating chronic pain is recommended when patients present with significant psychosocial concerns, particularly when the patient's prescribing physician is unable to offer sufficient guidance. Attention should be paid to the recognition and prevention of any withdrawal symptoms from unknown medications, management of short-term analgesics, short-term use of higher than average doses in some cases, and addition of adjunctive agents. Other issues can arise such as the concern about the worsening of opioid-induced hyperalgesia if the patient is already using high-dose opioids, particularly in cases in which the patient's chronic pain has been poorly controlled on the current chronic opioid regimen.

The research provides limited guidance with respect to postoperative management of the opioid tolerant patient in dentistry, particularly when active substance abuse is present. The overall goal of providing adequate acute pain management should be the same for all patients, whether they have an active addiction or are receiving of high-dose opioids. The at-risk patient may fear receiving inadequate pain relief, thereby increasing anxiety and complicating treatment. Avoiding the use of opioids in an opioid-dependent patient also may not be possible or advisable if the goal is to assure effective pain relief. Nonetheless, there may be a role for additional prudence in selecting the treatment regimen. For example, there may be an important role for adjuvant and alternative agents. The clinician also should be aware that anesthesia or nerve blocks remain the standard of care. In general, a single drug may not be optimal, whereas a multimodal drug approach may be needed to achieve sufficient analgesia due to synergistic effects between the agents. Specific strategies can include the addition of nonsteroidal antiinflammatory drugs (NSAIDs) before and after a procedure, use of the mild analgesics such as acetaminophen, antiepileptic agents (eg, gabapentin), or considering stronger drugs such as tramadol. The use of NSAIDs also has been shown to decrease postoperative nausea and vomiting compared with placebo, and they are well established with respect to producing opioid dose-sparing effects.[53] Topical agents at the extraction site might also be considered.

Physicians and dentists face a challenge when the patient has already been provided with care but there is suspicion of ongoing substance abuse and/or evidence of diversion. If there is a suspicion of substance abuse after a risk assessment, it is reasonable to require consultation with an addiction-medicine specialist before writing opioids. If the patient is undergoing treatment of current substance use, the treating addiction medicine clinician should also be consulted. In cases of clear evidence for diversion, a prescription should not be written for controlled substances. Instead, proper authorities should be notified.

During or after surgery, other challenging events may arise with the at-risk patient. In cases in which the patient is showing withdrawal signs, respiratory depression, or other emergencies, the situation should be dealt with by standard patient care protocols. The patient may have been inaccurate or dishonest regarding their medication or illicit drug regimen, increasing the likelihood of such risks.

Problematic postprocedure situations could involve the patient's immediate request for stronger analgesics or emergency phone calls in cases in which the patient escalates use of analgesics, loses the prescription, or complains of inadequate pain relief. If a problematic course is anticipated, booking an earlier than usual return appointment is always advisable. Postoperative opioid analgesics are limited to a specific number of days and legislative efforts are now being considered to mandate prescriptions for maximum limited time such as 3 or 5 days. Of course, there are occasions in which the patient may complain of persistent pain despite adequate healing and apparent resolution of the underlying nociception. When the problem is dental, consultation with an orofacial pain specialist or other oral surgeon may lead to a resolution. When there is an indication of substance misuse and/or mediating psychosocial factors, an expeditious mental health or addiction medicine referral should be arranged (see previous discussion). The major difficulty results when the dentist continues to explore the underlying cause of the patient's pain complaint for weeks or months, fails to seek consultation, and continues to prescribe opioids with an unclear rationale for this treatment.

Tamper-resistant formulations for short-acting analgesics may reduce some risk in the future, although they are not yet in widespread use.[54] Aside from their expense, the tamper-resistant approach to risk mitigation solves only part of the problem because patients can still abuse prescription medications by increasing their dose or combining the drug with other controlled substances for reasons other than pain relief.

The woman of child-bearing age or the pregnant patient present other unique issues with respect to care and the screening for substance use risk is particularly relevant for this population. The relative medical risks for short-term exposure to opioids may be low for the pregnant patient and the fetus during dental procedures. Guidelines are available for the care of these patients.[55] In contrast, little effort has been made to address the woman who is pregnant or planning on pregnancy and actively abusing substances. Across the United States, cases of drug withdrawal in newborn infants exposed to opioids in utero (eg, neonatal abstinence syndrome [NAS]) have dramatically increased in the past several years, which leads to a marked increase in length of hospital stay and charges for affected newborns.[56]

Maternal opiate use during pregnancy increased from 1.19 per 1000 births in 2000 to 5.63 in 2009.[57] Consequences of untreated NAS include serious morbidity such as seizure disorder, as well as death. Care of the neonate typically includes extended hospitalization of the infant and prolonged pharmacologic management and extended outpatient care for the infant and mother. The pregnant patient, as well as all other women of childbearing age, is frequently encountered in dental settings. Although the patient's condition may dictate a nonopioid approach to care, in some cases, an adequate assessment of substance use risk also requires attention and provides a unique opportunity for referral.

SUMMARY

Many dentists have already responded to the national opioid crisis. Fewer prescriptions are being written, a behavior that likely reduces illicit drug availability on the street. Limiting opioid quantities, counseling proper storage and disposal, and awareness of adjunctive or alternatives analgesics may assist. It is also the dentist's obligation to provide adequate acute pain care, an outcome deserved by all patients. Concurrent to this goal, integrating a concise risk-assessment protocol into a dental practice is encouraged. The multimodal approach is optimal. Necessary components include a brief screening questionnaire, relevant medical and psychosocial history, direct communication with the patient about risk factors, arranging appropriate referrals, using information from cotreating colleagues, and accessing the prescription monitoring program. Efforts to adequately assess, manage, and refer the at-risk patient with a substance use comorbidity may be a daunting task but most professionals think that it is now within the scope and obligation of the practicing dentist.

REFERENCES

1. Okie S. A flood of opioids, a rising tide of deaths. N Engl J Med 2010;363(21):1981–5.
2. Rasubala L, Pernapati L, Velasquez X, et al. Impact of a mandatory prescription drug monitoring program on prescription of opioid analgesics by dentists. PLoS One 2015;10(8):e0135957.
3. Burris JL, Evans DR, Carlson CR. Psychological correlates of medical comorbidities in patients with temporomandibular disorders. J Am Dent Assoc 2010;141(1):22–31.
4. Curran SL, Carlson CR, Okeson JP. Emotional and physiologic responses to laboratory challenges: patients with temporomandibular disorders versus matched control subjects. J Orofac Pain 1996;10(2):141–50.
5. Burris JL, Cyders MA, de Leeuw R, et al. Posttraumatic stress disorder symptoms and chronic orofacial pain: an empirical examination of the mutual maintenance model. J Orofac Pain 2009;23(3):243–52.
6. Berger M, Oleszek-Listopad J, Marczak M, et al. Psychological aspects of temporomandibular disorders – literature review. Curr Issues Pharm Med Sci 2015;28(1):55–9.
7. Wiger D. The psychotherapy documentation primer. 3rd edition. Hoboken (NJ): Wiley; 2011. p. 252.
8. Correll DJ, Vlassakov KV, Kissin I. No evidence of real progress in treatment of acute pain, 1993-2012: scientometric analysis. J Pain Res 2014;7:199–210.
9. Tracy SM. Under the looking glass. Pain Manag Nurs 2014;15(2):437–8.
10. Fields HA. Nation in pain: healing our biggest health problem (Book Review). [Internet]. 2014. Available at: http://www.painresearchforum.org/forums/discussion/40153-book-review-nation-pain-healing-our-biggest-health-problem. Accessed December 7, 2015.
11. Institute of Medicine (US) Committee on Advancing Pain Research, Care, and Education. Relieving pain in America: a blueprint for transforming prevention, care, education, and research [Internet]. Washington, DC: National Academies Press (US); 2011. Available at: http://www.ncbi.nlm.nih.gov/books/NBK91497/. Accessed December 7, 2015.
12. Ashrafioun L, Edwards P, Bohnert A, et al. Nonmedical use of pain medications in dental patients. Am J Drug Alcohol Abuse 2014;40(4):312–6.
13. Combating misuse and abuse of prescription drugs: Q&A with Michael Klein, PhD [Internet]. FDA Consumer Health Information; 2010. Available at: http://www.fda.gov/downloads/ForConsumers/ConsumerUpdates/UCM220434.pdf.
14. Passik SD. Tamper-resistant opioid formulations in the treatment of acute pain. Adv Ther 2014;31(3):264–75.
15. Injury prevention & control: prescription drug overdose [Internet]. Centers for Disease Control and Prevention; 2015. Available at: http://www.cdc.gov/drugoverdose/epidemic/.
16. Deaths from prescription opioid overdose [Internet]. Centers for Disease Control and Prevention; 2015. Available at: http://www.cdc.gov/drugoverdose/data/overdose.html.
17. Levy B, Paulozzi L, Mack KA, et al. Trends in opioid analgesic-prescribing rates by specialty, U.S., 2007-2012. Am J Prev Med 2015;49(3):409–13.
18. The NIDA quick screen. [Internet]. Available at: http://www.drugabuse.gov/publications/resource-guide-screening-drug-use-in-general-medical-settings/nida-quick-screen. Accessed December 7, 2015.
19. America's addiction to opioids: heroin and prescription drug abuse. [Internet]. National Institute on Drug Abuse. Available at: http://www.drugabuse.gov/about-nida/legislative-activities/testimony-to-congress/2015/americas-addiction-to-opioids-heroin-prescription-drug-abuse. Accessed December 7, 2015.
20. Denisco RC, Kenna GA, O'Neil MG, et al. Prevention of prescription opioid abuse: the role of the dentist. J Am Dent Assoc 2011;142(7):800–10.
21. Parish CL, Pereyra MR, Pollack HA, et al. Screening for substance misuse in the dental care setting: findings from a nationally representative survey of dentists. Addiction 2015;110(9):1516–23.
22. Keith D. The prescription monitoring program in Massachusetts and its use in dentistry. J Mass Dent Soc 2015;64(3):18–20.
23. O'Neil M. The ADA practical guide to substance use disorders and safe prescribing. 1st edition. Hoboken (NJ): Wiley-Blackwell; 2015. p. 240.
24. SAMHSA. Substance use disorders [Internet]. Substance Abuse and Mental Health Services Administration (SAMHSA); 2014. Available at: http://www.samhsa.gov/disorders/substance-use. Accessed December 7, 2014.
25. American Psychiatric Association, American Psychiatric Association, DSM-5 Task Force. Diagnostic and statistical manual of mental disorders: DSM-5. Arlington (VA): American Psychiatric Association; 2013.
26. Definitions related to the use of opioids for the treatment of pain: consensus statement of the American Academy of Pain Medicine, the American Pain Society, and the American Society of Addiction Medicine [Internet]. American Society of Addiction Medicine; 2001. Available at: http://www.asam.org/docs/publicy-policy-statements/1opioid-definitions-consensus-2-011.pdf?sfvrsn=0. Accessed December 7, 2015.
27. Ballantyne JC, Mao J. Opioid therapy for chronic pain. N Engl J Med 2003;349(20):1943–53.

28. Lee M, Silverman SM, Hansen H, et al. A comprehensive review of opioid-induced hyperalgesia. Pain Physician 2011;14(2):145–61.

29. Commonly abused drugs charts [Internet]. National Institute on Drug Abuse; 2015. Available at: http://www.drugabuse.gov/drugs-abuse/commonly-abused-drugs-charts. Accessed December 7, 2015.

30. Starrels JL, Becker WC, Weiner MG, et al. Low use of opioid risk reduction strategies in primary care even for high risk patients with chronic pain. J Gen Intern Med 2011;26(9):958–64.

31. Zedler B, Xie L, Wang L, et al. Development of a risk index for serious prescription opioid-induced respiratory depression or overdose in veterans' health administration patients. Pain Med 2015;16(8):1566–79.

32. Irvine JM, Hallvik SE, Hildebran C, et al. Who uses a prescription drug monitoring program and how? Insights from a statewide survey of Oregon clinicians. J Pain 2014;15(7):747–55.

33. HHS.gov [Internet]. HHS.gov; 2005. Available at: http://www.hhs.gov/ocr/privacy/hipaa/faq/disclosures/482.html. Accessed December 8, 2015.

34. Palmieri JJ, Stern TA. Lies in the doctor-patient relationship. Prim Care Companion J Clin Psychiatry 2009;11(4):163–8.

35. Holmes OW. Medical essays, 1842–1882. New York: Houghton, Mifflin & Co; 1891.

36. Greenfield SF, Brooks AJ, Gordon SM, et al. Substance abuse treatment entry, retention, and outcome in women: a review of the literature. Drug Alcohol Depend 2007;86(1):1–21.

37. Jamison RN, Edwards RR. Risk factor assessment for problematic use of opioids for chronic pain. Clin Neuropsychol 2013;27(1):60–80.

38. Butler SF, Budman SH, Fernandez K, et al. Validation of a screener and opioid assessment measure for patients with chronic pain. Pain 2004;112(1–2):65–75.

39. Butler SF, Fernandez K, Benoit C, et al. Validation of the revised screener and opioid assessment for patients with pain (SOAPP-R). J Pain 2008;9(4):360–72.

40. Butler SF, Budman SH, Fernandez KC, et al. Cross-validation of a screener to predict opioid misuse in chronic pain patients (SOAPP-R). J Addict Med 2009;3(2):66–73.

41. Butler SF, Budman SH, Fernandez KC, et al. Development and validation of the Current Opioid Misuse Measure. Pain 2007;130(1–2):144–56.

42. Butler SF, Budman SH, Fanciullo GJ, et al. Cross validation of the current opioid misuse measure to monitor chronic pain patients on opioid therapy. Clin J Pain 2010;26(9):770–6.

43. Webster LR, Webster RM. Predicting aberrant behaviors in opioid-treated patients: preliminary validation of the Opioid Risk Tool. Pain Med 2005;6(6):432–42.

44. Finkelman MD, Kulich RJ, Zacharoff KL, et al. Shortening the Screener and Opioid Assessment for Patients with Pain-Revised (SOAPP-R): A Proof-of-Principle Study for Customized Computer-Based Testing. Pain Med 2015;16(12):2344–56.

45. Dugdale DC, Epstein R, Pantilat SZ. Time and the patient-physician relationship. J Gen Intern Med 1999;14(Suppl 1):S34–40.

46. Koyyalagunta D, Bruera E, Aigner C, et al. Risk stratification of opioid misuse among patients with cancer pain using the SOAPP-SF. Pain Med 2013;14(5):667–75.

47. Finkelman MD, Kulich RJ, Zoukhri D, et al. Shortening the current opioid misuse measure via computer-based testing: a retrospective proof-of-concept study. BMC Med Res Methodol 2013;13(1):126.

48. NIDA drug screening tool. [Internet]. Available at: http://www.drugabuse.gov/nmassist/?q=qm_json&pageId=questions_1&pageName=QuickScreen&token_id=104033. Accessed December 11, 2015.

49. National Institute on Drug Abuse. Screening for drug use in general medical settings: resource guide. [Internet]. Available at: http://www.drugabuse.gov/publications/resource-guide/preface. Accessed December 9, 2015.

50. SAMHSA behavioral health treatment services locator. [Internet]. Available at: https://findtreatment.samhsa.gov/. Accessed December 9, 2015.

51. Granot M, Ferber SG. The roles of pain catastrophizing and anxiety in the prediction of postoperative pain intensity: a prospective study. Clin J Pain 2005;21(5):439–45.

52. Theunissen M, Peters ML, Bruce J, et al. Preoperative anxiety and catastrophizing: a systematic review and meta-analysis of the association with chronic postsurgical pain. Clin J Pain 2012;28(9):819–41.

53. Maund E, McDaid C, Rice S, et al. Paracetamol and selective and non-selective non-steroidal anti-inflammatory drugs for the reduction in morphine-related side-effects after major surgery: a systematic review. Br J Anaesth 2011;106(3):292–7.

54. Moorman-Li R, Motycka CA, Inge LD, et al. A review of abuse-deterrent opioids for chronic nonmalignant pain. Pharmacol Ther 2012;37(7):412–8.

55. Kurien S, Kattimani VS, Sriram RR, et al. Management of pregnant patient in dentistry. J Int Oral Health 2013;5(1):88–97.

56. Patrick SW, Davis MM, Lehmann CU, et al. Increasing incidence and geographic distribution of neonatal abstinence syndrome: United States 2009 to 2012. J Perinatol 2015;35(8):650–5.

57. Patrick SW, Schumacher RE, Benneyworth BD, et al. Neonatal abstinence syndrome and associated health care expenditures: United States, 2000-2009. JAMA 2012;307(18):1934–40.

Intraoral Pain Disorders

Mary Hil Edens, DDS, Yasser Khaled, BDS, MDSc, MMSc,
Joel J. Napeñas, DDS, FDSRCS(Ed)*

KEYWORDS

- Pulpitis • Alveolar osteitis • Aphthous stomatitis • Candidiasis • Cracked tooth syndrome
- Lichen planus • Vesiculobullous disorders • Medication related osteonecrosis of the jaw

KEY POINTS

- Dental providers should be aware of the vast range of common causes for intraoral pain.
- Pain of dental origin can range from a short, sharp pain that can progresses to a persistent, dull pain, depending on the severity of disease.
- Pain caused by chronic periodontal conditions may be mild, persistent, or episodic dull pain, whereas acute periodontal conditions can be continuous or intermittent of increased severity.
- Pain of mucosal origin is continuous, usually described as raw, stinging, aching, and burning.
- Inflammatory and infectious processes of bone may be characterized by continuous pain, swelling, reduced jaw mobility, bony destruction, and purulent drainage.
- Salivary gland disorders may have localized pain in the area of the affected gland with swelling and intermittent pain associated with gland stimulation.

INTRODUCTION

Those experiencing intraoral pain associated with dental and oral diseases of various causes are likely to pursue treatment from medical and dental providers. A range of causes for intraoral pain include odontogenic, periodontal, oral mucosal, or contiguous hard and soft tissue structures to the oral cavity. Providers should be vigilant when diagnosing these, as they should be among the first in their differential diagnoses to be ruled out. Accordingly, this review provides brief overviews of frequently encountered oral/dental diseases that cause intraoral pain, originating from the teeth, the surrounding mucosa and gingivae, tongue, bone and salivary glands and their causes, features, diagnosis, and management strategies.

DENTAL AND PULPAL

Dental and pulpal pain occurs when there is noxious stimulation of the teeth or disease affecting the enamel, dentin, or pulpal structures. This pain may be attributable to trauma, attrition, abrasion, erosion, or iatrogenic or bacteria causing caries. There is typically a continuum of symptoms based on the severity of disease ranging from short, sharp pain that can progresses to a persistent, dull pain indicating the presence of inflammation, infection, and disease. Because enamel is avascular, noninnervated, and nonporous, loss of structure due to demineralization, mechanical means, or caries isolated in the enamel is usually painless. However, once lesions breach the dentinoenamel junction, pain can be experienced through stimuli affecting the dentinal tubules. Myelinated (Aδ) and unmyelinated (C) fibers innervate the pulp. If there is sufficient stimulation with temperature or pressure, fluid movement in the dentinal tubules activates the low-threshold Aδ fibers, producing a quick, sharp, localized pain. An injured tooth with local inflammation lowers the pain threshold of Aδ fibers; as the pulpal involvement and inflammation persists,

Funding Sources and Conflict of Interest: None.
Oral Medicine Residency Program, Department of Oral Medicine, Carolinas Healthcare System, PO Box 32861, Charlotte, NC 28232, USA
* Corresponding author.
E-mail address: joel.napenas@carolinashealthcare.org

Oral Maxillofacial Surg Clin N Am 28 (2016) 275–288
http://dx.doi.org/10.1016/j.coms.2016.03.008

the C fibers are stimulated producing a more pro-longed, dull, and diffuse pain.

Caries

Bacterial invasion leads to subsequent acid metabolite formation on tooth structures, leading to damage of tooth structure. Symptoms are a result of lost enamel and exposure of dentin, cementum, and pulp.

- Symptoms and features: Patients may report sensitivity to thermal changes, sweet, or acidic foods. Pain is sharp, localized, and dissipates immediately after removal of the stimuli.
- Diagnosis: Caries are detected both clinically and radiographically (**Fig. 1**).
- Management: If a lesion is asymptomatic and incipient involving only the enamel, monitoring and topical fluoride placement are usually adequate. However, if the lesion is symptomatic, extends into dentin, and is not arrested, removal of the decayed tooth structure and placement of a dental restoration is indicated.

Exposed Cementum or Dentin

Gingival recession leading to exposed cementum (**Fig. 2**) commonly results from heavy

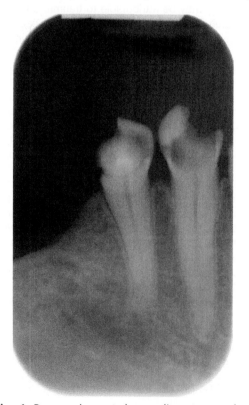

Fig. 1. Deep caries noted on adjacent premolars radiographically.

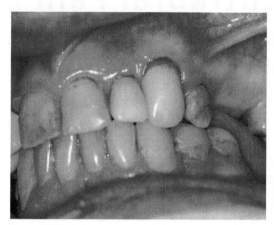

Fig. 2. Exposed cementum of the upper left canine due to gingival recession.

pressure from aggressive tooth brushing. Abrasion of enamel leading to exposed dentin can also occur from aggressive tooth brushing, bruxism, or abnormal or traumatic occlusion.

- Symptoms and features: Tooth sensitivity to thermal stimuli generally results in pain that is sharp, localized, and dissipates immediately after removal of the stimuli.
- Diagnosis: Diagnosis is made clinically through evaluation and testing exposure of cold stimuli to the exposed root surface.
- Management: Treatment measures are directed toward limiting dentinal fluid movement by covering the exposed dentin or cementum with desensitizing agents or restorations.[1] Oral hygiene instruction is also important to improve toothbrushing technique and prevent further recession.

Pulpal Disease

Caries, trauma, fracture, exposed dentin or cementum, or premature or traumatic occlusal contact can all result in inflammation with or without infection that causes pulpal pain.

- Symptoms and features: There may be continuous, dull, aching pain and episodes of pulsing, throbbing, and sharp pain, representing stimulation of the C fibers and Aδ fibers, respectively. Intermittent pulpal pain can be stimulated by heat, cold, pressure, and head positioning. Teeth that only have pulpal disease are not sensitive to percussion of the affected tooth.

Characteristics and management strategies for specific pulpal disease states are as follows:

- Normal pulp
  - Symptoms and features include a short response to cold stimuli that is mildly uncomfortable and subsides almost immediately on removal.
  - Diagnosis is made clinically, as there is no evidence of loss of tooth structure or periapical abnormalities (eg, widened periodontal ligament [PDL] or periapical radiolucencies) on radiographs.
  - Management: In the absence of tooth abnormality, no treatment indicated.
- Reversible pulpitis
  - Symptoms and features include an exaggerated quick, sharp response to cold stimuli, followed by a dull ache that dissipates. There is no complaint of spontaneous pain.
  - Diagnosis is primarily made based on clinical features and pulp testing to cold and heat stimuli. There usually is not any radiographic evidence of periapical abnormalities.
  - Management entails removal of the pain-causing stimulus, usually removal of carious lesion, and/or restoration of lost tooth structure.
- Irreversible pulpitis
  - Symptoms and features include spontaneous, lingering dull ache or a constant, severe, unrelenting pain; increased pain intensity to noxious stimuli; and positive response to cold and heat stimuli (ie, sharp response followed by dull ache that persists).
  - Diagnosis: Radiographically, there may or may not be a thickening of the PDL or periapical radiolucencies at the tooth's apex.
  - Management: Treatment requires either root canal therapy (RCT) or tooth extraction.
- Pulpal necrosis
  - Symptoms and features: There is no pain or response to heat, cold, or electronic pulp testing.
  - Diagnosis: Radiographs may or may not reveal the presence of a widened PDL at the apex or periapical radiolucency. If the infection has extended beyond the apex of the tooth in the surrounding bone, a percussion test may be positive.
  - Treatment requires either RCT or extraction.

Cracked Tooth Syndrome

Cracked tooth syndrome is when tooth fractures become symptomatic[2] and is defined as incomplete fracture of the dentin that may or may not extend to the pulp.[3]

- Symptoms and features: Complaints include sharp, transient pain that is stimulated by biting or releasing or resulting from exposure to cold food or drinks that can be easily localized. Pain may sometimes linger minutes after chewing.
- Diagnosis: Transillumination on the tooth is best performed with the use of magnification to better illustrate color changes and clinically significant cracks. Detection of a cracked tooth on a radiograph is rare. Tooth percussion seldom elicits pain with percussion in the apical direction. Pain on biting is more commonly noted with release of biting, owing to fluids within dentinal tubules moving toward the pulp.
- Management: Treatment of cracked tooth syndrome may include stabilization with an orthodontic band, a crown, or onlay. RCT or extraction of the tooth may be indicated depending on the extent of the crack or lack of resolution or severity of symptoms.[4]

PERIODONTAL

Periodontal pain is a localized pain, owing to the mechanoreceptors and proprioceptors in the periodontium. Pain caused by chronic periodontal conditions may be mild, persistent, or episodic dull pain. Periodontal pain caused by local factors is localized to affected teeth in which there is inflammation or infection involving the gingiva, periodontium, alveolar bone, or pericoronal tissue.[5] Further discussion later concerns acute pain of periodontal origin.

Gingival/Periodontal Abscess

This abscess is a localized collection of pus within the tissues of the gingiva and periodontium adjacent to a vital tooth. This abscess occurs when bacteria within a periodontal pocket continually finds their way into the soft tissues, with abscess formation representing a decreased local or systemic resistance of the host.

- Symptoms and features: The main symptom is sudden onset of pain, which is made worse by biting on the involved tooth. The tooth may be mobile, and the lesion may contribute to destruction of the PDL and alveolar bone, noted radiographically (**Fig. 3**). The pain is deep and throbbing, and the surface may be shiny because of stretching of the mucosa. Before pus has formed, the lesion will not be fluctuant and there will be no purulent discharge. There may be regional lymphadenitis. Such abscesses are classified primarily by location[6]:

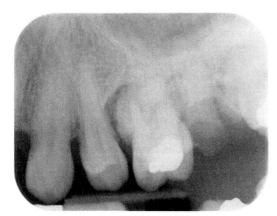

Fig. 3. Periodontal bone loss noted radiographically.

- Gingival abscess is a localized, purulent infection that involves only the soft tissue near the marginal gingiva or the interdental papilla.
- Periodontal abscess is a localized, purulent infection involving a greater dimension of tissue, extending apically and adjacent to a periodontal pocket.
- Pericoronal abscess is a localized, purulent infection within the tissue surrounding the crown of a partially or fully erupted tooth.
- Combined periodontal/endodontic abscess is a periodontal abscess that occurs in conjunction with a tooth that has infected pulp.
- Diagnosis: Clinical features as described earlier, in addition to radiographic evidence of periodontal disease (see **Fig. 3**), are sufficient to obtain a diagnosis.
- Management: The initial management of a periodontal abscess involves pain relief and control of the infection. This management entails obtaining drainage, either through incision at the area of fluctuance or in the gingival margin or through the socket if the tooth is extracted.[7] Removal of the source of infection is indicated whether it is bacteria or a foreign body, which can be accomplished through root debridement in the cases of periodontal abscesses. A history of recurrent periodontal abscesses and significantly compromised periodontal support indicate that the prognosis for the involved tooth is poor and it should be extracted.

Periapical Inflammatory Lesions

- Periapical periodontitis
  - This lesion is an acute or chronic inflammatory lesion around the apex of a tooth root, representing the bacterial invasion from a

necrotic tooth.[8,9] This lesion can be considered a sequela in the natural history of dental caries, irreversible pulpitis, and pulpal necrosis. The type of periapical periodontitis is classified according to whether it is an acute/symptomatic process and includes the following:
- Acute periapical periodontitis
- Chronic periapical periodontitis
- Periapical granuloma
  - Symptoms and features: In acute periapical periodontitis, pain may be continuous, aching, and/or throbbing or only elicited through percussion of the involved tooth. Chronic periapical periodontitis and periapical granuloma may be painless.
- Periapical abscess
  - Periapical periodontitis may develop into a periapical abscess whereby a collection of pus forms at the tooth apex, with the consequence of spread of infection from the tooth pulp.
  - Symptoms and features: Symptoms are similar to that described for gingival and periodontal abscesses earlier. Pain may be continuous, aching, and/or throbbing, with percussion sensitivity of the involved tooth. The associated tooth is necrotic and nonvital.
- Diagnosis: The radiographic features of periapical inflammatory lesions vary depending on the time or course of the lesion. Because very early lesions may not show any radiographic changes, diagnosis of these lesions relies solely on the clinical symptoms. More chronic lesions may show lytic (radiolucent) or sclerotic (radiopaque) changes or both (**Fig. 4**).
- Management: Definitive treatment is targeted toward addressing the source of infection, which is the necrotic tooth, through RCT, or extraction.[10]

Alveolar Osteitis (Dry Socket)

Alveolar osteitis is an inflammation with or without infection of the alveolar bone, which occurs as a postoperative complication of tooth extraction. This complication is a result of bare alveolar bone being exposed to bacteria and/or debris.

- Symptoms and features: Signs may include an empty socket, which is partially or totally devoid of blood clot or shows denuded (bare) bone walls.[11] Symptoms may include dull, aching, throbbing pain in the area of the socket that is moderate to severe and may radiate to other parts of the head, such as

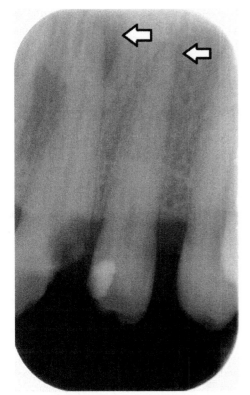

Fig. 4. Periapical radiolucencies (*arrows*) noted radiographically on adjacent teeth.

the ear, eye, temple, and neck. Intraoral halitosis and bad taste in the mouth may also occur.[12]

- Diagnosis: Diagnosis is made clinically, in conjunction with the history of a recent tooth extraction.
- Management: Treatment is usually symptomatic with analgesic medications and removal of debris from the socket by irrigation with saline or chlorhexidine, with local anesthetic. Medicated dressings are also commonly placed in the socket. Although there is concern that these will act as a foreign body and prolong healing, they are usually needed because of the severe pain.[13]

Pericoronitis

Pericoronitis, also known as operculitis, is inflammation of the soft tissues surrounding the crown of a partially erupted tooth, including the gingiva and the dental follicle.[14] This inflammation may occur as a result of trauma or bacterial infection and commonly occurs in impacted third molars.

- Symptoms and features: Pain is in the affected is continuous and often severe. Other

signs and symptoms depend on the severity and include the following:
  - ○ Halitosis
  - ○ Bad taste
  - ○ Pus exudate
  - ○ Signs of trauma on the operculum
  - ○ Dysphagia
  - ○ Cervical lymphadenitis
  - ○ Facial swelling[15]
- Diagnosis: Diagnosis is made based on clinical features, associated with an impacted tooth.
- Management: Initial treatment involves prescription of analgesic and antibiotics. Prevention and/or definitive treatment can be achieved by extraction of the associated impacted tooth.[16]

ORAL MUCOSAL PAIN

Oral pain related to mucosal disorders is a direct manifestation of changes of the mucosal epithelium. These changes are seen intraorally as vesicle formation, ulcerations, erosions, erythema, pseudomembranous, and/or hyperkeratosis, with hyperalgesia of the affected mucosal tissue. Pain of mucosal origin is continuous and usually described as raw, stinging, aching, and burning. Painful oral mucosal disorders may develop as a result of infection, reactive processes, systemic disorders, or dysplasia,[17] some of which are reviewed in this article.

Oral Candidiasis

Oral candidiasis is a mycosis of *Candida* species occurring on the oral mucosal surfaces. Causes of fungal proliferation are thought to be multiple, attributed to one or a combination of hyposalivation, change in oral bacterial flora (eg, through antibiotic use), immune compromise, immune suppression, diabetes, or topical corticosteroid use.[18]

- Symptoms and features: A continuous burning sensation in affected areas may occur in the presence or absence of lesions. Three main clinical appearances of candidiasis are generally recognized: *pseudomembranous, erythematous,* and *hyperplastic* (**Fig. 5**). Other specific variants include the following:
  - ○ Angular cheilitis is inflammation at the corners (angles) of the mouth, very commonly involving *Candida* species, when sometimes the terms "*Candida*-associated angular cheilitis"[19] or, less commonly, "monilial perlèche" are used.[20]

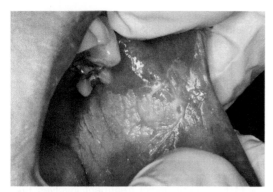

Fig. 5. Hyperplastic oral candidiasis of the left buccal mucosa.

- ○ Denture-related stomatitis refers to a mild inflammation and erythema of the mucosa beneath the denture surface.
- ○ Median rhomboid glossitis is an elliptical or rhomboid lesion in the center of the dorsal tongue, just anterior (in front) of the circumvallate papillae. The area is depapillated, reddened (or red and white), and rarely painful.[21]
- ○ Linear gingival erythema is a localized or generalized linear band of erythematous gingivitis. It was first observed in human immunodeficiency virus (HIV)–infected individuals and termed *HIV-gingivitis*, but the condition is not confined to this group.[21]
- Diagnosis: Diagnosis is mostly made based on clinical features, history, and symptoms. Low-grade fungal infections in the absence of clinical signs can sometimes be misdiagnosed as burning mouth syndrome. If diagnosis is uncertain, a cytologic smear or culture may be performed.
- Management: Oral candidiasis can be treated with topical antifungal drugs, such as nystatin, clotrimazole, or miconazole.[20] In cases of persistent recurrent oral candidiasis, antifungal therapy alone does not permanently resolve these lesions, but rather the underlying predisposing factors (eg, hyposalivation, immunosuppression, immunocompromised, diabetic control) must also be addressed.[22]

Herpes Simplex Virus

Herpes simplex virus 1 and 2 (HSV-1 and HSV-2) are two members of the herpes virus (Herpesviridae) family.[23] The ubiquitous and contagious HSV-1 and HSV-2 are associated with oral and genital lesions, respectively, but not exclusively. They can be transmitted when an infected person is producing and shedding the virus during active episodes and can be spread through contact with saliva, such as sharing drinks.

- Symptoms and features: Reactivation and recurrent lesions typically present as painful vesicle eruptions on keratinized tissue (**Fig. 6**), often preceded by prodromal tingling or burning sensations in the affected area. Vesicles are short lived, quickly rupturing, resulting in a yellow ulceration with erythematous borders. Healing occurs within 1 to 4 days.
- Diagnosis: Diagnosis is often based on clinical presentation and history. If the diagnosis is uncertain, viral cultures are obtained by swabbing a fresh (nonruptured) vesicle.
- Management: No method completely eradicates herpes virus, as it remains latent or dormant in the trigeminal ganglion; but antiviral medications can reduce the frequency, duration, and severity of outbreaks. Several systemic antiviral drugs are effective for treating herpes, including acyclovir, valacyclovir, famciclovir, and penciclovir.[24] Several topical antivirals are effective for herpes labialis, including acyclovir, penciclovir, and docosanol.[25] Certain dietary supplements and alternative remedies are claimed to be beneficial.[26] Systemic analgesics and topical anesthetic treatments (eg, prilocaine, lidocaine, benzocaine, or tetracaine) are used to relieve pain.[27]

Herpes Zoster (Shingles)

Herpes zoster is an infection resulting from reactivation of the varicella-zoster virus that affects peripheral or cranial nerves, usually occurring years after primary infection with the varicella (chickenpox) virus or receipt of the live, attenuated varicella vaccine.[28]

- Symptoms and features: The disease manifests as painful vesicular eruptions over a

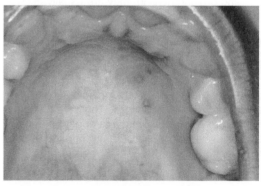

Fig. 6. Herpes simplex lesions of the palate.

single dermatome or 2 or more contiguous dermatomes in the mucous membranes and/or skin. They are invariably unilateral and do not cross the midline.[29] Concern after resolution of condition is postherpetic neuralgia, which is a continuous, intractable, burning pain in the previously involved affected sites.

- Diagnosis: Diagnosis is usually made by history and clinical presentation.
- Management: Treatment is with higher doses and extended regimens of systemic antiviral medications, such as acyclovir, valacyclovir, and famciclovir. Systemic steroids are have been noted to decrease the severity and duration of pain[30] and are also used as a prophylactic measure to prevent postherpetic neuralgia.

Necrotizing Periodontal Diseases

Necrotizing periodontal diseases are inflammatory periodontal diseases thought to be caused by bacteria (spirochetes, fusiform bacteria) and triggered by other factors (eg, stress, impaired immunity).

- Symptoms and features: These diseases usually have a sudden onset and are characterized by continuous moderate pain, fetid odor, and systemic symptoms (eg, malaise, low-grade fever).
  - Necrotizing ulcerative gingivitis is characterized by erythematous and edematous gingiva, with punched-out papillae.
  - Necrotizing ulcerative periodontitis (NUP) has soft tissue necrosis, rapid bone loss involving the gingiva, PDL, and alveolar bone.
  - Necrotizing stomatitis occurs when NUP progresses into the tissue beyond the mucogingival junction.[31]
- Diagnosis: Diagnosis is made based on history and clinical features.
- Management: Treatment entails local debridement, topical antimicrobials (eg, chlorhexidine rinse), analgesics, and oral antibiotic therapy in the event of systemic manifestations.

Recurrent Aphthous Stomatitis

Aphthous stomatitis is a relatively common condition characterized by the repeated formation of benign and noncontagious oral ulcers (aphthae) in otherwise healthy individuals, with no detectable systemic symptoms or signs outside the mouth.[32]

- Symptoms and features: Generally, symptoms may include prodromal sensations such as burning, itching, or stinging, which

may precede the appearance of any lesion by some hours; and pain, which is often out of proportion to the size of the ulceration. It is worsened by physical contact especially with certain foods and drinks (eg, acidic). Ulcerations are yellow with erythematous borders (**Fig. 7**), typically appearing on nonkeratinized mucosa. A more common method of classifying aphthous stomatitis is into 3 variants, distinguished by the size, number and location of the lesions, the healing time of individual ulcers and whether a scar is left after healing. *Minor aphthae* is the most common type of aphthous stomatitis, accounting for about 80% to 85% of all cases.[33] *Major aphthae*, making up about 10% of all cases of aphthous stomatitis, are similar to minor aphthous ulcers but are more than 10 mm in diameter and the ulceration is deeper. *Herpetiform ulceration* is a subtype of aphthous stomatitis so named because the lesions resemble a primary infection with HSV.

- Diagnosis: Diagnosis is made based on history and clinical presentation. Other potential underlying causes for similar lesions (eg, hematinic deficiency, Behçet disease, celiac disease, inflammatory bowel disease) are ruled out through laboratory studies.
- Management: Treatment is palliation (eg, with topical anesthetics or topical or systemic analgesics) until lesions resolve. Topical anti-inflammatory medications (eg, steroids, chlorhexidine rinse, tetracyclines) may be used, with immune modulators (eg, oral steroids, pentoxifylline, dapsone, colchicine) used for severe, refractory cases or in the immunocompromised.

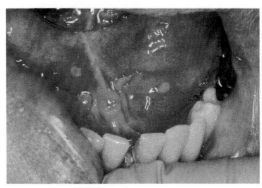

Fig. 7. Recurrent aphthous stomatitis lesions on the floor of mouth.

Lichen Planus

Lichen planus (LP) is an inflammatory disease of the skin and/or mucous membranes thought to be the result of a T cell–mediated immune process targeting an unknown self-antigen in the epithelium, with an unknown initial trigger.

- Symptoms and features: Six clinical forms of oral LP are recognized:
  - Reticular: The most common variant is characterized by the classic netlike or spider weblike appearance of lacy white lines, known as Wickham striae. This variant is usually asymptomatic and painless.
  - Erosive/ulcerative: This form is characterized by oral ulcers presenting with persistent, irregular areas of redness, ulcerations, and erosions covered with a yellow slough (**Fig. 8**). Ulcerations are usually continuously significantly painful, with sensitivity to acidic or mechanical stimuli.
  - Papular: This form is characterized by white papules that are usually asymptomatic.
  - Plaquelike: This form appears as white patches that may resemble leukoplakia and are usually painless.
  - Atrophic: Atrophic oral LP may also manifest as desquamative gingivitis, with some areas of pain and sensitivity.
  - Bullous: This form appears as fluid-filled vesicles that project from the surface and are painful.
- Diagnosis: Diagnosis may be made clinically for the reticular variant. Other variants may resemble other mucosal disorders, thus biopsy of representative tissue may provide a histopathologic diagnosis.
- Management: There is no cure, but many different medications and procedures have been used to control the symptoms. Treatment is only required if lesions are symptomatic, usually involving topical corticosteroids and analgesics. If these are ineffective and the condition is severe, intralesional or systemic corticosteroids may be used. Calcineurin inhibitors (eg, tacrolimus) are sometimes used.

Vesiculobullous Diseases

A vesiculobullous disease is a type of mucocutaneous disease that is characterized by vesicles and bullae.[34] These diseases occur when autoantibodies target components of the epithelium and underlying connective tissue. Examples of vesiculobullous diseases include pemphigus vulgaris (**Fig. 9**), cicatricial (mucous membrane) pemphigoid (**Fig. 10**), dermatitis herpetiformis, linear immunoglobulin A disease, and epidermolysis bullosa.[35]

- Symptoms and features: These diseases are characterized by blisters, erosions, and ulcerations affecting the oral mucosa, with some exhibiting extraoral manifestations (eg, skin, eyes, genitals). Affected intraoral areas may be continuously painful, sensitive to foods, or only mildly painful.
- Diagnosis: Diagnosis is made by biopsy of lesional and perilesional tissue and serum studies, with the last two being used for direct immunofluorescence and indirect immunofluorescence, respectively, for autoantibodies.
- Management: Treatment is varied depending on the exact diagnosis and composed of one or a combination of topical steroids, systemic steroids, or other systemic immune modulators.

Squamous Cell Carcinoma

Squamous cell carcinoma (SCC) accounts for upwards of 90% of intraoral malignancies.[36] Risk

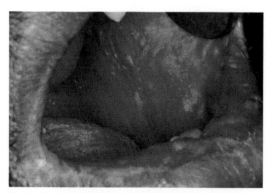

Fig. 8. Erythema, white plaques, and ulcerative lesions on the left buccal mucosa and lips due to erosive LP.

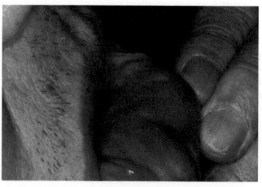

Fig. 9. Pemphigus vulgaris lesions of the lower lip.

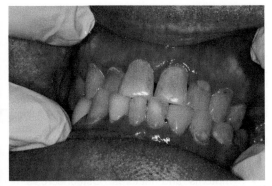

Fig. 10. Cicatricial (mucous membrane) pemphigoid lesions involving the gingiva.

factors for the development of oral SCC include chronic exposure of oral mucosa to tobacco and/or alcohol.

- Symptoms and features: Lesions initially present as areas of leukoplakia, erythroplakia, exophytic lesions, and/or ulceration that persists (**Fig. 11**). There may or may not be the presence of pain; but when present, it is continuous in the affected areas. Pain can be due to the ulcerations themselves, secondary infection, and/or encroachment of adjacent peripheral nerves. Hypoesthesia and/or paresthesia may also accompany lesions.
- Diagnosis: Diagnosis is made histopathologically. Incisional biopsies should be made of indurated leukoplakic lesions, erythroplakic lesions, and/or long-standing ulcerations in the absence of apparent sources of irritation or trauma.
- Management: Specific and detailed discussion of management strategies (composed of one or a combination of surgical removal, chemotherapy, and radiation therapy) is beyond the scope of this overview.

Oral Mucositis Related to Cancer Therapy

Patients may develop oral mucositis as a result of therapies targeted toward treating cancer due to radiation or chemotherapy or hematopoietic stem cell transplantation for hematologic malignancies.

- Symptoms and features: This condition is characterized by erythema, edema, pseudomembrane formation, mucosal shedding, and ulcer formation (**Fig. 12**). Mucosal pain usually coincides with the onset of erythema and ulceration.
- Diagnosis: Diagnosis is made based on the appearance of lesions coinciding with treatment. For radiation therapy, severity is dose dependent, with erythema and ulceration occurring after a cumulative dose of 30 Gy. In chemotherapy with mucotoxic regimens, changes begin 2 to 4 days after initiation of chemotherapy, with ulceration occurring 5 to 8 days after initiation.
- Management: Treatment is generally for analgesia, composed of topical analgesics, oral and parenteral analgesics, in addition to nutritional and fluid support. Signs and symptoms persist for 2 to 6 weeks following the completion of radiation therapy[37] and 7 to 10 days during chemotherapy, as long as patients do not develop secondary infection or remain granulocytopenic or immunocompromised.

Immunocompromised States (Transplantation Medicine, Human Immunodeficiency Virus)

Oral lesions occurring in the immunocompromised, either due to an inherent condition

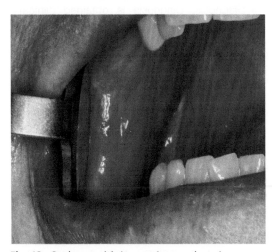

Fig. 12. Oral mucositis in a patient undergoing cancer chemotherapy.

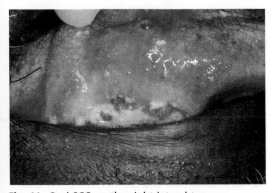

Fig. 11. Oral SCC on the right lateral tongue.

(eg, HIV) or due to immunosuppressive medications (ie, after transplantation), are due to opportunistic oral infections, such as HSV, oral candidiasis, and other uncommon viral and fungal infections. In addition, aphthous ulcers may form.

- Symptoms and features: Clinical appearance and symptoms are dependent on the actual condition; however, infectious lesions may present with a more atypical or severe appearance than those found in immunocompetent patients.
- Diagnosis: Diagnosis is based on clinical appearance. If the actual nature is unclear, culture through swab or with tissue samples or biopsy for histopathologic analysis may be performed.
- Management: In addition to analgesia, management is specific to the exact nature of the lesion, with systemic antimicrobials for fungal and viral lesions and topical and/or systemic steroids for ulcerative (noninfectious) lesions.

BONE
Osteomyelitis

Osteomyelitis occurs when an infectious inflammatory process spreads through the medullary spaces of the bone.

- Symptoms and features: An acute osteomyelitis causes significant pain and swelling in the affected area of the jaw, along with fever, lymphadenopathy, and leukocytosis. They may also present with paresthesia and exfoliation of bony sequestra. Chronic osteomyelitis may present with swelling, pain, sinus formation, and intermittent periods of pain.
- Diagnosis: Diagnosis is obtained clinically and radiographically with ill-defined radiolucencies evident in the affected bone.
- Management: Treatment entails abscess drainage if present and antibiotic therapy. For refractory chronic osteomyelitis, surgical intervention is required, involving removal of affected bone through curettage and, in more severe cases, resection.

Osteonecrosis

Osteonecrosis occurs as formation of necrotic bone in the oral cavity from hypoxia, hypovascularity, and hypocellularity. Osteoradionecrosis (ORN) occurs as a result of radiation therapy exposure. The risk for ORN increases with radiation doses greater than 60 Gy, dental disease, postradiation dental extractions, and previous cancer resection.[38] Medication-related osteonecrosis of the jaw (MRONJ) is associated with various medications used for osteoporosis or cancer therapy (eg, bisphosphonates, antiangiogenics, and Receptor activator of nuclear factor kappa-B ligand receptors). The risk for bisphosphonate-associated MRONJ is increased by intravenous administration of the medication, longer duration periods of treatment, compromised immune status, concomitant steroid therapy, dental disease, and invasive oral procedures.[39]

- Symptoms and features: Osteonecrosis is typically characterized by the presence of nonhealing areas of exposed bone present for at least 6 months (**Fig. 13**). Affected areas may remain painless, with clinical symptoms including continuous pain, swelling, reduced jaw mobility, bony destruction, and purulent drainage when there is a secondary osteomyelitis.
- Diagnosis: Diagnosis is made by clinical findings and history of previous exposure to radiation therapy to affected areas or implicated medications.
- Management: Treatment of both ORN and MRONJ is challenging because of the nonhealing nature, and there is no established effective treatment regimen. Analgesia, long-term topical and systemic antibiotic therapy for secondary infections, pentoxifylline, and hyperbaric oxygen therapy are current treatment options. Surgical considerations include removal of affected bone by curettage or resection and vascularized bone containing a pedicle flap, although surgery may exacerbate the condition.

Maxillary Sinusitis

The most common causes of maxillary sinusitis are upper respiratory tract infections and allergic

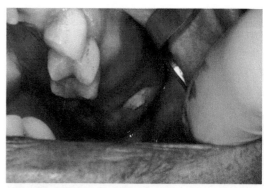

Fig. 13. MRONJ involving the right maxillary buccal plate with exposed necrotic bone.

rhinitis. Most common bacteria implicated are *Streptococcus pneumoniae* and *Haemophilus influenza*.[40] As the maxillary sinus is in close proximity to the maxillary posterior teeth, 10% of maxillary sinusitis cases may result from odontogenic sources, including infection of manipulation of posterior teeth.

- Symptoms and features: Patients with acute sinusitis may present with headache, fever, facial pain over affected sinus, nasal or pharyngeal discharge, pain over cheekbone, toothache and tenderness to percussion of multiple maxillary teeth, periorbital pain, and pain during positional changes. Patients with chronic sinusitis may experience facial pressure and pain, sensation of obstruction, headache, sore throat, lightheadedness, and generalized fatigue.
- Diagnosis: Clinical features and imaging studies (eg, computed tomography [CT] or Water's view radiograph) showing increased radio-opacities in the sinus aid in obtaining a diagnosis.
- Management: Symptom relief is typically the goal of treatment and includes decongestants, antihistamines, mucolytic agents, α-adrenergic agents, corticosteroids, analgesics, and antibiotics for cases of more than 1-week duration.

SALIVARY GLAND ABNORMALITIES
Oral Sialoliths

Sialolithiasis is a condition whereby a calcified mass or *sialolith* forms within a salivary gland, usually in the duct of the submandibular gland. Less commonly, the parotid gland or rarely the sublingual gland or a minor salivary gland may develop sialoliths. Sialadenitis (infectious and noninfectious) of the gland may develop as a result. Although, in many cases, the cause is idiopathic, sialolithiasis may develop because of existing chronic infection of the glands, dehydration, hyposalivation, and changes in fluid and electrolyte makeup in the gland, such as increased local levels of calcium.

- Symptoms and features: Usual symptoms are pain and swelling of the affected salivary gland, both of which get worse when salivary flow is stimulated (eg, with the sight, thought, smell, or taste of food or with hunger or chewing). Signs and symptoms are variable and depend largely on whether the obstruction of the duct is complete or partial and how much resultant pressure is created within the gland. The development of infection in the gland also influences

the signs and symptoms, which include intermittent swelling of the gland, tenderness of the involved gland, palpable hard lump (**Fig. 14**), lack of saliva coming from the duct, erythema of the duct, purulence discharge from the duct, and cervical lymphadenitis.
- Diagnosis: Diagnosis is usually made by characteristic history and physical examination and can be confirmed by radiographic imaging, sialogram, or ultrasonography.
- Management: The condition is usually managed by removing the sialolith. Other treatments include includes hydration, moist heat therapy, analgesics, Shock-wave therapy, and sialendoscopy.[41]

Bacterial Sialadenitis

Bacterial sialadenitis occurs when there is bacterial infection of the salivary gland. Hyposalivation due to various causes (eg, dehydration, medications, or Sjögren's syndrome [SS]) may lead to increased bacterial colonization of salivary gland ducts.

- Symptoms and features
  - Acute
    - Painful swelling
    - Reddened skin
    - Edema of the cheek
    - Low-grade fever
    - Malaise
    - Serum studies showing raised erythrocyte sedimentation rate, raised C-reactive protein, leukocytosis
    - Purulent exudate from duct openings
  - Chronic
    - Unilateral
    - Mild pain/swelling
    - Symptoms common after meals
    - Parotid or submandibular gland enlargement

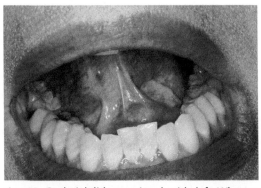

Fig. 14. Oral sialolith associated with left Wharton duct on the floor of mouth.

- Intermittent recurrent painful swelling associated with salivary flow stimulation
- Diagnosis: Diagnosis is primarily made through observation of clinical features as noted earlier.
- Management: For acute bacterial sialadenitis, initial management involves empirical antibiotic therapy for oral flora coverage, with appropriate cultures obtained. In chronic recurrent sialadenitis or chronic sclerosing sialadenitis, symptomatic periods are managed with conservative therapies, such as hydration, analgesics, sialogogues to stimulate salivary secretion, and regular, gentle gland massage. If episodes occur more than 3 times per year or are severe, surgical excision of the affected gland may be considered.[40]

Mumps

Mumps (paramyxovirus) primarily affects both parotid glands and is highly contagious and can spread rapidly, transmitted by respiratory droplets or direct contact with an infected person.[42] Viral parotitis may also be a result of infection due to HIV, Epstein-Barr virus, coxsackievirus, and influenza A and parainfluenza viruses.

- Symptoms and features: Prodromal symptoms include low-grade fever, headache, and malaise, followed by swelling of one or both parotid glands. Patients may also have a sore face and ears and difficulty talking.[43] In the case of mumps, symptoms typically occur 16 to 18 days after exposure.
- Diagnosis: Diagnosis is mostly based on clinical symptoms, with blood testing showing leukopenia with relative lymphocytosis and elevated serum amylase.
- Management: Treatment is symptomatic and involves analgesics and antipyretics. Symptoms resolve after 7 to 10 days.

Sjögren's Syndrome

SS is a chronic autoimmune inflammatory disorder primarily affecting exocrine glands, such as salivary and lacrimal glands, due to lymphocytic infiltration but can also have extraglandular organ involvement.

- Symptoms and features: In addition to primary complaints of xerostomia and/or dry eyes, pain symptoms in patients may vary, with patients with SS showing a higher incidence of burning mouth, glossodynia, and bilateral distal neuropathies.[44] Other features include fatigue, myalgia, and mild cognitive

dysfunction; some may present with parotitis. To obtain a diagnosis, some may use the American-European Consensus Group and the American College of Rheumatology classification criteria for SS.

- Diagnosis: Diagnosis is based on clinical symptoms, specific answers to a set of validated questions on symptoms, and serology for anti-Sjögren's antibodies (anti-Ro/SSA and/or anti-La/SSB). Other tests may include scintigraphy and minor salivary gland lip biopsy to evaluate for lymphocytic infiltrate.
- Management: Treatment measures are targeted toward alleviating individual symptoms. For oral symptoms, focus is on moistening of the mouth, measures for salivary stimulation (both local and systemic), and analgesia for pain.

Salivary Gland Neoplasms

Salivary gland neoplasms, both of the benign and malignant varieties, are relatively rare. Most common benign tumors include pleomorphic adenoma and papillary cystadenoma lymphomatosum. Among the most common malignant salivary gland neoplasms are mucoepidermoid carcinoma and adenoid cystic carcinoma.

- Symptoms and features: Most major salivary gland neoplasms arise as a slowly enlarging painless mass in an otherwise normal-appearing gland. Minor salivary gland tumors vary in presentation, with painless masses on the palate or floor of mouth being the most common presentation (**Fig. 15**). Pain may be a feature of both benign and malignant salivary gland tumors. Pain, numbness, and nerve paralysis may be a feature in adenoid cystic carcinoma because of its nature of infiltrating around nerves.
- Diagnosis: If suspicion for such neoplasms arises through signs and symptoms, imaging

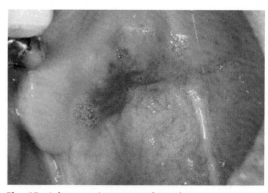

Fig. 15. Adenocarcinoma on the palate.

studies (eg, CT, MRI, ultrasound) and biopsy to obtain definitive histologic diagnosis are warranted.

- Management: Detailed management strategies for these are beyond the scope of this article. In the case of both benign and malignant tumors, surgical excision is indicated. Malignant tumors may require subsequent radiation and/or chemotherapy depending on the staging and type of tumor.

REFERENCES

1. Orchardson R, Gillam DG. The efficacy of potassium salts as agents for treating dentin hypersensitivity. J Orofac Pain 2000;14(1):9–19.

2. Turp JC, Gobetti JP. The cracked tooth syndrome: an elusive diagnosis. J Am Dent Assoc 1996;127: 1502–7.

3. Mathew S, Thangavel B, Mathew CA, et al. Diagnosis of cracked tooth syndrome. J Pharm Bioallied Sci 2012;4(Suppl 2):S242–4.

4. Berman LH, Hartwell GR. Diagnosis. In: Cohen S, Hargreaves K, editors. Pathways of the pulp. 9th edition. St Louis (MO): Mosby; 2006. p. 1–39.

5. Hupp JR, Ellis E, Tucker MR. Contemporary oral and maxillofacial surgery. 5th edition. St Louis (MO): Mosby Elsevier; 2008. p. 293.

6. American Academy of Periodontology. Consensus report: abscesses of the periodontium. Ann Periodontol 1999;4(1):83.

7. Abrams H, Jasper SJ. Diagnosis and management of acute periodontal problems. In: Falace DA, editor. Emergency dental care: diagnosis and management of urgent dental problems. Baltimore (MD): Williams & Wilkins; 1995. p. 137–42.

8. American Academy of Periossdontology. Parameter on acute periodontal diseases. American Academy of Periodontology. J Periodontol 2000;71(Suppl 5): 863–6.

9. Segura-Egea JJ, Castellanos-Cosano L, Machuca G, et al. Diabetes mellitus, periapical inflammation and endodontic treatment outcome. Med Oral Patol Oral Cir Bucal 2012;17(2):e356–61.

10. Hargreaves KM, Cohen S, Berman LH, editors. Cohen's pathways of the pulp. 10th edition. St Louis (MO): Mosby Elsevier; 2010. p. 529–55.

11. Neville BW, Damm DD, Allen CA, et al. Oral & maxillofacial pathology. 2nd edition. Philadelphia: W.B. Saunders; 2002. p. 113–24, 393–5.

12. Douglass AB, Douglass JM. Common dental emergencies. Am Fam Physician 2003;67(3):511–6.

13. Tucker MR, Hupp JR, Ellis E, editors. Contemporary oral and maxillofacial surgery. 5th edition. St Louis (MO): Mosby Elsevier; 2008. p. 198.

14. Fragiskos FD, editor. Oral surgery. Berlin: Springer; 2007. p. 122–99.

15. Newman MG, Takei HH, Klokkevold PR, et al, editors. Carranza's clinical periodontology. 11th edition. St Louis (MO): Elsevier/Saunders; 2012. p. 103–33, 331–3, 440, 447.

16. Daly B, Sharif MO, Newton T, et al. Local interventions for the management of alveolar osteitis (dry socket). Cochrane Database Syst Rev 2012;(12):CD006968.

17. Greenberg MS, Glick M, Ship JA, editors. Burket's oral medicine. 11th edition. Hamilton (Canada): BC Decker; 2008. p. 89–97.

18. Barnes L, editor. Surgical pathology of the head and neck. 3rd edition. New York: Informa Healthcare; 2008.

19. Thongprasom K, Carrozzo M, Furness S, et al. Interventions for treating oral lichen planus. Cochrane Database Syst Rev 2011;(7):CD001168.

20. Asch S, Goldenberg G. Systemic treatment of cutaneous lichen planus: an update. Cutis 2011;87(3): 129–34.

21. Sharma A, Białynicki-Birula R, Schwartz RA, et al. Lichen planus: an update and review. Cutis 2012; 90(1):17–23.

22. Lewis MAO, Jordan RCK, editors. Oral medicine. 2nd edition. London: Manson Publishing; 2012. p. 66–72.

23. Genital herpes - CDC fact sheet. Available at: cdc. gov. Accessed December 31, 2014.

24. Mosby. Mosby's medical dictionary. 9th edition. Amsterdam (Netherlands): Elsevier Health Sciences; 2013. p. 836–7.

25. Wu IB, Schwartz RA. Herpetic whitlow. Cutis 2007; 79(3):193–6.

26. Steiner I, Benninger F. Update on herpes virus infections of the nervous system. Curr Neurol Neurosci Rep 2013;13(12):414.

27. Balasubramaniam R, Kuperstein AS, Stoopler ET. Update on oral herpes virus infections. Dent Clin North Am 2014;58(2):265–80.

28. Stephenson-Famy A, Gardella C. Herpes simplex virus infection during pregnancy. Obstet Gynecol Clin North Am 2014;41(4):601–14.

29. Elad S, Zadik Y, Hewson I, et al. A systematic review of viral infections associated with oral involvement in cancer patients: a spotlight on herpesviridea. Support Care Cancer 2010;18(8): 993–1006.

30. Eaglestein WH, Katz R, Brown JA. The effects of early corticosteroid therapy in the skin eruption and pain of herpes zoster. J Am Med Assoc 1970; 211:1681–3.

31. Lindhe J, Lang NP, Karring T, editors. Clinical periodontology and implant dentistry. 5th edition. Copenhagen: Blackwell Munksgaard; 2008. p. 413–59.

32. Brocklehurst P, Tickle M, Glenny AM, et al. Systemic interventions for recurrent apthous stomatitis (mouth ulcers). Cochrane Database Syst Rev 2012;(9):CD005411.

33. Millet D, Welbury R, editors. Clinical problem solving in orthodontics and paediatric dentistry. Edinburgh (United Kingdom): Churchill Livingstone; 2004. p. 143–4.

34. Magro CM, Roberts-Barnes J, Crowson AN. Direct immunofluorescence testing in the diagnosis of immunobullous disease, collagen vascular disease, and vascular injury syndromes. Dermatol Clin 2012; 30(4):763–98.

35. Rao R, Prabhu SS, Sripathi H, et al. Vesiculobullous lesions in lipoid proteinosis: a case report. Dermatol Online J 2008;14(7):16.

36. Barasch A, Safford M, Eisenberg E. Oral cancer and oral effects of anticancer therapy. Mt Sinai J Med 1998;65(5–6):370–7.

37. Spijkervet FK, van Saene HK, Panders AK, et al. Scoring irradiation mucositis in head and neck cancer patients. J Oral Pathol Med 1989;18(3):167–71.

38. Katsura K, Sasai K, Sato K, et al. Relationship between oral health status and development of osteoradionecrosis of the mandible: a retrospective longitudinal study. Oral Surg Oral Med Oral Pathol Oral Radiol Endod 2008;105:731–8.

39. Migliorati CA, Woo SB, Hewson I, et al. A systemic review of bisphosphonate osteonecrosis (BON) in cancer. Support Care Cancer 2010;18(8):1099–106.

40. Lee KC, Lee SJ. Clinical features and treatments of odontogenic sinusitis. Yonsei Med J 2010;51(6):932.

41. Capaccio P, Torretta S, Ottavian F, et al. Modern management of obstructive salivary diseases. Acta Otorhinolaryngol Ital 2007;27(4):161–72.

42. Rubin S, Carbone KM. Mumps. In: Kasper DL, Braunwald E, Fauci AS, et al, editors. Harrison's principles of internal medicine. 18th edition. New York: McGraw-Hill Professional; 2011.

43. Davis NF, McGuire BB, Mahon JA, et al. The increasing incidence of mumps orchitis: a comprehensive review. BJU Int 2010;105(8):1060–5.

44. Olney RK. Neuropathies associated with connective tissue disease. Semin Neurol 1998;18:63–72.

Myofascial Pain
Mechanisms to Management

James Fricton, DDS, MS

KEYWORDS

- Pain • Muscles • Spasm • Myofascial pain • Trigger point • Soft tissue • Chronic pain
- Tender muscles

KEY POINTS

- Chronic pain is the main reason for seeking health care, the most common reason for disability and addiction, and the highest driver of health care costs, and it is most often caused by myopain conditions.
- Myofascial pain (MFP) is the most common cause of persistent regional pain such as back pain, headaches, and facial pain.
- MFP is readily diagnosed through identifying differential clinical characteristics and soft tissue palpation.
- Treatments of myopain conditions include:
  - Stretching, postural, relaxation, strengthening, and conditioning exercises
  - Reduction of all contributing factors that strain the muscles and heighten peripheral and central sensitization
  - Counterstimulation treatments to desensitize soft tissues
- Use of a transformative care model that integrates patient training in reducing risk factors and enhancing protective factors with evidence-based treatments using an integrative team of health professionals enhances long-term outcomes.

INTRODUCTION

More than 100 million adults in the United States are affected by chronic pain conditions, costing more than $500 billion annually in medical care and lost productivity.[1–4] Several studies have found that myopain conditions such as myofascial pain (MFP) and fibromyalgia (FBM) are the most common chronic pain condition leading to nearly all chronic pain conditions, including back pain, headaches, neck pain, and jaw pain.[5–10] This finding makes them one of the top reasons for seeking health care, the most common reason for disability and addiction, and the highest driver of health care costs, costing more than cancer, heart disease, dementia, and diabetes. The personal impact of chronic pain in terms of suffering, disability, drug use, depression, and conflict is incalculable. In hopes of improving the condition, medical care often involves expensive and high-risk passive interventions, such as polypharmacy, opioid analgesics, high-tech imaging, implantable stimulators, and surgery. However, more than half of the persons seeking care for pain conditions still have pain 5 years later and many develop long-term disability.[11–19] Because nearly one-third of the population has chronic pain to some extent, most people assume chronic pain is intractable. However, that is not the case. Myopain conditions can be successfully managed in most patients and any poor long-term outcomes are often caused by the lack of recognition and adequate care.[20–26] Thus,

Disclosures: None.

HealthPartners Institute for Education and Research, University of Minnesota School of Dentistry, 4700 Dale Drive, Edina, MN 55424, USA

E-mail address: frict001@umn.edu

Oral Maxillofacial Surg Clin N Am 28 (2016) 289–311
http://dx.doi.org/10.1016/j.coms.2016.03.010

the principals of cause, diagnosis, and management of myopain conditions are relevant for all health care professionals.

Most Common Chronic Pain Conditions

Everyone, at some point in their lives, has experienced acute muscle pain associated with muscle spasm or repetitive strain. However, when acute pain becomes chronic, patients and their health care professionals often become confused and overlook the muscle in favor of treating other conditions, such as depression, osteoarthritis, or neuropathic conditions. This lack of understanding leads to misdiagnosis, inadequate care, mistreatment, and progression of an acute problem to chronic pain. When behavioral and psychological factors are evident, myopain conditions often become misunderstood, assuming the patient's experience of pain is imagined or exaggerated or caused by the psychosocial issues. However, MFP is a physical pain condition that can be successfully managed.

MFP is the most common cause of persistent regional pain such as back pain, shoulder pain, tension-type headaches, and facial pain, whereas FBM is the most common widespread pain.[20] MFP is a regional muscle pain disorder characterized by localized muscle tenderness, limited range of motion, and regional pain, whereas FBM is associated with soft tissue tenderness, fatigue, stiffness, nonrefreshed sleep, and widespread physical pain.[24] Two prior studies of clinic populations found that MFP conditions were cited as the most common cause of pain, responsible for 54.6% of chronic head and neck pain[6] and 85% of back pain.[7] Another study, in a general internal medicine practice, found that, among those patients who presented with pain, MFP was present in 29.6% of the population and was the most common cause of pain.[8] Symptoms of FBM also seem to be prevalent in the general population, with up to 5% having FBM, and are more prevalent in patients with chronic fatigue (estimated as at least 20%).[4,5,27]

CLINICAL PRESENTATION
Clinical Characteristics

The clinical characteristics of MFP include hard, palpable, discrete, localized nodules, called trigger points (TrPs), which are located within taut bands of skeletal muscle (**Box 1**). TrPs are painful on compression and associated with pain in predictable regional patterns within a referral zone. The pain in the zone of reference is usually located over the tender point (TeP) or spreads out in a referral pattern to distant sites (**Fig. 1**). This tenderness is often referred to as a TrP because palpation

---

Box 1
Clinical characteristics of MFP

TrPs in taut band of muscle

Tenderness on palpation

Consistent points of tenderness

Palpation alters pain locally or distally

Associated symptoms

Otologic

Paresthesias

Gastrointestinal distress

Visual disturbances

Dermatographia

Pain in zone of reference

Constant dull ache

Fluctuates in intensity

Consistent patterns of referral

Alleviation with extinction of TrP

Contributing factors

Traumatic and whiplash injuries

Occupational and repetitive strain injuries

Physical disorders

Parafunctional muscle tension producing habits

Postural and repetitive strains

Disuse

Metabolic/nutritional

Sleep disturbance

Psychosocial and emotional stressors (direct)

---

of the TeP in the muscle alters the pain in the zone of reference, and, if treated, it resolves the resultant pain.[24] MTrPs can be either active or latent.[24] An active TrP is associated with spontaneous pain in which pain is present without palpation. This spontaneous pain can be at the site of the TrP or referred to more distant sites. However, firm palpation of the active TrP (A-TrP) increases pain locally and usually reproduces the patient's remote pain. A latent MTrP (L-TrP) is not associated with spontaneous pain, although pain can often be elicited in an asymptomatic patient by a mechanical stimulus such as finger pressure over the L-TrP. There are generally no neurologic deficits associated with the disorder unless a nerve entrapment syndrome with weakness and diminished sensation coincides with the muscle TrPs.[6] Blood and urine studies are generally normal unless the pain is caused by a concomitant disorder.[7] Imaging studies, including radiographs

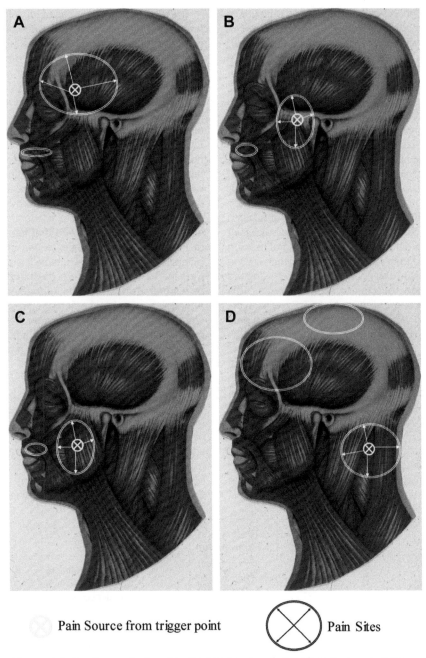

Pain Source from trigger point   Pain Sites

Fig. 1. TrPs with associated patterns of referral in the head and neck. (*A*) The pain source is the anterior temporalis TrP. The pain sites include temple, frontal, and retro-orbital headaches and pain in the maxillary anterior teeth. These muscles are activated by clenching, bruxism, and other oral parafunctional habits. (*B*) The pain source is the deep masseter TrP. The pain sites include preauricular pain, earaches, and pain in the maxillary posterior teeth. These muscles are also activated by clenching, bruxism, and other oral parafunctional habits. (*C*) The pain source is the middle masseter TrP. The pain sites include temple, frontal, and retro-orbital headaches and pain in the maxillary anterior teeth. These muscles are also activated by clenching, bruxism, and other oral parafunctional habits. (*D*) The pain source is the splenius capitis TrP in the posterior cervical area. The pain sites include posterior cervical, vertex headache, and frontal headaches. These muscles are also activated by clenching and forward head posture.

and MRI, do not reveal any pathologic changes in the muscle or connective tissue.

The affected muscles may also have increased fatigability, stiffness, subjective weakness, pain in movement, and slightly restricted range of motion.[5–7,27] The muscles are painful when stretched, causing the patient to protect the muscle through poor posture, bracing, and sustained contraction resulting in persistence of the pain.[8] For example, in a study of jaw range of motion in patients with MFP and no joint abnormalities, the patients showed a slightly diminished range of motion (approximately 10%) compared with normal individuals and pain in full range of motion,[8] which is considerably less limitation than is found with joint locking caused by a temporomandibular joint (TMJ) internal derangement. This postural bracing may also lead to the development of other TrPs in the same muscle and agonist muscles causing the pain to spread to broader regional areas. This development can cause multiple TrPs with overlapping areas of pain referral and changes in pain patterns as TrPs are inactivated.

Although routine clinical electromyographic (EMG) studies show no significant abnormalities associated with TrPs, some specialized EMG studies reveal differences.[28–31] Needle insertion into the TrP can produce a burst of electrical activity that is not produced in adjacent muscle fibers.[31] In 2 experimental EMG studies of TrPs, Simons[30] and Fricton and colleagues[28] found abnormal electrical activity associated with the local muscle twitch response when specifically snapping the tense muscle band containing a myofascial TrP.

The mechanical properties of muscles, including firm consistency, stiffness, and lack of elasticity of muscles containing the TrPs, has also been documented and found to be different from adjacent muscles.[32,33] For example, elastography with ultrasonography imaging confirms these significant tissue abnormalities and that morphologic changes are associated with MTrPs (**Fig. 2**). Changes in elasticity and stiffness of MTrP compared with the surrounding tissue suggest a disruption of normal muscle fiber structure. The increase in local tissue density in the form of contraction knots may result from increased muscle fiber contraction and recruitment and local injury. Furthermore, this possibility was confirmed with magnetic resonance elastography, which showed that the propagation of induced vibration shear waves in TrP bands differs from that in normal muscle tissue. Skin overlying the TrPs in the masseter muscle also seems to be warmer, as measured by infrared emission.[34,35] Although most of these findings are from solitary studies, they provide preliminary evidence of a broad range of objective characteristics that are important in understanding the diagnosis and cause of MFP.

Association with Other Pain Conditions

MFP, particularly in the head and neck, is frequently overlooked as a diagnosis because it is often accompanied by signs and symptoms in addition to pain as well as other pathologic pain conditions.[24] MFP seems to not only mimic many other conditions, such as joint disorders, migraine headaches,

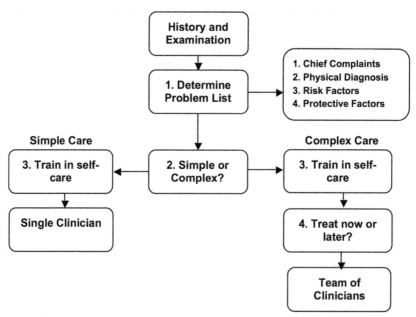

Fig. 2. A decision tree for triaging patients and enhancing outcomes and successful care.

neuralgias, temporal arteritis, TMJ disorders, spinal disk disease, sinusitis, dental pain, and other disorders, but also accompanies other pain disorders.[36–41] For example, TrPs coincide with 14 of 18 TeP sites in diagnostic criteria for FBM.[42,43] TrPs also develop in association with joint disorders such as disc derangements, osteoarthritis, and subluxation.[43–48] MFP is also reported to be found with systemic or local infections of viral or bacterial origin; with lupus erythematosus, scleroderma, and rheumatoid arthritis; and along segmental distribution of nerve injury, nerve root compression, or neuralgias.[44] These findings suggest that muscles may serve as part of the alarm system for regional disorders and may lead to confusion regarding diagnosis of MFP as the primary cause of pain.

Relationship to Other Muscle Pain Disorders

In addition to MFP, there are several other distinct muscle disorder subtypes affecting the masticatory system, including myositis, muscle spasm, muscle contracture, and FBM.[40,41] Perhaps the most pragmatic taxonomy related to differentiating muscle pain disorders is in the Academy of Orofacial Pain's Guidelines for Diagnosis and Management of Orofacial Pain.[40] In this classification, different muscle disorders are descriptively defined by their characteristics and classified as MFP (regional pain and localized tender TrPs), FBM (widespread pain with localized TePs), myositis (regional pain and diffuse tenderness), muscle spasm (brief painful contraction with limited range of motion), contracture (longstanding limited range of motion), and muscle splinting (regional pain and localized tenderness accompanying a joint problem).

Myositis

Myositis is an acute condition with localized or generalized inflammation of the muscle and connective tissue and associated pain and swelling overlying the muscle. Most areas in the muscle are tender, with pain in active range of motion. The inflammation usually has a local cause, such as overuse, excessive stretch, a drug, local infection from pericoronitis, trauma, or cellulitis. This condition is also termed delayed-onset muscle soreness in cases of acute overuse.

Muscle spasm

Muscle spasm is also an acute disorder characterized by a brief involuntary tonic contraction of a muscle. It can occur as a result of overstretching of a previously weakened muscle, protective splinting of an injury, as a centrally mediated phenomenon such as Compazine-induced spasm of the lateral pterygoid muscle, or overuse of a muscle. A muscle in spasm is acutely shortened, painful, and with joint range of motion limited. Lateral pterygoid spasm on one side can also cause a shift of the occlusion to the contralateral side.

Muscle contracture

Muscle contracture is a chronic condition characterized by continuous gross shortening of the muscle with significant limited range of motion. It can begin as a result of factors such as trauma, infection, or prolonged hypomobility. If the muscle is maintained in a shortened state, muscular fibrosis and contracture may develop over several months. Pain is often minimal in the process but it can occur as a result of reactive bracing or clenching to protect the muscle.

Fibromyalgia

FBM is a common rheumatic pain syndrome that resembles MFP but is more widespread and centrally generated. It consists of widespread pain, fatigue, unrefreshed sleep, and cognitive dysfunction such as confusion, forgetfulness, inability to concentrate, and impaired memory. In addition, most patients have tenderness on palpation at definable classic locations on the neck, trunk, and extremities (**Box 2**). The prevalence of FBM in the general population has ranged from 3.7% to 20%.[19,20] Other characteristics of FBM are divided into the frequency that they occur. The characteristics that occur in more than 75% of patients with FBM include chronic fatigue, stiffness, and sleep disturbance, whereas the variety of associated symptoms that occur in less than 25% of patients with FBM include irritable bowel, headaches, psychological distress, Raynaud phenomena, swelling, paresthesias, and functional disabilities.[21,22] It has been shown that central nervous system (CNS)–modulating factors such as stress, sleep disorders, and depression play some role in FBM.[23] Sleep abnormalities have been well documented, but it is unproved whether these are the primary abnormality or an associated or secondary abnormality. More than 75% of patients with FBM are female between the ages of 30 and 60 years.[45] Because FBM commonly occurs with other medical conditions, it is possible that the reported age of onset is artificially high. Therefore, FBM should be suspected in any person presenting with widespread pain because the consequences of prolonged, undiagnosed pain can be considerable.

Examination Findings

Tenderness in the soft tissues is the primary clinical and diagnostic characteristic in MFP and

---

Box 2
Clinical characteristics of Fibromyalgia (FBM) as defined by the American College of Rheumatology 2010 criteria

1. Widespread Pain Index (WPI) score. History of widespread pain in the past week (0–19): shoulder girdle (left or right), upper arm (left or right), lower arm (left or right), hip (buttock; left or right), upper leg (left or right), lower leg (left or right), jaw (left or right), chest, abdomen, neck, upper back, or lower back

2. Symptom Score (SS) includes adding both primary and secondary symptoms (0–6)

   a. Primary SS (0–9): 1, fatigue; 2, unrefreshed sleep; and 3, cognitive symptoms such as confusion, forgetfulness, inability to concentrate. For each of 3 problems, a score of 0 = no problem; 1 = slight, mild, or intermittent problems; 2 = moderate (considerable problems are often present at a moderate level); and 3 = severe: pervasive, continuous, and life-disturbing problems.

   b. Secondary SS (0–3): 0 = 0 symptoms, 1 = 1 to 10 symptoms, 2 = 11 to 24 symptoms, and 3 = 25 or more symptoms.

Diagnosis of FBM is present if the following 3 conditions are met:

1. (a) The WPI score (part 1) is greater than or equal to 7 and the SS score (parts 2a and b) is greater than or equal to 5 or; (b) the WPI score (part 1) is from 3 to 6 and the SS score (parts 2a and b) is greater than or equal to 9.

2. Symptoms have been present at a similar level for at least 3 months.

3. The person does not have a disorder that would otherwise explain the pain.

Adapted from Wolfe, F, Clauw DJ, Fitzcharles MA, et al. The American College of Rheumatology Preliminary Diagnostic Criteria for Fibromyalgia and Measurement of Symptom Severity. Arthritis Care Res (Hoboken) 2010;62(5):600–10.

---

other muscle disorders. Tender areas in FBM are termed TePs, whereas in MFP they are termed TrPs. TrPs in MFP are 2-mm to 5-mm diameter points of increased hypersensitivity in palpable bands of skeletal muscle, tendons, and ligaments with decreasing hypersensitivity as the band is palpated further away from the TrP. As noted earlier, TrPs may be active or latent.[30] Active TrPs are hypersensitive and have continuous pain in the zone of reference that can be altered with compression, whereas latent TrPs have only hypersensitivity with no continuous pain. This localized tenderness, elicited with both manual palpation and pressure algometers, has been found to be a reliable indicator of the presence and severity of MFP.[32,33] However, the presence of taut bands seems to be a characteristic of skeletal muscles in all people regardless of the presence of MFP.[34]

Palpating the active TrP with sustained deep single-finger pressure on the taut band elicits an alteration of the pain (intensification or reduction) in the zone of reference (area of pain complaint) or cause radiation of the pain toward the zone of reference. This pain can occur immediately or be delayed a few seconds. The pattern of referral is both reproducible and consistent with patterns of other patients with similar TrPs (see **Fig. 1**). This pattern enables clinicians to use the zone of reference as a guide to locate the TrP for purposes of treatment. In contrast, TePs require a

standardized palpation at 18 predefined sites, as noted in **Fig. 2** and **Box 2**.

Many of the TePs in the diagnosis of FBM are in similar locations to many TrPs. For example, Simons[49] points out that 16 of the 18 TeP sites in FBM are at well-known TrP sites. Many of the clinical characteristics of FBM, such as fatigue, morning stiffness, and sleep disorders, can also accompany MFP. Bennett[5] compares these 2 disorders and concludes that they are 2 distinct disorders but may have the same underlying pathophysiology. FBM is characterized by more common CNS-generated contributing factors such as sleep disorders, depression, and stress. In contrast, MFP is distinguished by more common regional contributing factors like localized trauma, posture, and muscle tension habits. MFP generally had a better prognosis for treatment than FBM.

The patient's behavioral reaction to this firm palpation is a distinguishing characteristic of MFP and FBM and is termed a jump sign. This reaction may include withdrawal of the head, wrinkling of the face or forehead, or a verbal response such as "That's it" or "Oh, yes." The jump sign should be distinguished from the local twitch response in MFP, which can also occur with palpation. This latter response can be elicited by placing the muscle in moderate passive tension and snapping the band containing the TrP briskly with firm pressure from a palpating finger moving perpendicularly across the muscle band at its most tender point. This pressure can produce a reproducible shortening of the muscle band (visible in larger muscles) and associated electromyographic changes characteristic of the local twitch response described later. In locating an active TrP, the jump sign should be elicited and, if possible, alteration of the patient's complaint by the palpation.

In FBM, TePs require direct pressure of about 4 kg/cm² over the site instead of the snapping palpation with TrPs. In both TrPs and TePs, palpating pressure over neutral areas such as the middle of the forehead can help the patient distinguish between dull pressure and overt tenderness. This distinction gives the examiner an appreciation of the individual's pain threshold and provides a standard pressure to be placed directly over the sites. TePs often elicit a pain directly over the site of the tenderness without the radiation of pain that is often characteristic of TrPs.

Pain Symptoms

The regional pain found with MFP needs to be distinguished from the widespread muscular pain associated with FBM (**Table 1**). In both cases, the pain is often described as a chronic, dull, aching pain and this is central to the diagnosis. These 2 disorders have many similar characteristics and may represent 2 ends of a continuous spectrum, MFP being generated by regional factors and

FBM being generated by centrally mediated factors.

There is evidence that supports the pain of MFP being related to and/or generated by the TrP, particularly if it is distant from the TrP. For example, clinical examination of TrPs shows that in accessible muscles palpation of the active TrPs alters, usually intensifying, the referred pain. In addition, injections of local anesthetic into the active TrP reduce or eliminate the referred pain and the tenderness.[50–52] Treatments such as spray and stretch, exercise, or massage directed at the muscle with the TrP also predictably reduce the referred pain.[53] Other evidence to confirm the relationship includes the use of pressure algometry to show a positive correlation between the scope of tenderness and the severity of pain.[54] In addition, the change in scope of tenderness in response to treatment positively correlates with the change in symptom severity ($r = .54$).[55]

Pain in FBM is stable and consistent, in contrast with MFP, which can vary in intensity and location depending on which muscles are involved. Patients with FBM most often have pain in the low back, neck, shoulders, and hips.[44,45,56] However, these are areas that frequently affect MFP, reflecting the overlap between the two disorders. These studies have also shown that the pain in FBM is considerably more severe over a larger body area than the pain experienced by patients with other nonlocalized rheumatic disease syndromes.

Contributing Factors

As with all chronic pain conditions, concomitant social, behavioral, and psychological disturbances often precede or follow the development of MFP and other masticatory muscle pain disorders.[54] Patients report psychological symptoms such as frustration, anxiety, depression, and anger if acute cases become chronic. Maladaptive behaviors such as pain verbalization, poor sleep and dietary habits, lack of exercise, poor posture, bruxism, other tension-producing habits, and medication dependencies can also be seen when pain becomes prolonged. Each of these may complicate the clinical picture by perpetuating the pain, preventing compliance with the treatment program, and causing self-perpetuating chronic pain cycles to develop.

Parafunctional muscle tension–producing habits such as back bracing, neck tensing, and teeth clenching can be generated as a form of tension release as well as a learned behavioral response. The relationship between stress and MFP is difficult to assess because stress is difficult to define and major methodological problems exist

Table 1 Differences between FBM and MFP		
	FBM	**MFP**
Gender	Female/male: 10:1	Female/male: 1:2
Pain	3 of 4 quadrants	Regional related to muscle involved
General fatigue	Yes	No
Unrefreshed sleep	Yes	Situational
Cognitive symptoms (confusion, forgetfulness, inability to concentrate)	Yes	No
TeP distribution	Widespread	Regional in muscle involved
Stiffness and other symptoms	Widespread	Regional
Prognosis	Moderate	Excellent

in studying stress. Although no evidence suggests a direct causal relationship between stress and MFP, some studies suggest that a correlation does exist between them. There is a higher than normal incidence of psychophysiologic disorders such as migraine headaches, backache, neck pain, nervous asthma, and ulcers in patients with MFP and other muscle disorders, which suggests similar causal factors.[57–62] Also, higher than normal levels of urinary concentrations of catecholamines and 17-hydroxysteriods, which are commonly associated with a high number of stressful events, were found in a group of patients with MFP dysfunction syndrome compared with controls.[63] In addition, stress management interventions frequently provide significant benefit for patients with MFP and other muscle disorders.

Poor muscle health caused by lack of exercise, muscle disuse, or poor posture has also been suggested to predispose the muscle to the development of TrPs and TePs,[64,65] and often arises after muscles have been weakened through immobilization caused by the prolonged use of cervical collars or extended bed rest, for example. Postural discrepancies may also contribute to joint displacement and abnormal functional patterns, which can contribute to abnormal proprioceptive input and sustained muscle contraction in an attempt to correct the poor postural relationships and allow better compensated neuromuscular function. Poor posture caused by a unilateral short leg, small hemipelvis, increased cervical or lumbar lordosis, noncompensated scoliosis, occlusal abnormalities, and poor positioning of the head or tongue have also been implicated.[66]

CAUSE AND PATHOPHYSIOLOGY

The results of this research suggest that an explanatory model can account for the mechanisms in the development of myalgia from its onset to increasing severity found with clinical and chronic cases. It is apparent that both central and peripheral mechanisms are associated with this process but peripheral sensitization may have more prominence in MFP, whereas central sensitization may occur more in FBM.[9]

Peripheral and Central Sensitization

Peripheral strain to the muscles from sustained muscle tension habits, repetitive strain, and injury contribute to localized progressive increases in oxidative metabolism and depleted energy supply (decrease in the levels of ATP, ADP, and phosphoryl creatine, and abnormal tissue oxygenation). This situation results in an increase in muscle nociception, particularly with type I muscle fiber types associated with static muscle tone and posture.[22–24] The muscle tenderness and pain are mediated by type III and IV muscle nociceptors, which may be activated by locally released noxious substances such as potassium, histamine, kinins, or prostaglandins, causing tenderness.[67–69] Phasic modulation of excitatory and inhibitory interneurons supplied by the high-threshold sensory afferents may also become involved, ramping up the peripheral sensitization. Tonic muscular hyperactivity and bracing may be normal protective adaptations to the pain instead of its cause but can still perpetuate the peripheral sensitization. Likewise, interventions that provide counterstimulation to the muscle TrPs, such as massage, temperature change, stretching, electrical stimulation, dry needling, and local anesthetic injections, can decrease peripheral sensitization.

Multiple afferent inputs from the muscle and other visceral and somatic structures in the orofacial area, such as joints, dentition, and periodontal ligaments, converge in lamina I or V of the dorsal horn on the way to the cortex, which can result in both local and referred regional pain.[22] Multiple peripheral and central factors, such as oral habits, anxiety, and stress, may facilitate central input through the modulatory influence of the brain stem, which supports the central biasing mechanism and central sensitization.[56–65] In addition, similar to what happens in the periphery, the central modulatory influences can also decrease central input and inhibit central sensitization. This process may explain the diverse factors that can either exacerbate or alleviate the pain, such as stress, repetitive strain, poor posture, and muscle tension, to increase sensitization; or interventions such as relaxation, medications, counseling, and mindful-based stress reduction that can reduce central sensitization.

Peripheral Changes

The nature of the peripheral neuropathologic and/or dysfunctional processes of MFP TrPs or FBM TePs and the peripheral changes associated with the pain are still not fully understood. Several histologic and biochemical studies have been completed on biopsies of tender muscle sites in patients with both generalized and regional muscle complaints. These studies suggest that there are localized progressive increases in oxidative metabolism, particularly in muscle fiber type I with depleted energy supply, increases in metabolic by-products, and resultant muscle nociception at the periphery. This condition results in local and referred pain in the CNS that can be altered by a central biasing mechanism that either amplifies or suppresses the pain.

Injury to Muscle Fiber Type I

Each skeletal muscle has different proportions of muscle fiber types that group into 3 broad categories: type I, type IIA, and type IIB (Table 2).[70] Type IIC and IIM are involved in development and are not frequently seen in the adult masticatory muscles. Type I muscle fibers are functionally associated with static muscle tone and posture. They are slow-twitch, fatigue-resistant fibers with a high number of mitochondria needed for oxidative phosphorylation used in energy metabolism. Type II fibers are functionally associated with increased velocity and force of contraction over brief periods. They are fast-twitch fibers that fatigue easily, are rich in glycogen, and use anaerobic glycolysis for energy metabolism. These fibers can transform from one type to another depending on the demands placed on the muscle. For example, Uhlig and colleagues[70] found signs of fiber transformation from type I to type IIc in cervical muscles associated with pain and dysfunction after spondylodesis. This finding is consistent with the transformation associated with prolonged inactivity caused by the injury. Furthermore, Mayo and colleagues[71] found decreases in the cross-sectional diameter of muscle fiber types I and II in the masticatory system in rhesus monkeys undergoing maxillomandibular fixation.

Thus, transformation caused by inactivity and pain can decrease both the percentage and size of type I fibers available to maintain normal postural and resting muscle activity. In contrast, an increase in demands of postural muscle activity may result in an increase in type I fibers and a decrease in type II fibers, as found by Bengsston and colleagues[72] in patients with muscle pain.[73] If the increased demand placed on the type I fibers by repetitive strain from activities such as clenching or shoulder tensing is beyond normal physiologic parameters, the intracellular components of these fibers will be damaged. This damage will result in hyperpolarization outside the muscle caused by high levels of K^+ from sustained motor unit activity and K^+ pump damage, damage to the actin and myosin myofilaments, disruption of the sarcoplasmic reticulum and the calcium pump, and decrease in local blood flow. Specific factors that are important in initiating this process included both direct macrotrauma and indirect microtrauma from repetitive muscle strain factors.

Metabolic Distress at the Motor End Plates

In explaining the local nature of MFP TrPs, Simons[74,75] suggested that the damage to the muscle occurs primarily at the motor endplates creating an energy crisis at the TrP. He suggested that this crisis occurs from a grossly abnormal increase in acetylcholine release at the endplate and generation of numerous miniature endplate potentials. This situation results in an increase in energy demand, sustained depolarization of the postjunction membrane, and mitochondrial changes.[50] Hubbard and Berkoff[75] found spontaneous EMG activity at the TrP.[76] Hong[77] and Torigoe found that the EMG characteristics of the local twitch response are generated locally without input from the CNS. Also, botulinum toxin A injections, which act on the neuromuscular junction only, have also been shown to be effective in MFP TrPs.[78]

Histologic studies also provide some support to this mechanism.[67,68,79–82] They have shown myofibrillar lysis, moth-eaten fibers, and ragged red type I fibers with deposition of glycogen and abnormal mitochondria, but little evidence of cellular inflammation hypothesis.[22,68] Studies of muscle energy metabolism found decreases in the levels of ATP, ADP, and phosphoryl creatine and abnormal tissue oxygenation in muscles with TrPs.[73] El-Labban and colleagues[79] showed histologically that TMJ ankylosis results in degenerative changes in masseter and temporalis muscles. It has been hypothesized that these changes represent localized progressive increases in oxidative metabolism and depleted energy supply in type I fibers, which may result in progressive abnormal muscle changes that initially include reactive dysfunctional changes occurring within the muscle, particularly muscle fiber type I and surrounding connective tissue.[80]

Activation of Muscle Nociceptors

The resulting metabolic by-products of this damage, whether by high potassium concentration and hyperpolarization outside the muscle caused by K^+ pump damage, high calcium concentration caused by damage to the sarcoplasmic reticulum, or inflammatory mediators from tissue damage, peripheral sensitization of nociceptors in the muscle, fatigue, and disuse can result.[81] Localized tenderness and pain in the muscle involve type III and IV muscle nociceptors and have been shown to be activated by noxious substances, including K^+, bradykinin, histamine, or prostaglandins, that can be released locally from the damage and trigger tenderness.[67–69,82–84] Note that the K^+ activated a higher percentage of type IV muscle

Table 2
Characteristics of muscle fiber types I, IIA, and IIB in skeletal muscles. Type IIC and IIM are primarily involved in growth and development and are not often seen in skeletal muscles

	Major Fiber Types		
	Type I (Red)	Type IIA (Pink)	Type IIB (White)
Staining	Weak: ATPase (light pink) Strong NADH-TR (dark pink)	Strong: ATPase (light pink) Strong NADH-TR (dark pink)	Strong: ATPase (light pink) Weak NADH-TR (dark pink)
Contraction speed and fatigue	Slow twitch Without fatigue Gradual recruitment to maximal force	Fast twitch Fatigue resistant Higher threshold to recruitment	Slow twitch Fatigue resistant Develops highest muscle tension
Cellular characteristics	Low glycogen High number of mitochondria High oxidative enzyme levels Slow myosin	Low glycogen Low number of mitochondria Low oxidative enzyme levels Fast myosin	Rich in glycogen Low number of mitochondria Low oxidative enzyme levels Fast myosin
Morphology	1. Less in deep masseter with short face 2. More with loss of teeth	1. More in deep masseter with short face 2. Less with loss of teeth	1. Hypertrophy with long face 2. Less with loss of teeth
Function	Posture Sustained low-force contraction Increased muscle length does not alter function or morphology	Long-term use Sustained high-force contraction Increased muscle length does not alter function or morphology	Strength Brief high-force contraction Increased muscle length does not alter function or morphology
Response to electrical stimulation	At 50 Hz: Type I to II Increase glycogen level Decreased mitochondria	At 10 Hz: Type II to I Decrease glycogen level Increased mitochondria	At 10 Hz: Type II to I Decrease glycogen level Increased mitochondria
Metabolism	Oxidative phosphorylation	Glycolytic	Glycolytic

Data from Graff-Radford SB, Reeves JL, Jaeger B. Management of chronic head and neck pain: effectiveness of altering factors perpetuating myofascial pain. Headache 1987;27(4):186–90.

nociceptors than other agents, providing support that localized increases in K^+ concentration at the neuromuscular junction may be responsible for sensitization of nociceptors. This peripheral sensitization is thought to play a major role in local tenderness and pain, which, together with central sensitization, produces hyperalgesia in patients with persistent muscle pain.

Central Nervous System Changes

The afferent inputs from type III and IV muscle nociceptors in the body are transmitted to the CNS through cells such as those of the lamina I, V, and possibly IV of the dorsal horn on the way to the cortex, resulting in perception of local pain.[85,86] In the trigeminal system, these afferent inputs project to the second-order neurons in the brain stem regions, including the superficial lamina of trigeminal subnucleus caudalis, as well as its more rostral laminae such as interpolaris and oralis.[87,88] These neurons can then project to neurons in higher levels of the CNS such as the thalamus, cranial motor nuclei, or the reticular formation.[88] In the thalamus, the ventrobasal complex, the posterior group of nuclei, and parts of the medial thalamus are involved in receiving and relaying somatosensory information.[89] These inputs can also converge with other visceral and somatic inputs from tissues such as the joint or skin and be responsible for referred pain perception.[90]

Central Biasing of Nociceptive Input

Both FBM and MFP need to be considered as a primary disorders of central pain perception. Although nociceptive input from the periphery do occur, they have been shown to be modified by multiple factors in their transmission to the CNS. For example, low-intensity and high-intensity electrical stimulation of sensory nerves or noxious stimulation of sites remote from site of pain suppress nociceptive responses of trigeminal brain stem neurons and related reflexes.[88] This finding provides support that afferent inputs can be inhibited by multiple peripherally or centrally initiated alterations in neural input to the brain stem through various treatment modalities such as cold, heat, analgesic medications, massage, muscular injections, and transcutaneous electrical stimulation.[68]

Likewise, persistent peripheral or central nociceptive activity can result in an increase in abnormal neuroplastic changes in cutaneous and deep neurons. These neuroplastic changes may include prolonged responsiveness to afferent inputs, increased receptive field size, and spontaneous bursts of activity.[76,89–92] Thus, peripheral inputs from muscles may also be facilitated or accentuated by multiple peripherally or centrally initiated alterations in neural input with further sustained neural activity such as persistent joint pain, sustained muscle activity habits, or postural tension, or CNS alterations such as depression and anxiety that can support the central sensitization, further perpetuating the problem. This sensitization may be subserved by several neuropeptides; for example, substance P, serotonin, acetylcholine, and endorphins. Serotonin, or 5-hydroxytryptamine, is a CNS neurotransmitter that has been shown to have an inverse relationship to the pain of FBM and, with substance P, has been shown to be at increased levels in the cerebral spinal fluid of patients with FBM.[72,73]

These biochemical changes underlie an integrated central biasing mechanism in the CNS that dampens or accentuates peripheral input.[59] This mechanism may explain many of the characteristics of MFP and other muscle disorders, including the broad regions of pain referral, the recruitment of additional muscles in chronic cases, the interrelationship between muscle and joint pain, and the ability of many treatments, including medication, spray and stretch, massage, and TrP injections, to reduce the pain for longer than the duration of action.

There is evidence that patients with FBM may also have an abnormality associated with the immune system that may distinguish patients with FBM from patients with MFP and support the more systemic nature of FM. Several studies have found that most patients with chronic fatigue and immune dysfunction syndrome fulfill the criteria for FBM and that they may have several serum abnormalities of immune function.[67–69] It is suggested that, in some patients with FBM, a herpes simplex viral infectious process initiates the symptoms that lead to a chronic disturbances in both immune system functioning and the mechanisms of sleep and small fiber neuropathic pain. Thus, an antiviral, valacyclovir, in combination with an antiinflammatory medication, such as celecoxib, has been initially shown to be helpful for FM.[83,84]

EVIDENCE-BASED MANAGEMENT

Treatment of MFP can range from simple cases with transient single-muscle syndromes to complex cases involving multiple pain areas and many interrelating contributing factors, including the presence of FBM. Many systematic reviews and randomized controlled trials (RCTs) have shown success in treatment of MFP using a wide variety of techniques, such as exercise, TrP injections, myotherapy, vapocoolant spray and stretch, transcutaneous electrical nerve stimulation, biofeedback, posture correction, tricyclic antidepressants, muscle relaxants and other medications, and addressing perpetuating factors.[4,6,7,27,78,93–103] For the masticatory muscles, the use of intraoral appliance therapy has also been helpful.[104–110]

However, the difficulty in management lies not in the selection of which treatment to use but in how to educate, engage, and empower patients to reduce the lifestyle risk factors that contribute to its persistence and treatment failure. Results from clinical studies reveal that many patients with MFP have seen many clinicians, and have received numerous medications and multiple other singular treatments for years without receiving more than temporary improvement.[111,112]

These and other studies of chronic pain suggest that, regardless of the pathogenesis of chronic pain, a major characteristic of some of these patients is the failure of traditional biomedical approaches to resolve the problem. Several new strategies are needed in the care model to improve outcomes of chronic pain, including:

- Using an inclusive problem list (physical diagnoses, protective factors, and risk factors) to personalize the care strategy
- Determining the complexity of the patient with risk assessment and using a decision process (tree) to stratify care based on complexity to increase the potential for successful management
- Use a transformative care model that provides patient training on an equal and integrated basis with evidence-based treatment
- Recognizing the role of the health care provider as an agent of change and shift to new chronic illness paradigms

Each of these is discussed later.

Determine a Complete Problem List

The first step in helping patients shift their understanding of their illness so they learn to achieve health and wellness is to establish a complete problem list. The problem list includes both the physical diagnoses (the physical problem responsible for the chief complaint and its associated symptoms) and the list of contributing factors that initiate, perpetuate, or result from the disorder and complicate the problem. Multidimensional risk assessment helps to determine which contributing factors are present. Specific risk factors for chronic pain are included in **Table 3**. These risk factors may range from peripheral factors, such repetitive stress-strain and postural habits, to central mediating factors, such as anxiety and depression, comorbid conditions, somatization, and catastrophizing. Protective factors, such as level of exercise, healthy diet, sleep, coping, self-efficacy, patient beliefs (eg, perceived control over pain), and social support, reduce vulnerability to chronic pain and can create more positive outcomes.

Match the Complexity of Management to the Complexity of the Patient

High treatment failure rates dictate the critical need to match the level of complexity of the management program with the complexity of the patient; the more risk factors and training needed, the more complex the care team. **Fig. 2** describes a hierarchical approach from acute to simple to complex management. Failure to address the entire problem, including all involved muscles, concomitant diagnoses, and risk factors, may lead to failure to resolve the pain, delayed recovery, and perpetuation of the pain. In addition, managing only those patients whose complexity matches the care strategy available to the clinician improves success. Simple cases with minimal behavioral and psychosocial involvement can typically be managed by a single clinician. Complex patients with many risk factors should be managed within an interdisciplinary pain clinic setting that uses a team of clinicians to address different aspects of the problem in a concerted fashion. In both simple and complex cases, each clinician needs to recognize and address the whole problem and use a transformative care model to maximize the potential for a successful outcome.

The difficulty in long-term management of chronic pain often lies not in treating the muscle but in the complex task of training the patient to change the identified risk factors because they can be integrally related to the patient's physical characteristics, attitudes, emotions, lifestyles, and social and physical environment. Interdisciplinary teams integrate various health professionals in a supportive environment to accomplish both long-term treatment of illness and modification of these contributing factors. Many approaches, such as habit reversal techniques, biofeedback, and stress management, have been used to achieve this result within a transformative care approach.

Transformative Care Model

Combining evidence-based biomedical treatments with robust patient training to reduce risk

Table 3
The 7 realms of risk factors and protective factors involved in management of MFP

Realm	Description	Protective Factors that Protect from Delayed Recovery and Chronic Pain	Risk Factors that Increase Risk of Chronic Pain
Body	Physical and physiologic structures of the body	Balanced relaxed posture, stretching, strengthening, and conditioning exercise	Poor posture, tight weak muscles, hypomobile or hypermobile joints, poor conditioning, injury, genetic risk, and comorbidities
Lifestyle	Regular lifestyles and behaviors	Protective diet, good pacing, reduce repetitive strain, staying active, restful sleep, chemical free, and compliance with protective actions	Poor diet, sedentary life, prolonged sitting, poor sleep, hurrying, repetitive strain habits, high-risk behaviors, chemical use
Emotions	Positive and negative feelings and affect	Sustained positive emotions, such as feelings of joy, excitement, calmness, confidence, happiness, and contentment	Prolonged negative emotional experiences: anger, anxiety, sadness, fear, guilt, and depression
Society	Relationships with others	Positive relationships with family, friends, colleagues, community, social support, helping others, work wellness, rewarding recovery	Poor relationships, routine conflict, loss, abuse, posttraumatic stress, low social support, secondary and tertiary gain
Spirit	Beliefs and purpose in life	Purpose, direction, beliefs, faith, hope, self-compassion, self-esteem, inner strength, determination	Stress, feeling lost, burnout, disbelief, cynicism, doubt, hopelessness, resignation
Mind	Thoughts and attitudes	Broad understanding of conditions, resilience, self-efficacy and self-control, accepting responsibility, having realistic expectations, and engaging in active coping	Ignorance or limited understanding of broader problem, low resilience, low self-efficacy/control, refusal of responsibility, poor compliance, unrealistic expectations, and passive coping
Environment	Physical environment	Clean, organized, safe environment and interaction with the environment that is protective, cautious, and careful	Living within an unclean, chaotic, disorganized, negligent, and dangerous environment increases risk of injury and accident

From Preventing chronic pain. International MYOPAIN Society. Available at: https://www.preventingchronicpain.org/drupal/pcpnet/rsrch_cause; with permission.

factors and enhance protective factors can transform a person's life from one beset by illness to one characterized by health and wellness.[14,15] This principle is the basis for a transformative model of care. When self-management is combined with these evidence-based biomedical treatments, outcomes can be dramatically improved and patients are less dependent on the health care system. Transformative care includes the use of risk assessments to identify risk factors as part of the problem list. Personalized care strategies include integrative teams that can be supported by health coaches, social support networks, on-line and in-person patient training programs, and dashboards to document patient engagement and patient-centered outcomes. A transformative care management strategy for masticatory MFP includes 2 components:

1. Treatment with intraoral appliance therapy, medication, physical therapy, and other treatments to reduce the pain and muscle dysfunction.
2. Training on exercises to improve flexibility, function, and pain with cognitive behavior therapy to reduce risk factors and promote protective factors (see **Box 1**).

The short-term goal is to reduce pain by reducing muscle strain and restoring the muscle to normal length, posture, and full joint range of motion. The long-term goal is to prevent delayed recovery by developing a daily exercise routine, such as yoga; maintaining balanced, relaxed postures; and making changes in risk factors permanent. Thus, patient compliance with a new daily routine is important. This outcome can best be achieved if the health care provider becomes an agent of change.

The Health Care Provider as an Agent of Change

Health care providers need to recognize that they are part of the patient's system of health and/or illness. In some cases, dependency on medications, repeated use of interventions and surgery, secondary gain from care-seeking behavior, and rebound pain from drugs can be part of the patient's cycle of problems. If clinicians understand their integral role in the cycle of self-perpetuating illness, they can be part of the solution and help initiate change. Because of the long history of the biomedical model of care, patients often expect to have a passive role in care. To change this, new paradigms described in **Table 4** need to be conveyed to the patient as part of the evaluation. Embracing patient-centered health care paradigms that foster responsibility, education, motivation, self-efficacy, social support, strong provider-patient relationships, and long-term change encourages a passive, dependent patient to become an empowered, engaged, and educated patient.[1,2]

Muscle exercises

The most useful exercise techniques for muscle rehabilitation include muscle stretching;

Table 4
Shifting clinical paradigms associated with transformative care involves each member of the team following the same concepts by conveying the same messages implicit in their dialogue with the patient

New Paradigm	Statement that Shifts to New Paradigm
Understand the whole patient	We will help you identify all diagnoses, risk factors, and protective factors associated with your condition
Each patient is complex	Multiple conditions and interrelated contributing factors may initiate, result from, and increase or decrease risk of illness. Each needs to be addressed as part of management strategy
Self-responsibility is key to recovery	You have more influence on the problem than any treatment provided. Will you take ownership and control of the condition?
Self-care	You will need to make daily changes to improve your condition
Education and training	We will teach you how to make changes to improve your condition
Long-term change	Change only occurs over time, and it may take months for the changes to have a large impact on reducing pain and symptoms
Strong provider-patient partnerships	We as health professionals will support you as you make changes to improve your pain condition
Personal motivation	Will you be able to make the changes needed to achieve wellness?
Social support	You may need help to make the changes required for recovery
Fluctuation of progress	Expect ups and downs during the recovery process

posture; strengthening exercises; and, particularly for FBM, cardiovascular fitness. In patients with both MFP and other muscle disorders, a home program of active and passive muscle stretching exercises reduces the muscle tenderness, whereas postural exercises reduce its susceptibility to flare-ups caused by physical strain. Strengthening and cardiovascular fitness exercises improve circulation, strength, and endurance of the muscles.[6,99,113]

Evaluating the present range of motion of muscles is the first step in prescribing a set of exercises to follow. For example, in the head and neck, range of motion should be determined for the jaw and neck at the initial evaluation. A limited mandibular opening in the jaw indicates whether there are any TrPs within the elevator muscles: temporalis, masseter, and medial pterygoid. If mandibular opening is measured as the interincisal distance, the maximum range of opening is generally between 42 and 60 mm, or approximately 3 knuckle widths (nondominant hand). A mandibular opening with TrPs in the masseter is approximately between 30 mm and 40 mm or 2 knuckle widths. If contracture of masticatory muscles is present, the mandibular opening can be as limited as 10 to 20 mm. Other causes of diminished mandibular opening include structural disorders of the TMJ, such as ankylosis, internal derangements, and gross osteoarthritis.

Passive and active stretching of the muscles increases the opening to the normal range as well as decreasing the pain. Passive stretching of the masticatory muscles during counterstimulation of the TrP can be accomplished through placing a properly trimmed and sterile cork, tongue blades, or other object between the incisors while the spray-and-stretch technique is accomplished. Rapid, jerky stretching or overstretching of the muscle must be avoided to reduce potential injury to the muscle.

Postural exercises are designed to teach patients mental reminders to hold the body in a balanced, relaxed position and to use body positions that afford the best mechanical advantage. This approach includes static postural problems such as unilateral short leg, small hemipelvis, occlusal discrepancies, and scoliosis, or functional postural habits such as forward head, jaw thrust, shoulder phone bracing, and lumbar lifting. In a study of postural problems in 164 patients with head and neck MFP, Fricton and colleagues[103] found poor sitting/standing posture in 96%, forward head in 84.7%, rounded shoulders in 82.3%, lower tongue position in 67.7%, abnormal lordosis in 46.3%, scoliosis in 15.9%, and leg length discrepancy in 14.0%. In improving posture, specific skeletal conditions such as structural asymmetry or weakness of certain muscles need to be considered. In the masticatory system, patients should be instructed to place the tongue gently on the roof of the mouth and keep the teeth slightly apart. In the cervical spine, a forward or lateral head posture must be corrected by guiding the chin in and the head vertex up. The shoulders naturally fall back if the thorax is positioned up and back with proper lumbar support. Patients need to be instructed in proper posture for each position (sitting, standing, and lying down), as well as in movements that are done repetitively throughout the day, such as lifting or turning the head to the side. Sleeping posture on the side or back is particularly important for patients who wake up with soreness. Improved posture is also facilitated by regular physical conditioning. Patients need to be placed on a conditioning program to facilitate increased aerobic capacity and strength. Aerobic programs, such as exercise classes, regular running, walking, biking, or swimming, improve comfort, endurance, and functional status of patients with MFP.

Muscle treatments

There are many methods suggested for providing repetitive stimulation to tender muscles. Massage, acupressure, and ultrasonography provide noninvasive mechanical disruption to inactivate the TrPs. Moist heat applications, ice pack, Fluori-Methane, and diathermy provide skin and muscle temperature change as a form of counterstimulation. Transcutaneous electrical nerve stimulation, electroacupuncture, and direct current stimulation provide electric currents to stimulate the muscles and TrPs. Acupuncture, TrP injections of local anesthetic, corticosteroids, or saline cause direct mechanical or chemical alteration of TrPs. However, the 2 most common techniques for treating TrPs are the spray-and-stretch technique and TrP injections, and these are discussed here.

With the spray-and-stretch technique, an application of a vapocoolant spray such as Fluori-Methane over the muscle with simultaneous passive stretching can provide immediate reduction of pain, although lasting relief requires a full management program.[24,53] The technique involves directing a fine stream of Fluori-Methane spray from the finely calibrated nozzle toward the skin directly overlying the muscle with the TrP. A few sweeps of the spray are first passed over the TrP and zone of reference before adding sufficient manual stretch to the muscle to elicit pain and discomfort. The muscle is put on a progressively increasing passive stretch while the jet stream of spray is directed at an acute angle 30 to 50 cm (1–1.5 feet) away. It is applied in

1 direction from the TrP toward its reference zone in slow, even sweeps over adjacent parallel areas at a rate of about 10 cm/s. This sequence can be repeated up to 4 times if the clinician warms the muscle with a hand or warm moist packs to prevent overcooling after each sequence. Frosting the skin and excessive sweeps should be avoided because these may reduce the underlying skeletal muscle temperature, which tends to aggravate TrPs. The range of passive and active motion can be tested before and after spraying as an indication of responsiveness to therapy. Failure to reduce TrPs with spray and stretch may be caused by (1) inability to secure full muscle length because of bone or joint abnormalities, muscle contracture, or the patient avoiding voluntary relaxation; (2) incorrect spray technique; or (3) failure to reduce perpetuating factors. If spray and stretch fails with repeated trials, direct needling with TrP injections may be effective.

TrP injections have also been shown to reduce pain, increase range of motion, increase exercise tolerance, and increase circulation of muscles.[50–52] The pain relief may last from the duration of the anesthetic to many months, depending on the chronicity and severity of TrPs, and the degree of reducing perpetuating factors. Because the critical factor in relief seems to be the mechanical disruption of the TrP by the needle, precision in needling of the exact TrP and the intensity of pain during needling seem to be the major factors in TrP inactivation. TrP injections with local anesthetic are generally more effective and comfortable than dry needling or injecting other substances, such as saline, although acupuncture may be helpful for patients with chronic TrPs in multiple muscles. The effect of needling can be complemented with the use of local anesthetics in concentrations less than those required for a nerve conduction block, which can markedly lengthen the relative refractory period of peripheral nerves and limit the maximum frequency of impulse conduction. Local anesthetics can be chosen for their duration, safety, and versatility. Three percent chloroprocaine (short acting) and 5% procaine (medium acting) without vasoconstrictors are suggested.

Intraoral appliance therapy

Several systematic reviews of RCTs have found that stabilization appliances, when adjusted to be comfortable and used daily, have good evidence of efficacy in the treatment of masticatory MFP compared with nonoccluding appliances and no treatment. They are also at least equally effective in reducing MFP compared with physical therapy, behavioral therapies, and pharmacologic treatment. Other types of appliances, including soft stabilization appliances, anterior positioning appliances, and anterior bite appliances, have some RCT evidence of efficacy in reducing pain from TMJ disorders. However, the potential for adverse events with these appliances is higher and close monitoring is suggested in their use. There are no studies that suggest maxillary or mandibular appliances have more efficacy than the other; this depends on patient and clinician preference and comfort.

Hard acrylic full-coverage intraoral appliances are intended to reduce MFP and dysfunction by producing orthopedically comfortable jaw positions, reducing masticatory muscle activity and TMJ loading, and increasing patients' awareness of oral parafunctional habits. They also can prevent tooth wear and periodontal trauma. In most cases, stabilization appliances are comfortable to wear unless they are bulky, tight, or ill-fitting, so they need to be well adjusted to facilitate patient comfort, stability, and compliance. Although the percentage of adverse events was not provided in most of these studies, patients should be monitored regularly for evidence of mucosal ulceration or inflammation, tooth pain, mouth odors, speech difficulties, dental caries, tooth mobility, and occlusal changes. Soft, resilient, full-coverage appliances may be less expensive than hard stabilization appliances but need to be adjusted similarly to hard appliances to allow comfort and efficacy.[51,52]

Pharmacotherapy

Pharmacotherapy is a useful adjunct to initial treatment of MFP and other muscle disorders. The most commonly used medications for pain are classified as nonnarcotic analgesics (nonsteroidal antiinflammatories), narcotic analgesics, muscle relaxants, tranquilizers (ataractics), sedatives, and antidepressants. Analgesics are used to allay pain; muscle relaxants and tranquilizers are used for anxiety, fear, and muscle tension; sedatives for enhancing sleep; and antidepressants for pain, depression, and enhancing sleep.[85] Randomized clinical trials on nonsteroidal antiinflammatory drugs (NSAIDs) such as ibuprofen or piroxicam suggest that, for myalgia, short-term use of these medications for analgesic and/or antiinflammatory effects can be considered as a supplement to overall management.[114] Chronic, long-term use requires caution because of the long-term systemic and gastrointestinal effects. However, cyclooxygenase-2 inhibitors (Rofecoxib, Vioxx) have recently become available and these may prove to be safer NSAIDs for long-term use with less gastrointestinal toxicity. If some therapeutic result is not apparent after 7 to 10 days or if the patient develops any side effects, especially gastrointestinal symptoms, the medication should be discontinued.

For MFP, especially with limited range of motion, benzodiazepines, including diazepam and clonazepam, have been shown to be effective.[115] Experience suggests that these are best used before bedtime to minimize sedation while awake. Cyclobenzaprine (Flexeril) has been shown, in clinical trials of myalgia, to be efficacious in reducing pain and improving sleep.[112,114,115] These medications, with or without NSAIDs, can also be considered for a 2-week to 4-week trial with minimal dependency potential. However, long-term use has not been adequately tested.

For chronic pain conditions that are resistant to interventions, short-term use of opioids can be considered but this is discouraged as a long-term solution because of the adverse events, increasing pain, and abuse potential. Tramadol has been shown to be effective in FBM.[112] However, there are no RCTs evaluating the appropriateness of opioids in the long-term treatment of chronic MFP pain. At this time, chronic opioid use is mainly indicated for patients with chronic, intractable, severe pain conditions that are refractory to all other reasonable treatments. Despite the advantages of medications for pain disorders, there exists an opportunity for problems to be caused by their misuse. The problems that can occur from use of medications include chemical dependency, behavioral reinforcement of continuing pain, inhibition of endogenous pain relief mechanisms, side effects, and adverse effects from the use of polypharmaceuticals. For this reason, use of medication should proceed with caution with MFP.

Training to reduce risk factors

One of the common causes of failure in managing MFP and other muscle disorders is failure to recognize and subsequently control risk factors that may perpetuate muscle restriction and tension. As noted earlier, postural factors, whether behavioral or biological, perpetuate muscle pain if not corrected. In general, a muscle is more predisposed to developing problems if it is held in sustained contraction in the normal position and, especially, if it is in an abnormally shortened position. Such a situation exists with structural problems such as loss of posterior teeth, an excessive lordosis of the cervical spine, a unilateral short leg, or a small hemipelvis. An occlusal imbalance can be corrected with an occlusal stabilization splint, also termed a flat-plane or full-coverage splint. Other postural factors that can

be corrected include a foot lift for a unilateral leg length discrepancy, a pelvic lift for a small hemipelvis, and proper height of arm rests in chairs for short upper arms.

Behavioral risk factors causing sustained muscle tension can also occur with habits such as a receptionist cradling a phone between the head and shoulder for hours each day, a student typing on a computer for hours at a time, or day or nighttime oral parafunctional habits. Correcting poor habits through education, training, and long-term reinforcement is essential to preventing MFP from returning. Biofeedback, meditation, stress management, psychotherapy, antianxiety medications, antidepressants, and even placebos have been reported to be effective in treating MFP and other muscle disorders.[92–95] Many of these treatments are directed toward reducing muscle tension–producing habits such as bruxism or bracing of muscles. Teaching control of habits is a difficult process because of the relationship that muscle tension may have to psychosocial factors. Simply telling patients to stop the habits may be helpful with some but with others may result in noncompliance, failure, and frustration. An integrated transformative care approach involving education, increased awareness, and patient training such as cognitive behavior therapy, biofeedback, and mindfulness-based stress reduction has the best potential for success.

Interdisciplinary team management

Although each clinician may have limited success in managing whole patients alone, a team approach can address different aspects of the problem with different health professionals in order to enhance the overall potential for success.[94,116–120] Although these programs provide a broader framework for treating complex patients, they have added another dimension to the skills needed by clinicians: working as part of a coordinated team. Failure to adequately integrate care may result in poor communication, fragmented care, distrustful relationships, and eventually confusion and failure in management. However, team coordination can be facilitated by a well-defined evaluation and management system that clearly integrates team members. **Fig. 3** provides a patient flow from evaluation to assessment to treatment to follow-up.

A prerequisite to a team approach is an inclusive medical model and conceptual framework that places the physical, behavioral, and psychosocial aspects of illness on an equal and integrated basis.[12,14–17] With an inclusive theory of human systems and their relationship to illness, patients can be assessed as whole persons by different

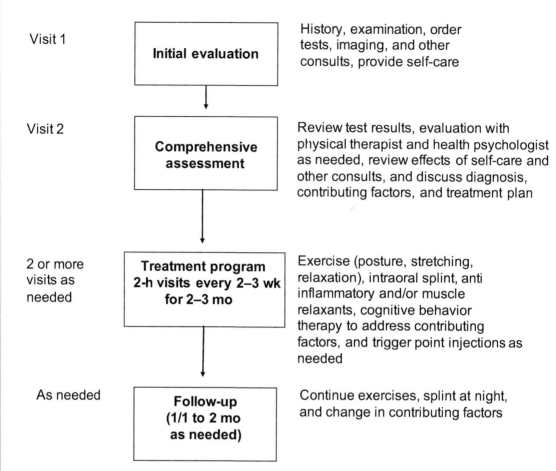

Fig. 3. Patient flow from evaluation to assessment to treatment includes many components. The key to successful management lies in matching the patient's needs with the unique combination of active treatment, education on contributing factors, and self-care appropriate for that patient.

clinicians from diverse backgrounds. Although each clinician understands a different part of the patient's problem, these can be integrated with other clinicians' perspectives to see how each part is interrelated in the whole patient. For example, a physician or dentist evaluates the physical diagnosis, a physical therapist evaluates poor postural habits, and a psychologist evaluates behavioral problems or social stressors. Each factor becomes part of the problem list to be addressed in the treatment plan. In the process, the synergism of each factor in the cause of the disorder can become apparent to clinicians. For example, social stressors can lead to anxiety, anxiety can lead to poor posture and muscle tension, and the poor posture and muscle tension can lead to MFP syndrome; the pain then contributes to more anxiety, and a cycle continues. Likewise, a reduction of each factor works synergistically to improve the whole problem. Treatment of only 1 factor may improve the problem, but relief may

be partial or temporary. Treatment of all factors simultaneously can have a cumulative effect that is greater than the effects of treating each factor individually.

As noted, the problem list for a patient with a specific chronic illness includes both a physical diagnosis and a list of risk factors and protective factors. In establishing the problem list, the clinician needs to determine whether the patient is complex and requires a team approach. Recommended criteria for determining complexity include any of the following: multiple diagnoses, persistent pain longer than 6 months in duration, significant emotional problems (depression, anxiety), frequent use of health care services or medication, daily oral parafunctional habits, and significant lifestyle disturbances. The use of a screening instrument can readily elicit the degree of complexity of a case at initial evaluation (see www.preventingchronicpain.org). The more complex the case is, the greater the need for a team approach. The decision to use a team must be made at the time of evaluation and not part way through a failing singular treatment plan. If a team is needed, the broad understanding of the patient is then used to design a long-term management program that both treats the physical diagnosis and helps reduce these contributing factors.

The primary goals of the program include reducing the pain and dysfunction while helping the patient return to normal daily activities without the need for future health care. The dentist or physician is responsible for establishing the physical diagnosis, providing short-term treatment, and monitoring patient progress. The health psychologist is responsible for providing training on reducing risk factors and enhancing protective factors; diagnosing, managing, or referring for primary psychological disturbances. A health coach can also provide support to the patient and family in making changes. The physical therapist is responsible for providing support, training, and a management program specifically designed to improve protective factors, such as an exercise and posture program. Depending on the therapist's background and the patient's needs, this person may also provide special care, such as physical therapy modalities or occupational therapy. Each clinician is also responsible for establishing a trusting, supportive relationship with the patient while reaffirming the self-care philosophy of the program, reinforcing change, and ensuring compliance. The patient is viewed as responsible for making the changes (see **Table 4**).

SUMMARY

MFP is a regional muscle pain disorder characterized by localized muscle tenderness and pain and is the most common cause of persistent regional pain. FBM is a widespread pain disorder characterized by sleep disturbance, fatigue, cognitive symptoms, and often psychological distress. The affected muscles in both disorders may also have increased fatigability, stiffness, subjective weakness, pain in movement, and slightly restricted range of motion that is unrelated to joint restriction. They are frequently overlooked as diagnoses because they are often accompanied by signs and symptoms in addition to pain, coincidental disorders, and behavioral and psychosocial problems. As these disorders persist, chronic pain characteristics often precede or follow their development.

Management of both disorders includes exercise, therapy to the TrPs, training the patient in reducing risk factors and strengthening protective

factors, and selective treatments. The difficulty in management lies in the need to integrate training with treatments to educate, engage, and empower patients to reduce the lifestyle risk factors that contribute to their persistence. This requirement dictates the critical need to match the level of complexity of the management program with the complexity of the patient; the more risk factors and training needed, the more complex the care team. Failure to address the entire problem through a team approach if needed may lead to failure to resolve the pain and the perpetuation of chronic pain.

REFERENCES

1. Institute of Medicine. Relieving pain in America: a blueprint for transforming prevention, care, education, and research. Washington, DC: National Academies Press; 2011.
2. US Department of Health and Human Services. National Institutes of Health PA-13-118. Available at: http://grants.nih.gov/grants/guide/pa-files/PA-13-118.html. Accessed June 29, 2016.
3. Stewart WF, Ricci JA, Chee E, et al. Lost productive time and cost due to common pain conditions in the US workforce. JAMA 2003;290:2443–54.
4. Kato K, Sullivan PF, Evengard B, et al. Chronic widespread pain and its co-morbidities: a population-based study. Arch Intern Med 2006;166(15):1649–54.
5. Bennett R. Myofascial pain syndromes and the fibromyalgia syndrome: a comparative analysis. In: Fricton J, Awad EA, editors. Myofascial pain and fibromyalgia. New York: Raven Press; 1990. p. 43–66.
6. Fricton J, Kroening R, Haley D, et al. Myofascial pain syndrome of the head and neck: a review of clinical characteristics of 164 patients. Oral Surg Oral Med Oral Pathol 1985;60(6):615–23.
7. Rosomoff HL, Fishbain DA, Goldberg M, et al. Physical findings in patients with chronic intractable benign pain of the neck and/or back. Pain 1989;37:279–87.
8. Skootsky S, Jaeger B, Oye RK. Prevalence of myofascial pain in general internal medicine practice. West J Med 1989;151(2):157–60.
9. Fricton J. Masticatory myofascial pain: an explanatory model integrating clinical, epidemiological, and basic science research. Bull Group Int Rech Sci Stomatol Odontol 1999;41:14–25.
10. Fricton JR, Kroening R. Practical differential diagnosis of chronic craniofacial pain. Oral Surg Oral Med Oral Pathol 1982;54(6):628–34.
11. Hestbaek L, Leboeuf-Yde C, Manniche C. Low-back pain: what is the long-term course? A review

of studies of general patient populations. Eur Spine J 2003;12(2):149–65.

12. Deyo RA, Mirza SK, Turner JA, et al. Over-treating chronic back pain: time to back off? J Am Board Fam Med 2009;22(1):62–8.

13. McGreevy K, Bottros MM, Raja SN. Preventing chronic pain following acute pain: risk factors, preventive strategies, and their efficacy. Eur J Pain Suppl 2011;11:365–72.

14. Fricton JR, Anderson K, Clavel A, et al. Preventing chronic pain: a human systems approach—results from a massive open online course. Glob Adv Health Med 2015;4(5):23–32.

15. Fricton JR. The need for preventing chronic pain. Glob Adv Health Med 2015;4(1):6–7.

16. Fricton JR, Gupta A, Weisberg MB, et al. Can we prevent chronic pain? Pract Pain Management 2015;15(10):1–9.

17. Aggarwal VR, Macfarlane GJ, Farragher TM, et al. Risk factors for onset of chronic oro-facial pain-results of the North Cheshire oro-facial pain prospective population study. Pain 2010;149(2):354–9.

18. Scher AI, Stewart WF, Ricci JA, et al. Factors associated with the onset and remission of chronic daily headache in a population-based study. Pain 2003;106(1–2):81–8.

19. Cote P, Cassidy JD, Carroll LJ, et al. The annual incidence and course of neck pain in the general population: a population-based cohort study. Pain 2004;112:267–73.

20. Bonica JJ. Management of myofascial pain syndrome in general practice. JAMA 1957;164:732–8.

21. Simons DG. Muscle pain syndromes–Part I [review]. Am J Phys Med 1975;54(6):289–311.

22. Simons DG. Myofascial trigger points: a need for understanding. Arch Phys Med Rehabil 1981;62(3):97–9.

23. Travell J. Myofascial trigger points: clinical view. In: Bonica JJ, Lindblom U, Iggo A, et al, editors. Advances in pain research and therapy. New York: Raven Press; 1976. p. 919–26.

24. Travell J, Simons DG. Myofascial pain and dysfunction: the trigger point manual. Baltimore (MD): Williams & Wilkins; 1998.

25. Darlow LA, Pesco J, Greenberg MS. The relationship of posture to myofascial pain dysfunction syndrome. J Am Dent Assoc 1987;114(1):73–5.

26. Arroyo P Jr. Electromyography in the evaluation of reflex muscle spasm. Simplified method for direct evaluation of muscle-relaxant drugs. J Fla Med Assoc 1966;53(1):29–31.

27. National Center for Health Statistics. Health, United States, 2006, special feature on pain with chartbook on trends in Americans. Hyattsville (MD). Available at: http://www.cdc.gov/nchs/data/hus/hus06.pdf. Accessed June 28, 2016.

28. Fricton J, Auvinen MD, Dykstra D, et al. Myofascial pain syndrome: electromyographic changes associated with local twitch response. Arch Phys Med Rehabil 1985;66(5):314–7.

29. Lewit K. The needle effect in the relief of myofascial pain. Pain 1979;6(1):83–90.

30. Simons DG. Electrogenic nature of palpable bands and "jump sign" associated with myofascial trigger points. In: Bonica JJ, et al, editors. Advances in pain research and therapy. New York: Raven Press; 1976. p. 913–8.

31. Dexter JR, Simons DS. Local twitch response in human muscle evoked by palpation and needle penetration of trigger point. Arch Phys Med Rehabil 1981;62:521–2.

32. Fischer AA. Tissue compliance meter for objective, quantitative documentation of soft tissue consistency and pathology. Arch Phys Med Rehabil 1987;68(2):122–5.

33. Fischer A. Documentation of myofascial trigger points [review]. Arch Phys Med Rehabil 1988;69(4):286–91.

34. Berry DC, Yemm R. A further study of facial skin temperature in patients with mandibular dysfunction. J Oral Rehabil 1974;1(3):255–64.

35. Berry DC, Yemm R. Variations in skin temperature of the face in normal subjects and in patients with mandibular dysfunction. Br J Oral Surg 1971;8(3):242–7.

36. Shah, J, Heimur, J. New frontiers in pathophysiology of myofascial pain. Pain Practitioner 2012;2(2):26–33.

37. Shah JP, Danoff JV, Desai MJ, et al. Biochemicals associated with pain and inflammation are elevated in sites near to and remote from active myofascial trigger points. Arch Phys Med Rehabil 2008;89(1):16–23.

38. Shah JP, Phillips TM, Danoff JV, et al. An in vivo microanalytical technique for measuring the local biochemical milieu of human skeletal muscle. J Appl Physiol 2005;99(5):1977–84.

39. Chen Q, Bensamoun S, Basford JR, et al. Identification and quantification of myofascial taut bands with magnetic resonance elastography. Arch Phys Med Rehabil 2007;88(12):1658–61.

40. Okeson JP, editor. Orofacial pain: guidelines for assessment, diagnosis, and management. Chicago: Quintessence; 1996.

41. Okeson JP. Bell's orofacial pains. 5th edition. Chicago: Quintessence Publishing; 1995. p. 239–49.

42. Wolfe F, Ross K, Anderson J, et al. The prevalence and characteristics of fibromyalgia in the general population. Arthritis Rheum 1995;38(1):19–28.

43. Wolfe F, Smythe HA, Yunus MB, et al. The American College of Rheumatology 1990 criteria for the classification of fibromyalgia. Report of the Multicenter

Criteria Committee. Arthritis Rheum 1990;33(2): 160–72.

44. McCain GA, Scudds RA. The concept of primary fibromyalgia (fibrositis): clinical value, relation and significance to other chronic musculoskeletal pain syndromes [review]. Pain 1988;33(3): 273–87.

45. Wolfe F, Cathey MA. The epidemiology of tender points: a prospective study of 1520 patients. J Rheumatol 1985;12(6):1164–8.

46. Yunus MB, Masi AT, Aldag JC. Sleep disorders and fibromyalgia. J Rheumatol 1989;16(19):62–71.

47. Chung SC, Kim JH, Kim HS. Reliability and validity of the pressure pain thresholds (PPT) in the TMJ capsules by electronic algometer. Cranio 1993; 11(3):171–6 [discussion: 77].

48. Fricton J, Dall' Arancio D. Myofascial pain of the head and neck: controlled outcome study of an interdisciplinary pain program. J Musculoskelet Pain 1994;2(2):81–99.

49. Simons DG. Traumatic fibromyositis or myofascial trigger points. West J Med 1978;128:69–71.

50. Cifala J. Myofascial (trigger point pain) injection: theory and treatment. Int J Osteopath Med 1979;31–6.

51. Cooper AL. Trigger point injection: its place in physical. Arch Phys Med Rehabil 1961;42: 704–9.

52. Jaeger B, Skootsky SA. Double blind, controlled study of different myofascial trigger point injection techniques. Pain 1987;4(Suppl):S292.

53. Halkovich LR, Personius WJ, Clamann HP, et al. Effect of Fluori-Methane spray on passive hip flexion. Phys Ther 1981;61(2):185–9.

54. Fricton J. Psychosocial characteristics of patients with low back pain compared to patients with head and neck pain [abstract]. Am Congress Rehab Med 1987.

55. Schiffman E, Fricton JR, Haley D, et al. A pressure algometer for MPS: reliability and validity. Pain 1987;4(Suppl):S291.

56. Wolfe F, Cathey MA, Kleinheksel SM. Fibrositis (fibromyalgia) in rheumatoid arthritis. J Rheumatol 1984;11(6):814–8.

57. Bakal DA, Kaganov JA. Muscle contraction and migraine headache: psychophysiologic comparison. Headache 1977;17(5):208–15.

58. Flor H, Turk DC, Birbaumer N. Assessment of stress-related psychophysiological reactions in chronic back pain patients. J Consult Clin Psychol 1985;53(3):354–64.

59. Gamsa A. The role of psychological factors in chronic pain. I. A half century of study [review]. Pain 1994;57(1):5–15.

60. Haynes SN, Cuevas J, Gannon LR. The psychophysiological etiology of muscle-contraction headache. Headache 1982;22(3):122–32.

61. Kerns RD, Turk DC, Rudy TE. The West Haven-Yale Multidimensional Pain Inventory (WHYMPI). Pain 1985;23(4):345–56.

62. Gold S, Lipton J, Marbach J, et al. Sites of psychophysiological complaints in MPD patients: II. Areas remote from orofacial region [abstract]. J Dent Res 1975;480:165.

63. Evaskus DS, Laskin DM. A biochemical measure of stress in patients with myofascial pain-dysfunction syndrome. J Dent Res 1972;51(5):1464–6.

64. Glyn JH. Rheumatic pains: some concepts and hypotheses. Proc R Soc Med 1971;64(4):354–60.

65. Kendall HO, Kendall F, Boynton D. Posture and pain. Huntington (NY): RE Krieger Pub; 1970. p. 15–45.

66. Simons D. Muscular pain syndromes. In: Fricton J, Awad EA, editors. Myofascial pain and fibromyalgia. New York: Raven Press; 1990. p. 1–43.

67. Lim R, Guzman F, Rodgers DW. Note on the muscle receptors concerned with pain. In: Barker D, editor. Symposium on muscle receptors. Hong Kong: Hong Kong University Press; 1962. p. 215–9.

68. Melzack R. Myofascial trigger points: relation to acupuncture and mechanisms of pain. Arch Phys Med Rehabil 1981;62(3):114–7.

69. Mense S, Schmidt RF. Muscle pain: which receptors are responsible for the transmission of noxious stimuli? pp. 265–78. In: Rose FC, editor. Physiological aspects of clinical neurology, 102. Oxford (United Kingdom): Blackwell Scientific Publications; 1977. p. 575.

70. Uhlig Y, Weber BR, Grob D, et al. Fiber composition and fiber transformation in neck muscles of patients with dysfunction of the cervical spine. J Orthop Res 1995;13:240–9.

71. Mayo KH, Ellis E III, Carlson DS. Histochemical characteristics of masseter and temporalis muscles after 5 weeks of maxillomandibular fixation- an investigation in Macaca mulatta. Oral Surg Oral Med Oral Pathol 1988;66:421–6.

72. Bengtsson A, Henriksson KG, Jorfeldt L, et al. Primary fibromyalgia. A clinical and laboratory study of 55 patients. Scand J Rheumatol 1986;15(3): 340–7.

73. Bengtsson A, Henriksson KG, Larsson J. Reduced high-energy phosphate levels in the painful muscles of patients with primary fibromyalgia. Arthritis Rheum 1986;29(7):817–21.

74. Simons DG. Myofascial trigger points: the critical experiment. J Musculoskelet Pain 1997; 5(4):113–8.

75. Hubbard DR, Berkoff GM. Myofascial trigger points show spontaneous needle EMG activity. Spine 1993;18:1803–7.

76. Gerwin RD. Neurobiology of the myofascial trigger point [review]. Baillieres Clin Rheumatol 1994;8(4): 747–62.

77. Hong C-Z. Persistence of local twitch response with loss of conduction to and from the spinal cord. Arch Phys Med Rehabil 1994;75:12–6.

78. Cheshire WP, Abashian SW, Mann JD. Botulinum toxin in the treatment of myofascial pain syndrome. Pain 1994;59:65–9.

79. El-Labban NG, Harris M, Hopper C, et al. Degenerative changes in masseter and temporalis muscles in limited mouth opening and TMJ ankylosis. J Oral Pathol Med 1990;19:423–5.

80. Yunus M, Kalyan-Raman UP, Kalyan-Raman K, et al. Pathologic changes in muscle in primary fibromyalgia syndrome. Am J Med 1986;81(3A):38–42.

81. Mao J, Stein RB, Osborn JW. Fatigue in human jaw muscles: a review. J Orofac Pain 1993;7:135–42.

82. Kniffki K, Mense S, Schmidt RF. Responses of group IV afferent units from skeletal muscle to stretch, contraction and chemical stimulation. Exp Brain Res 1978;31(4):511–22.

83. Pomeranz B, Wall PD, Weber WV. Cord cells responding to fine myelinated afferents from viscera, muscle and skin. J Physiol 1968;199(3):511–32.

84. Selzer M, Spencer WA. Convergence of visceral and cutaneous afferent pathways in the lumbar spinal cord. Brain Res 1969;14(2):331–48.

85. Dubner R. Hyperalgesia in response to injury to cutaneous and deep tissues. In: Fricton J, Dubner R, editors. Orofacial pain and temporomandibular disorders. New York: Raven Press; 1995. p. 61–71.

86. Dubner R. Pain research in animals. Ann N Y Acad Sci 1983;406:128–32.

87. Sessle BJ, Dubner R. Presynaptic hyperpolarization of fibers projecting to trigeminal brain stem and thalamic nuclei. Brain Res 1970;22(1):121–5.

88. Sessle BJ. Masticatory muscle disorders: basic science perspectives. In: Sessle BJ, Bryant PS, Dionne RA, editors. Temporomandibular disorders and related pain conditions: progress in pain research and therapy. Seattle (WA): IASP Press; 1995. p. 47–61.

89. Willis WD. The pain system. Basel (Switzerland): Karger; 1985.

90. Sessle B. Brainstem mechanisms of orofacial pain. In: Fricton J, Dubner R, editors. Orofacial pain and temporomandibular disorders. New York: Raven Press; 1995. p. 43–60.

91. Guilbaud G. Central neurophysiological processing of joint pain on the basis of studies performed in normal animals and in models of experimental arthritis. Can J Physiol Pharmacol 1991;69:637–46.

92. Dubner R. Neuronal plasticity in the spinal dorsal horn following tissue inflammation. In: Inoki R, Shigenaga Y, Tohyama M, editors. Processing and inhibition of nociceptive information. Tokyo: Excerpta Medica; 1992. p. 35–41.

93. Clarke NG, Kardachi BJ. The treatment of myofascial pain-dysfunction syndrome using the biofeedback principle. J Periodontol 1977;48(10):643–5.

94. Fricton JR, Hathaway KM, Bromaghim C. Interdisciplinary management of patients with TMJ and craniofacial pain: characteristics and outcome. J Craniomandib Disord 1987;1(2):115–22.

95. Graff-Radford SB, Reeves JL, Jaeger B. Management of chronic head and neck pain: effectiveness of altering factors perpetuating myofascial pain. Headache 1987;27(4):186–90.

96. Brooke RI, Stenn PG, Mothersill KJ. The diagnosis and conservative treatment of myofascial pain dysfunction syndrome. Oral Surg Oral Med Oral Pathol 1977;44(6):844–52.

97. Cohen SR. Follow-up evaluation of 105 patients with myofascial pain-dysfunction syndrome. J Am Dent Assoc 1978;97(5):825–8.

98. Dalen K, Ellertsen B, Espelid I, et al. EMG feedback in the treatment of myofascial pain dysfunction syndrome. Acta Odontol Scand 1986;44(5):279–84.

99. Fricton JR. Management of masticatory myofascial pain [review]. Semin Orthod 1995;1(4):229–43.

100. Kerstein RB, Farrell S. Treatment of myofascial pain-dysfunction syndrome with occlusal equilibration. J Prosthet Dent 1990;63(6):695–700.

101. Vallerand WP, Hall MB. Improvement in myofascial pain and headaches following TMJ surgery. J Craniomandib Disord 1991;5(3):197–204.

102. Weinberg LA. The etiology, diagnosis, and treatment of TMJ dysfunction-pain syndrome. Part I: etiology. J Prosthet Dent 1979;42(6):654–64.

103. Fricton J. Myofascial pain: clinical characteristics and diagnostic criteria. J Musculoskelet Pain 1993;1(3–4):37–47.

104. Forssell H, Kalso E, Koskela P, et al. Occlusal treatments in temporomandibular disorders: a qualitative systematic review of randomized controlled trials. Pain 1999;83(3):549–60.

105. Fricton JR, Look JO, Wright E, et al. Systematic review and meta-analysis of randomized controlled trials evaluating intraoral orthopedic appliances for temporomandibular disorders. J Orofac Pain 2010;24(3):237–54.

106. Kreiner M, Betancor E, Clark GT. Occlusal stabilization appliances. Evidence of their efficacy. J Am Dent Assoc 2001;132(6):770–7.

107. Türp JC, Komine F, Hugger A. Efficacy of stabilization splints for the treatment of patients with masticatory muscle pain: a qualitative systematic review. Clin Oral Investig 2004;8:179–95.

108. Al-Ani Z, Gray RJ, Davies SJ, et al. Stabilization splint therapy for the treatment of temporomandibular

myofascial pain: a systematic review. J Dent Educ 2005;69(11):1242–50.

109. Fields HL, Liebeskind JC, editors. Pharmacological approaches to the treatment of chronic pain: new concepts and critical issues. Seattle (WA): IASP Press; 1994. Squibb B-M, editor. The Bristol-Myers Squibb Symposium on Pain.

110. Singer E, Dionne R. A controlled evaluation of ibuprofen and diazepam for chronic orofacial muscle pain. J Orofac Pain 1997;11(2):139–46.

111. Fricton JR, Velly A, Ouyang W, et al. Does exercise therapy improve headache? A systematic review with meta-analysis. Curr Pain Headache Rep 2009;13(6):413–9.

112. Aronoff GM, Evans WO, Enders PL. A review of follow-up studies of multidisciplinary pain units. Pain 1983;16(1):1–11.

113. Sturdivant J, Fricton JR. Physical therapy for temporomandibular disorders and orofacial pain [review]. Curr Opin Dent 1991;1(4):485–96.

114. Fricke JR Jr, Hewitt DJ, Jordan DM, et al. A double-blind placebo-controlled comparison of tramadol/acetaminophen and tramadol in patients with postoperative dental pain. Pain 2004;109(3):250–7.

115. Dionne RA. Pharmacologic treatments for temporomandibular disorders. Oral Surg Oral Med Oral Pathol Oral Radiol Endod 1997;83(1):134–42.

116. Fricton J. Temporomandibular disorders: a human systems approach. J Calif Dent Assoc 2014;42:523–36.

117. Halstead LS. Team care in chronic illness: a critical review of literature of the past 25 years. Arch Phys Med Rehabil 1976;61:507–11.

118. Rodin J. Biopsychosocial aspects of self management. In: Karoly P, Kanfer FH, editors. Self management and behavioral change: from theory to practice. New York: Pergamon Press; 1974. p. 60–92.

119. Schneider F, Kraly P. Conceptions of pain experience: the emergence of multidimensional models and their implications for contemporary clinical practice. Clin Psychol Rev 1983;3:61–86.

120. Fricton JR, Nelson A, Monsein M. IMPATH: microcomputer assessment of behavioral and psychosocial factors in craniomandibular disorders. Cranio 1987;5(4):372–81.

Internal Derangement of the Temporomandibular Joint
New Perspectives on an Old Problem

Howard A. Israel, DDS*

KEYWORDS

- Temporomandibular joint • Internal derangement • Classification system • Cause • Synovitis
- Osteoarthritis • Arthroscopy

KEY POINTS

- Internal derangement of the temporomandibular joint is not a disease, but a nonspecific sign of tissue failure leading to biomechanical dysfunction of the joint.
- Establishing the cause of the internal derangement is essential, because successful management must be based on the underlying cause of the pathologic process.
- Major categories of disease that cause temporomandibular joint internal derangement include inflammatory/degenerative arthropathy caused by joint overload, systemic arthropathy making the joint susceptible to tissue failure, atypical localized arthropathy (disorder localized to 1 temporomandibular joint), and false arthropathy (signs and symptoms that simulate internal derangement but are caused by extra-articular disorders).
- Minimally invasive operative arthroscopy is indicated when signs and symptoms persist, and often provides essential information on the cause of disease.
- Arthroscopic temporomandibular joint surgery permits biopsy of intra-articular disorders and is successful in reducing pain, increasing range of motion, and improving mandibular function, particularly in patients with inflammatory/degenerative arthropathies.

INTRODUCTION

Internal derangement of a synovial joint is not a disease. The biomechanical joint dysfunction that is associated with internal derangement represents a failure of the intra-articular tissues caused by the loss of the structure and function. Identifying the cause of the breakdown of the tissues within a synovial joint that leads to internal derangement is an important component of successful treatment. Clinicians must ask what disease process is causing the tissue breakdown. Is there a history of acute or chronic trauma to the joint? Is there a systemic disorder that is contributing to the breakdown of connective tissues? Is there an infection or a tumor present that is causing the nonspecific symptoms of internal derangement? A clear understanding of this concept by clinicians is essential and has significant implications on patient management and the outcome of therapy.

On review of the literature on temporomandibular joint disorders over the past 35 years, the problem of internal derangement of the temporomandibular

Disclosure: Dr H.A. Israel is the owner of Therapeutic Mobilization Devices, LLC, which manufactures and markets E-Z Flex II, a passive-motion jaw exerciser.
Division of Oral & Maxillofacial Surgery, Weill-Cornell Medical College, Cornell University, 525 East 68th Street, F2132, New York, NY 10065, USA
* 12 Bond Street, Great Neck, NY 11021.
E-mail address: drhowardisrael@yahoo.com

Oral Maxillofacial Surg Clin N Am 28 (2016) 313–333
http://dx.doi.org/10.1016/j.coms.2016.03.009
1042-3699/16/$ – see front matter © 2016 Elsevier Inc. All rights reserved.

joint is often the central focus of the diagnosis and management of patients with orofacial pain caused by temporomandibular disorders (TMDs). Clear guidelines for diagnosis and management of internal derangement of the temporomandibular joint are often elusive, although there has been much excellent research on the validation of classification systems, such as the Research Diagnostic Criteria for TMDs[1] (more recently updated to the Diagnostic Criteria [DC] for TMDs)[2,3] and the Wilkes Staging System[4] for temporomandibular joint disorders. For any given diagnosis, there are multiple management options that have been recommended, including no treatment, nonsurgical therapies, minimally invasive surgical procedures (arthrocentesis, arthroscopy), arthroplasty (repair of intra-articular tissues), discectomy, and total joint replacement. The main focus of this article the concept of internal derangement and temporomandibular joint disorders from a new perspective, based on clinical research, basic science research on synovial joint pathophysiology, and the principles of diagnosis and management from the perspective of the specialties of rheumatology and orthopaedics. This information ultimately leads to new concepts in the classification of internal derangement based on cause and pathophysiology, and leads to new perspectives on the management and treatment of internal derangement of the temporomandibular joint.

CURRENT CLASSIFICATION SYSTEMS FOR TEMPOROMANDIBULAR JOINT DISORDERS

The Research Diagnostic Criteria (RDC) for TMDs,[1] published in 1992, was an excellent first step in helping to standardize diagnostic categories of TMDs. The RDC have undergone extensive testing and much research has led toward validating this classification system for TMDs to enable clinical research investigators to use the same system. This progress has improved the overall ability to develop further insights into epidemiology, diagnostic categories, causes, and ultimately treatment/management of these disorders. The original investigators recognized that many of these patients had high levels of psychosocial stress along with the physical aspects of their disease, and so this diagnostic system included AXIS I, a classification system of the physical categories of TMDs, and AXIS II, a classification system of the psychosocial behavioral aspects of patients who develop these disorders. Following years of research involving validity testing of the RDC, more recently it became apparent that updates were necessary in this system to include a larger variety of disorders of the temporomandibular joint and surrounding structures. Thus recent changes in this classification system have been made, ultimately combining the RDC (recently changed to DC for TMD) with the American Association of Orofacial Pain (AAOP) Taxonomic Classification, which encompasses a larger and more accurate description of the variety of diseases affecting the temporomandibular joint and surrounding structures.[3] Although it is beyond the scope of this article to review the details of the most current DC/TMD and AAOP taxonomic classification systems (**Fig. 1**), many of the classification categories describe nonspecific signs and symptoms, and not a disease process.

The Wilkes Staging System[4] for internal derangement is frequently used by oral and maxillofacial surgeons and helps to provide a guide for treatment based on the severity of the damage to the joint. This system includes 5 stages with stage I being a painless disc displacement with reduction and stage V being an advanced disc displacement with severe degenerative changes, adhesions, subchondral bone changes, and disc perforation (**Box 1**). Because the main focus of the Wilkes

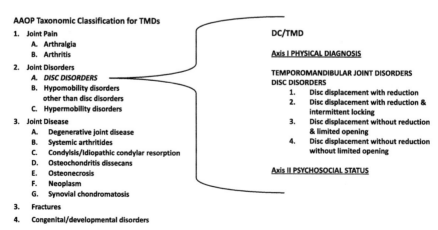

Fig. 1. AAOP taxonomic classification and DC for TMDs.

> **Box 1**
> **Wilkes staging of internal derangements**
>
> *Stage I: early*
>
> Painless clicking, anterior disc displacement with reduction
>
> *Stage II: early/intermediate*
>
> Clicking with intermittent pain and locking, anterior disc displacement with reduction
>
> *Stage III: intermediate*
>
> Pain, joint tenderness, frequent and prolonged locking, restricted motion, anterior disc displacement with or without reduction, no degenerative changes
>
> *Stage IV: intermediate/late*
>
> Chronic pain, restricted motion, no clicking, anterior disc displacement without reduction, degenerative bony changes, adhesions
>
> *Stage V: late*
>
> Variable pain, painful/reduced function, crepitus, anterior disc displacement without reduction, advanced degenerative bony changes, gross disc deformity and/or perforation, advanced adhesions
>
> *Adapted from* American Society of Temporomandibular Joint Surgeons. Guidelines for diagnosis and management of disorders involving the temporomandibular joint and related musculoskeletal structures. 2001.

system involves categorizing the extent of damage there is to joint tissues, it is useful to oral and maxillofacial surgeons in planning the operative procedure that they perceive will best treat the patient. However, in spite of the precise description of the various stages described for internal derangement, there is no corresponding information on the causal diagnosis associated with these stages.

From the standpoint of treating clinicians, there are flaws in these current classification systems that may further confuse diagnosis, cause, and ultimately treatment and management of these patients. For the most part, both of these systems are descriptive of a compilation of signs and symptoms and there is no useful categorization of cause and pathogenesis. For example, merely categorizing a patient with a disc displacement with or without reduction describes a sign of a disease process without any information as to the cause of the condition. The importance of this cannot be overstated, because many treatments over the past 35 years have focused on trying to recapture the disc. Oral repositioning appliances, mandibular manipulation, disc repositioning surgery, and disc replacement surgery have been the focus of most treatments for internal derangement. Without knowledge of the underlying cause, these treatments often fail, because causative factors persist. For example, if a patient has internal derangement associated with a systemic arthropathy, failure to treat and manage the systemic disorder is likely to result in persistent symptoms and treatment failure. Patients with excessive joint overload from

mandibular parafunction ultimately fail disc repositioning treatment because of the physiologic effects of joint overload on the intra-articular tissues. Further detailed discussion on the importance of identification and categorization of causal factors is provided later in this article.

Another intriguing factor in the development of the RDC for TMD is AXIS II, which is an essential component of the diagnosis. Clinicians must ask whether there is something unique about the temporomandibular joint that makes a psychosocial categorization model a component of the diagnosis. Do diagnostic classification systems for other synovial joints and musculoskeletal conditions include a psychosocial component as an integral part of the diagnosis?

A literature search of the orthopaedic and rheumatologic literature on diagnostic systems failed to find that AXIS II psychosocial classification is an integral part of disorders of the knee, hip, shoulder, patella-femoral pain and dysfunction, cervical spine, and lower back. The American College of Rheumatology has classification systems for osteoarthritis, systemic sclerosis, and other rheumatologic diseases[5,6] and a psychosocial component is not part of the diagnostic categorization of these conditions.

This is not to suggest that the psychosocial aspects of these diseases are not important. All chronic pain conditions have accompanying AXIS II diagnoses because chronic pain and loss of function affect quality of life. The impact of the disease and associated pain with loss of normal function must be an essential factor for clinicians to consider in the overall management of the patient. Perhaps the failures in appropriately and successfully treating many TMDs has led to patients with chronic pain, loss of function, and frustration because failed treatments have a profound effect on quality of life and result in psychological conditions such as depression and anxiety, which are common in those patients who seek treatment of TMDs. Regardless of whether preexisting psychosocial factors play an important role in causing the symptoms associated with TMDs or whether they are the result of the disease process itself, psychosocial factors must be addressed when considering the overall management of the patient. However, because psychosocial issues play an important role in most chronic disease entities, there is the need for primary treating clinicians to assess whether appropriate referral to specialists in psychology, psychiatry, and stress management is indicated.

INTERNAL DERANGEMENT OF THE TEMPOROMANDIBULAR JOINT: DEFINITION FROM AN ORTHOPAEDIC PERSPECTIVE

The most popular definition of internal derangement of the temporomandibular joint has generally alluded to joint dysfunction associated with an abnormal disc position. The Merck Manual[7] describes internal derangement of the temporomandibular joint as a condition with damage to the internal structures of the joint and "the most common form of internal temporomandibular joint derangement is anterior misalignment or displacement of the articular disc above the condyle." Molinari and colleagues[8] defined internal derangement as follows: "the term derangement refers to an alteration in the normal pathways of motion of the TMJ [temporomandibular joint] that largely involves the function of the articular disc." A definition of internal derangement of the temporomandibular joint that has been widely used by the dental profession for the past 4 decades describes a disruption of the internal aspects of the joint involving displacement of the disc from a normal functional relationship between the condyle of the mandible and the articular eminence of the temporal bone.[9] This definition has been widely accepted in the dental profession, but perhaps would not be accepted if temporomandibular joint disorders were treated by specialists in orthopaedics or rheumatology.

The specialties of orthopaedics and rheumatology have a much broader definition for internal derangement of a synovial joint. For example, these specialties describe knee internal derangement as an intra-articular disorder caused by damage to

internal structures within the joint. These conditions are usually caused by trauma and result in ongoing signs and symptoms of pain, instability, or abnormal mobility. Internal derangement is an old term that is nonspecific and requires a detailed history, physical examination, and diagnostic images to more clearly diagnose the condition. The classic textbook *Campbell's Operative Orthopaedics, 12th Edition*,[10] defines internal derangement of the knee as follows:

> The term internal derangement…loosely applied to a variety of intra-articular and extra-articular disturbances, usually of traumatic origin, that interfere with the function of the joint.

I choose to use a more orthopaedic and rheumatologic approach to the term, and thus all references to internal derangement of the temporomandibular joint in this article use the following definition.

A condition in which there are damaged intra-articular tissues leading to disturbances in the biomechanical functioning of the temporomandibular joint.

Based on this broader definition, anterior disc displacement is considered one type of internal derangement without exclusivity. Thus, a patient who has severely limited opening with decreased translation of the temporomandibular joint caused by adhesions, osteoarthritis, synovial inflammation, disc displacement, or other intra-articular disorder is also considered to have the clinical signs and symptoms of internal derangement.

IS INTERNAL DERANGEMENT A DISEASE?

Mosby's *Dictionary of Medicine, Nursing & Health Professions, Ninth Edition*, defines the term disease as follows: "a specific illness or disorder characterized by a recognizable set of signs and symptoms attributable to heredity, infection, diet or environment." A key aspect of this definition of disease is that there is an abnormal function or process involving an organ and/or system with characteristic symptoms that have a *specific cause*. Internal derangement of the temporomandibular joint represents signs and symptoms of altered biomechanical function (failure of translation, locking, intermittent locking, clicking) with damaged intra-articular tissues without alluding to a specific cause. The signs and symptoms associated with internal derangement are nonspecific and can be caused by a multitude of disease conditions. Therefore, internal derangement should not, by itself, be considered a disease, but should be considered a manifestation of a process in which there is damage to intra-articular tissues from a specific cause that must be identified by the clinician. The variety of disease categories that commonly cause internal derangement is further described later in this article.

Further complicating the understanding of internal derangement are the current diagnostic classification systems that are used in the staging of temporomandibular joint disorders. The DC/TMD classification system[2,3] uses physical diagnosis to further subclassify temporomandibular disease into muscle disorders, disc disorders, arthritic disorders, hypermobility disorders, and tension headaches. However, these disorders mostly represent signs and symptoms that are nonspecific and are not mutually exclusive.

The Wilkes classification system[4] also focuses on the progressive stages of internal derangement, ultimately leading to failure of normal joint function. These progressive changes leading to loss of the structure and function of the cartilage, synovium, and subchondral bone represent the end result of a disease process. Both of these classification systems are not based on the causal conditions that lead to failure of the joint tissues and loss of normal joint function.

Understanding the true cause of failure of the joint tissues is essential for proper treatment, prevention, and/or delay in the progression of joint disease. Stegenga[11] recognized this deficiency in the current classification of temporomandibular joint disorders and proposed a system based on the pathologic process that is causing the structural failure of the joint tissues. This proposed change in nomenclature emphasizes the importance of the diagnosis in providing the basis for treatment. Therefore, the author proposes control of risk factors that lead to pathologic intra-articular structural changes, reducing pain and improving function rather than attempting to control the position of the disc, as essential components of patient management. For clinicians to truly understand and manage the variety of disease conditions that affect the temporomandibular joint, it is important to understand that our current classification systems describe nonspecific stages of a disease process, without being specific for the true diagnosis that is responsible for the failure of the joint tissues.

The detailed review of the problem of internal derangement of the temporomandibular joint later in this article clearly shows that internal derangement is not a disease, but represents a variety of stages of biomechanical failure of the joint tissues, which can be caused by several specific disease entities.

DOES INTERNAL DERANGEMENT REQUIRE TREATMENT?
Historical Perspectives

A review of the history of treatment of internal derangement of the temporomandibular joint reveals changing perspectives on management. In the 1970s and 1980s, internal derangement was viewed as a mechanical problem, resulting in mechanical attempts at repositioning or replacing the disc. In 1979, McCarty and Farrar[9] published an article in the *Journal of Prosthodontics* that emphasized the importance of disc displacement as a major disorder of the temporomandibular joint. It was thought that the failure to have the disc in the proper position between the condyle and the articular eminence inevitably leads to severe degenerative joint disease. Thus, repositioning the disc became a central focus for many clinicians in the dental profession. Oral appliances designed to reposition the disc, as well as mandibular manipulations, were considered mainstays of conservative therapy. Patients who had persistent symptoms and internal derangement were often referred to oral and maxillofacial surgeons and there were a variety of surgeries designed to solve the problem of internal derangement of the temporomandibular joint. Discoplasty, involving disc repositioning surgery, was a common surgical procedure. Discectomy was often performed if there was a perforation in the disc. A variety of tissues were used for disc replacement, including ear cartilage, temporalis muscle, temporalis fascia, Silastic, and Proplast-Teflon. However, the use of Proplast-Teflon led to foreign body reaction and destruction of articular tissues.[12–14]

In the 1990s, the realization that arthroplasty with disc repositioning or disc replacement often resulted in degenerative changes and fibrosis and did not reliably maintain a repositioned disc[15] resulted in a significant change in the surgical management of patients with severe symptoms and internal derangement. Arthroscopic temporomandibular joint surgery was shown to be a safe and effective alternative to arthroplasty, which reliably reduced pain and improved maximum interincisal opening distance.[16–27] Excellent results were achieved with arthroscopic surgery without changing disc position. MRI studies[28–31] have shown a high percentage of disc displacement in asymptomatic patients (32%–38%) and this has raised further questions about the importance of internal derangement in patients with symptomatic temporomandibular joint disease.

Arthrocentesis[32-35] was introduced as another minimally invasive treatment of internal derangement and has been shown to be safe and effective. A major advance in the understanding of the pathogenesis of temporomandibular joint disease occurred as a result of arthroscopy and arthrocentesis and resulted in research on biochemical mediators in the synovial fluid. Mediators of inflammation, cartilage degradation, and adhesion formation have been identified, which represent the biochemical basis for destruction of joint tissues leading to internal derangement.[36-49] Synovial fluid research has continued since the 1990s and has offered promising strategies for the identification of biochemical markers of disease and the potential for new therapies designed to alter or block pathogenic mechanisms.

Internal Derangement Treatment: Clinical Research Results

Clinical research on the natural course of internal derangement without treatment[50-52] has shown the following:

- Most patients improve without any treatment
- The length of time for symptoms to resolve is variable, but generally a minimum of 1 year
- A percentage (25%–33%) of patients do not improve
- Older patients and those with MRI evidence of more advanced disease (osteoarthritis and advanced internal derangement) are at higher risk for not improving spontaneously

There have been a variety of good evidence-based literature reviews and studies[53-58] that compared the results of nonsurgical treatments of internal derangement. Nonsurgical therapies that have been studied include patient education, nonsteroidal antiinflammatory drugs (NSAIDs), muscle relaxants, hot/cold packs, mouth opening exercises, softer diet, and occlusal appliances.

Because *appliance therapy* is often the initial treatment intervention for patients who develop temporomandibular joint symptoms, knowledge of the evidence-based literature on occlusal appliances is necessary for clinicians. Lundh and colleagues[55] compared treatment outcomes on patients with anterior disc displacement without reduction who were placed into one of 2 groups. The first group was treated with an occlusal splint and the second group had no treatment. The results of treatment after 12 months were as follows:

- Pain disappeared in approximately 33% of patients in both groups

- Increased joint pain was experienced by 40% of the occlusal splint group, and 16% of the no-treatment group after 12 months

The investigators concluded that there was no significant benefit in occlusal splint therapy compared with no treatment.

Truelove and colleagues[56] evaluated treatment outcomes in 200 patients with anterior disc displacement with reduction, arthralgia, and myalgia. The patients were randomly assigned to one of 3 treatment groups:

- Usual treatment, which included self-care, education, NSAIDs, hot/cold packs, and passive stretching
- Hard flat plane splint and usual treatment (as described earlier)
- Soft splint and usual treatment

Treatment outcomes were evaluated at 3 months and 12 months, which revealed no significant difference in all 3 groups. The investigators concluded that self-care, low-cost therapy is as effective as occlusal splint therapy.

Clark and Minakuchi[57] provided an excellent review of the evidence-based literature on appliance therapy and their conclusions on occlusal stabilization appliances were:

- Occlusal stabilization appliances decrease symptoms of myalgia and arthralgia
- They protect the dentition from wear caused by parafunctional habits
- They are low risk as long as they are not worn 24 hours a day
- They do not change disc position

Clark and Minakuchi[57] also concluded that appliances that are designed to reposition the mandible do not change disc position.

Based on current research, clinicians should follow a common-sense approach concerning appliance therapy. Appliances should be designed to provide a buffer between the maxilla and the mandible, in theory to offset the forces of mandibular parafunction and to reduce the load on the temporomandibular joints. Therefore, occlusal stabilization appliances that equally distribute these forces throughout the arch should be considered as an appropriate initial treatment of myalgia and arthralgia. However, clinicians must continuously evaluate the patient's response to treatment. Some patients with a significant parafunctional habit develop increased parafunction with an appliance. Patients often tell clinicians that they find themselves clenching on the appliance and that their jaw muscles are more sore in the morning, following the nighttime use of an occlusal stabilization appliance. For patients with daytime clenching, an appliance can be used for 1 minute, to assist in self-awareness with the goal of breaking the habit. Continuous and/or excessive use of an appliance can contribute to the development of a malocclusion and must be avoided, particularly for appliances that provide partial coverage of the dentition, and thus these appliances are to be avoided. In addition, appliances that reposition the mandible in an attempt to recapture the disc in patients with arthralgia and/or internal derangement should be avoided, because the scientific literature does not support this. Most importantly, patients treated with appliance therapy must continuously be evaluated to determine whether the appliance is effective in reducing myalgia and arthralgia. If appliance therapy is not effective in reducing symptoms, the clinician must reevaluate the diagnosis and alter the therapeutic regimen.

Further complicating the understanding of response to treatment is the placebo effect of all therapeutic interventions. Greene and colleagues[59] studied placebo responses to orofacial pain and reported that "present knowledge suggests that every treatment for pain contains a placebo component, which sometimes is as powerful as the so-called active counterpart." A summary of the results of evidence-based studies on nonsurgical therapy for internal derangement is listed here[53–59]:

- Most patients have improvement in signs and symptoms with time
- No significant differences between treatment and nontreatment groups
- Palliative care (NSAIDs, education, diet modification, exercises) seem to be as effective as more costly appliance therapy
- Occlusal appliances do not change disc position
- Occlusal stabilization appliances may reduce myalgia and arthralgia
- Although patients with internal derangement improve with time, the length of time for symptoms to improve is not clearly identified
- All treatments have a powerful placebo effect

Patients with internal derangement with severe symptoms of pain and dysfunction who have failed nonsurgical therapy are often candidates for surgical treatment. Laskin[60] provided an excellent review of evidence-based research on the surgical management of internal derangement. Clinical research on the results of surgical treatment of internal derangement is summarized here:

- There are no prospective, randomized controlled, double-blinded trials; only case series, and comparison of preoperative and postoperative signs and symptoms
- Arthroscopy, arthrocentesis, discoplasty, and discectomy have all been reported to have reasonably good success with reduction in signs and symptoms in the range of 80% to 90%
- Surgical success is highest with the first surgery, and each surgical procedure reduces the success rate
- Surgical failure is often caused by lack of control of causal factors such as joint overload
- When surgery is indicated, the least invasive approach is recommended

Because of the lack of randomized controlled studies on surgical management of internal derangement, Reston and Turkelson[25] performed a meta-analysis of the results of surgical treatment of disc displacement without reduction. This biostatistical approach studied many reported surgical trials to help compensate for the lack of parallel control groups. The investigators concluded that only arthroscopic surgery and arthrocentesis showed effectiveness significantly greater than all assumed control group improvement rates. Al-Moraissi[27] performed a systematic review and meta-analysis comparing arthroscopy and arthrocentesis for management of internal derangement. The results suggested that arthroscopy yielded superior efficacy to arthrocentesis in increasing joint movement and decreasing pain.

Does Any Surgical Procedure Reposition and Maintain a Normal Disc Position?

The literature on surgical outcomes assess pain relief, improved function, and increased interincisal opening distance, but do not show the maintenance of normal disc position.[60–64] Zhang and colleagues[65] assessed the postoperative disc position following discoplasty and disc stabilization with bone anchors. The investigators reported 96% successful disc repositioning based on MRI scans taken 7 days postoperatively. However, conclusions based on a early postoperative MRI do not provide information about patients who function and load their temporomandibular joints. Therefore, based on a review of the literature, there does not seem to be any evidence that surgically repositioning a disc maintains the disc in a normal position; there does not seem to be any evidence that any procedure, treatment, or appliance repositions and maintains the disc in a normal position.

Thus the major goals of treatment of internal derangement should not be to reposition the disc, but should be to:

- Establish the diagnosis and the cause of the internal derangement
- Reduce inflammation
- Reduce pain
- Reduce joint overload
- Improve range of motion
- Restore mandibular function
- Identify and control causal factors

MANAGEMENT OF TEMPOROMANDIBULAR JOINT DISORDER BASED ON DISEASE CAUSE: NEW PERSPECTIVES ON INTERNAL DERANGEMENT AS A SIGN OF DISORDER

The DC for TMDs and the Wilkes staging of internal derangement are helpful for clinicians in assessing the extent to which a pathologic process has caused damage to the intra-articular tissues, resulting in biomechanical failure and/or compromise in joint function. However, these classification systems do not provide information on factors that cause damage and dysfunction of joint tissues leading to internal derangement. Thus, merely repositioning a disc ultimately leads to joint failure if the causal factors are not recognized and managed. The classification of intra-articular temporomandibular joint disease based on causal factors is discussed here, and is intended to provide clinicians with a different perspective in the management of temporomandibular joint internal derangements. Internal derangement should be viewed by clinicians as a sign of a disease process leading to biomechanical compromise or failure of the temporomandibular joint. The challenge for clinicians is to diagnose the condition that is causing the internal derangement. Once identified, the basis for treatment is to reduce the patient's symptoms while simultaneously identifying and managing the disease process. The following major categories of disease can cause internal derangement of the temporomandibular joint (**Fig. 2**):

1. Inflammatory/degenerative arthropathy: joint overload (acute and/or chronic) leading to inflammation and degeneration of intra-articular tissues
2. Systemic arthropathy: systemic disorder causing temporomandibular joint disease
3. Localized atypical arthropathy: intra-articular temporomandibular joint disorder that is atypical and not caused by joint overload
4. False arthropathy: extra-articular disorder simulating and/or causing temporomandibular joint symptoms

Inflammatory/Degenerative Arthropathy: Pathogenesis

Chronic joint overload is the most common cause of internal derangement of the temporomandibular joint. There is a significant body of research on temporomandibular joint synovial fluids and arthroscopic tissue morphology, which has shown that synovitis, osteoarthritis, and adhesions are the major tissue changes that occur in symptomatic patients requiring arthroscopic surgery.[36–49] Chronic joint overload, often caused by mandibular parafunction, results in a change in articular cartilage metabolism, with degradation of the cartilaginous matrix exceeding production. This overload of the cartilage upsets the balance between the buildup and degradation of the cartilage matrix, ultimately resulting in a breakdown of

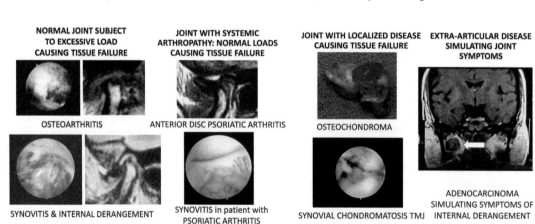

Fig. 2. Major categories of temporomandibular joint (TMJ) disease based on cause.

the cartilaginous surfaces. In the earliest stages of this pathologic process, fibrillation of articular cartilage is seen arthroscopically (**Fig. 3**). This fibrillation ultimately results in biomechanical failure impairing the sliding of articular surfaces. The clinical correlation with this early failure of articular cartilage is joint noise (clicking and/or crepitus). Tissue changes that occur in the cartilage impair the sliding ability of the joint, often resulting in a change in disc position (see **Fig. 3**). These early degenerative changes do not necessarily cause pain. If there is no associated inflammation, the patient may function with a clicking joint and no major functional disability. This possibility may explain why a significant percentage of the population (32%–38%) who are without complaints and totally functional have disc displacement, which can be seen on MRI.[28–31]

Individuals who have severe and persistent mandibular parafunction continue to load the intra-articular tissues beyond their adaptive capacity, leading to further changes in the structure and function of these tissues. Continued cartilage degradation results in significant osteoarthritis and can ultimately lead to a disc perforation (**Fig. 4**). The alteration in joint biomechanics often leads to loading of the synovial tissues, which is not what the synovium normally experiences. The synovium is a connective tissue that is very vascular and is well innervated, unlike articular cartilage. The major function of synovium is the production of synovial fluid, which is necessary for joint lubrication and also for nutrition of chondrocytes in the articular cartilage, which does not have a blood supply. Thus, loading of the synovial tissues results in a significant escalation in symptoms because:

1. The synovial membrane becomes inflamed, erythematous, and edematous, which results in the clinical appearance of synovitis (**Fig. 5**)

2. The abnormal loading of the synovial tissues causes pain, because this tissue has a nerve supply and does not normally undergo loading
3. Inflamed synovium impairs production of synovial fluid, impairing lubrication of the joint, further altering the biomechanics of the joint and reducing the ability of the temporomandibular joint to slide
4. Once synovitis develops in the temporomandibular joint, it is difficult to resolve, because this joint is constantly being used, resulting in further loading and further synovial inflammation

With the onset of an acute synovitis, patients have a noticeable increase in temporomandibular joint symptoms:

1. Acute pain localized to the temporomandibular joint
2. Reduced translation of the affected joint with limited maximum interincisal opening distance, deviation of the mandible to the affected side with opening, and reduced lateral excursion to the contralateral side
3. If there is significant intra-articular swelling associated with the synovitis, there may be an alteration in the occlusion with an ipsilateral posterior open bite and deviation of the mandibular midline to the contralateral side at rest
4. Myospasm of the surrounding muscles of mastication (masseter and temporalis become significantly tender to palpation) as the body attempts to splint the injured joint
5. MRI shows a synovial effusion best seen on the T2 images and anterior disc position (**Fig. 6**)

Patients who develop acute synovitis of the temporomandibular joint that does not resolve with nonsurgical therapies such as joint unloading (oral appliances, diet modification), anti-inflammatory medications, and muscle

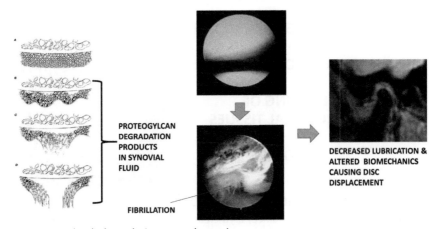

PROTEOGYLCAN DEGRADATION PRODUCTS IN SYNOVIAL FLUID

DECREASED LUBRICATION & ALTERED BIOMECHANICS CAUSING DISC DISPLACEMENT

FIBRILLATION

Fig. 3. Chronic joint overload: degradation exceeds repair.

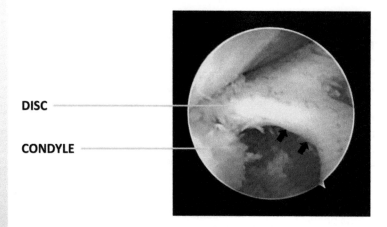

DISC

CONDYLE

Fig. 4. Arthroscopic view of left TMJ in patient with severe masticatory parafunction. Osteoarthritis with disc perforation and exposed condyle. *Black arrow* indicates disc perforation.

relaxant medications often transition to a chronic synovitis of the temporomandibular joint. The continued loading of inflamed synovial tissues combined with reduced mobilization often results in adhesions, which also affects the ability of the mandible to translate. Patients with chronic synovitis of the temporomandibular joint often present with a history of acute locking and pain, followed by a period of gradual reduction in pain and a slight increase in the maximum interincisal opening distance over several months. However, these chronic changes occur at the expense of greatly reduced masticatory function. Patients complain that they cannot open their mouths widely and they can only eat soft foods. If these patients do not pursue surgical treatment designed to reduce inflammation, remove adhesions, and increase mandibular mobility, they may eventually develop less pain, with reduced synovial inflammation, with persistent reduction in mandibular range of motion because of adhesions (**Fig. 7**).

The simultaneous occurrence of synovitis and reduced mobility leads to the development of adhesions in the synovial joint.[66] If the pathologic process continues with persistence of synovitis, cartilage degradation, reduced mobility, and adhesion formation, ultimately this may lead to a fibrous and/or bony ankylosis.

There are some patients with synovitis and internal derangement of the temporomandibular joint who do not progress to further joint disease and eventually return to normal masticatory function. However, clinicians do not have the capacity to predict which patients are likely to have a return to asymptomatic function and it is not clear why some patients have this healing capacity. Clinicians can speculate on those factors that may lead to a resolution of symptoms. Theoretically, if the clinician is successful in reducing joint overload, maximizing joint mobility, and reducing inflammation, this may create an intra-articular environment that is more likely to heal, given

JOINT OVERLOAD
⬇
ARTICULAR CARTILAGE DEGRADATION
⬇
IMPAIRED BIOMECHANICS
⬇
LOADING OF RETRODISCAL TISSUES
⬇
SYNOVITIS
⬇
IMPAIRED LUBRICATION & LIMITED MOBILITY

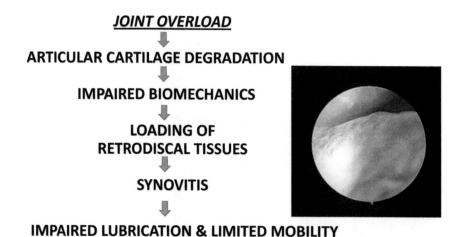

Fig. 5. The synovial membrane becomes inflamed, erythematous, and edematous, which results in the clinical appearance of synovitis.

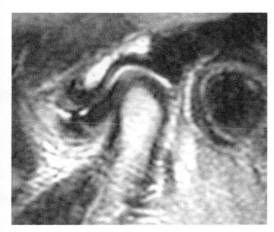

Fig. 6. MRI T2 images showing anterior disc position and a synovial effusion of the superior joint space. This important finding is consistent with synovitis.

enough time. Clinical arthroscopic observations have shown that some joints with anterior disc displacement have remodeled retrodiscal tissue that has the white appearance of cartilage but clearly is not disc, because of the presence of blood vessels that can be seen in the tissue (**Fig. 8**). Recent research showed that increased mechanical loading on the disc increased protein levels and proteoglycan messenger RNA expression in temporomandibular joint discs in a rat model.[67] It is likely that functional loading of the retrodiscal synovial tissues has the capacity to result in stimulation of the production of proteoglycans, leading to the formation of tissue that has the appearance and function of cartilage.

In patients with internal derangement caused by overload associated with a chronic inflammatory/degenerative arthropathy, it is also important to realize that the maintenance of the structure and function of synovial and cartilaginous tissues is

interdependent. Inflamed synovial tissues and adhesions lead to reduced joint motion, decreased pumping action of the synovial fluid, and a decrease in the nutrition of chondrocytes. Failure to maintain the viability and function of chondrocytes results in the loss of the matrix of the cartilage (collagen and proteoglycans), resulting in further cartilage degradation. This degradation leads to further progression of degenerative joint disease (osteoarthritis) within the joint. Joints with persistent degradation of articular cartilage have increased levels of degradation products (glycosaminoglycans) in the synovial fluid,[39,40,46] which can overwhelm the phagocytic function of the synovial membrane and lead to further synovial dysfunction and synovitis. It has been shown that osteoarthritis and synovitis occur simultaneously in symptomatic temporomandibular joints that have undergone arthroscopic surgery.[43] Thus the inflammatory and degenerative processes that occur in temporomandibular joints that are chronically overloaded occur simultaneously, resulting in the alteration of the intra-articular tissues, leading to biomechanical failure and internal derangement (**Fig. 9**).

Treatment of Inflammatory/Degenerative Arthropathy

A key principle in the management of internal derangement caused by an inflammatory/degenerative arthropathy is for clinicians to realize that the internal derangement is the end result of damaged intra-articular tissues usually caused by chronic overload. Therefore, identification and management of factors that contribute to the failure of the synovium and articular cartilage are essential for a favorable outcome. Once the diagnosis of inflammatory/degenerative arthropathy

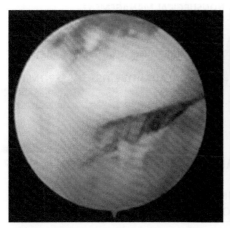
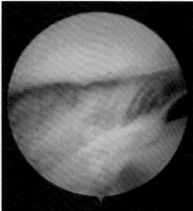

Fig. 7. Synovitis and adhesions in the posterior recess of the superior joint space in a right temporomandibular joint.

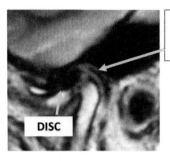 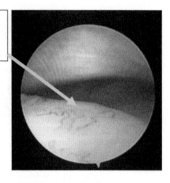

REMODELING OF RETRODISCAL TISSUE CAN BE SEEN ON MRI AND ARTHROSCOPICALLY IN PATIENTS WITH INTERNAL DERANGEMENTS

Fig. 8. Retrodiscal and other joint tissues have the capacity to adapt to functional loads.

with concurrent joint overload is established, essential principles of management include:

1. Reduction of joint loading
2. Maximizing joint mobility
3. Reduction of inflammation
4. Control of pain

Clinicians who treat these patients are well versed in nonsurgical therapies to accomplish these goals, including:

1. Diet modification
2. Awareness and control of mandibular parafunction
3. Passive-motion exercises
4. Physical therapy
5. Masticatory muscle massage and heat
6. Occlusal stabilization oral appliances (appliances that provide equal distribution of forces throughout the arch and do not attempt to reposition the mandible)
7. Antiinflammatory medications
8. Muscle relaxant medications
9. Pain management modalities
10. Improving sleep

Patient education is an essential part of management and it is important that these patients become partners in their care, focused on control of causal factors that are contributing to the disease process.

Patients often present to the oral and maxillofacial surgeon with symptoms associated with internal derangement. Clinicians must first approach these patients with an open mind with the realization that internal derangement is a nonspecific sign of intra-articular disorder that can have a variety of diagnoses. Thus, establishment of the diagnosis and the cause of the joint disorder is

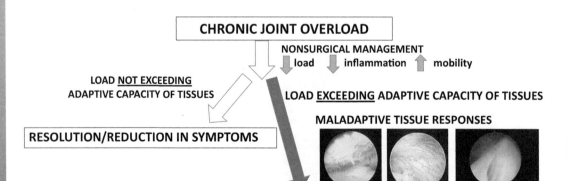

Fig. 9. The response (or lack thereof) to nonsurgical management determines whether the joint has adaptive capacity and dictates future treatment.

essential. If the patient has signs and symptoms caused by joint overload (chronic or acute) and if all other causal diagnoses are ruled out, an inflammatory/degenerative arthropathy is likely. These patients are placed on an intense 2-week to 3-week regimen of nonsurgical therapy as described earlier. If the symptoms begin to resolve, then nonsurgical management is continued (see **Fig. 9**). However, if the symptoms persist, minimally invasive surgical intervention is often required.

The least invasive procedure that will resolve the symptoms is the treatment of choice; therefore, arthroscopic surgery (or arthrocentesis) is performed.[25,27] A major advantage of arthroscopic surgery compared with arthrocentesis is the ability to directly see the disorder and to obtain specimens for histopathologic examination to further confirm the diagnosis. Furthermore, arthroscopic surgery involves the removal of pathologic tissue, lysis of adhesions, direct injection of medications into the synovium, and debridement of degenerative articular cartilage. Arthrocentesis requires less surgical skill and is performed at a lower cost but does not permit direct visualization and removal of pathologic tissue. Patients with symptoms of limited opening for greater than 3 months often have intra-articular adhesions, and arthrocentesis is not as effective as arthroscopy, which permits removal of these adhesions.

A major challenge to the specialty of oral and maxillofacial surgery is to properly train interested clinicians in the required skills necessary to perform arthroscopic surgery. Failure to train this specialty will ultimately prevent these patients from having access to minimally invasive temporomandibular joint surgery. Furthermore, clinicians in other fields, without advanced training in oral and maxillofacial surgery, will attempt to develop the skills for arthroscopic surgery, to the detriment of oral and maxillofacial surgery and of patients. The skills required for arthroscopic surgery are unique and thus it is necessary for experienced surgeons to train the next generation of oral and maxillofacial surgeons. Although many advanced education programs in oral and maxillofacial surgery do not provide training in arthroscopy, this should not be a justification for performing more invasive surgery when arthroscopy is indicated. Excellent hands-on training courses do exist for those oral and maxillofacial surgeons who want to provide arthroscopic temporomandibular joint surgery as an effective minimally invasive option for their patients.[68–70]

Regardless of which minimally invasive modality is performed, a postoperative rehabilitation regimen with control of causal factors is essential. This regimen is the same as the nonsurgical regimen that was prescribed before the decision to perform minimally invasive surgery. Aside from the reduction of joint loading, it is essential for patients to perform passive-motion exercises several times daily for a minimum of 2 months postoperatively. Mobilization of the mandible with gentle stretching prevents the formation of adhesions, which are removed during arthroscopic surgery, and helps to stimulate the synovial fluid to provide nutrition to articular cartilage chondrocytes. Passive mobilization exercises should be started within 24 hours of surgery and are repeated 3 to 4 times daily, with each session lasting 15 minutes. Physical therapy can be added to the postoperative regimen, but this must not be a replacement for the daily passive-motion exercises that the patient performs at home.

The treatment of an inflammatory/degenerative temporomandibular joint arthropathy varies based on the stage of the internal derangement and the disease process. The early stages of internal derangement (Wilkes I and II) can often be managed with nonsurgical therapy. More advanced stages of internal derangement with persistence of significant symptoms, in spite of appropriate nonsurgical therapy, are treated with minimally invasive surgery (arthroscopy or arthrocentesis) if diagnostic imaging confirms the presence of a joint space. Advanced stages of internal derangement leading to fibrosis and/or ankylosis with loss of joint space require arthrotomy. **Fig. 10** shows the treatment algorithm used for the various stages of internal derangement caused by inflammatory/degenerative arthropathies.

Systemic Arthropathy: Systemic Disorders Causing Temporomandibular Joint Disease

Systemic diseases can often contribute to temporomandibular joint disorders. In the case of an inflammatory/degenerative temporomandibular joint arthropathy, excessive joint loads exceed the adaptive capacity of the intra-articular tissues, resulting in cartilage degradation and synovial inflammation, which then cause internal derangement. Patients with a systemic arthropathy are those with joint tissues that will fail with normal joint loads, because the systemic disorder affects the structure and function of the intra-articular connective tissues. Therefore, internal derangement of the temporomandibular joint can be caused by a systemic disorder and it is essential for oral and maxillofacial surgeons to be aware of this when considering patient management. Examples of systemic disorders that can cause internal derangement include rheumatoid arthritis, psoriatic arthritis, juvenile idiopathic

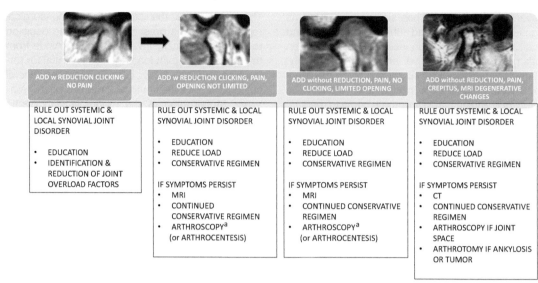

Fig. 10. Management of internal derangement caused by inflammatory/degenerative joint disease. [a] Arthroscopy is the minimally invasive treatment of choice.

arthritis, Lyme disease, polymyalgia rheumatica, chondrocalcinosis, Ehlers-Danlos syndrome, lupus, and other connective tissue disorders.

Arthroscopic surgery is often performed for obtaining pathologic tissue for diagnostic purposes, and is also helpful in managing symptoms. However, management of the systemic disorder is essential for prolonged control of the patient's symptoms and this frequently requires coordination of treatment with a rheumatologist (**Figs. 11–13**).

Localized Atypical Arthropathy: Intra-Articular Temporomandibular Joint Disorder that Is Atypical and Not Caused by Joint Overload or Systemic Disease

Because the temporomandibular joint is a synovial joint, it is subject to the same local disorders as other synovial joints. A localized atypical arthropathy is uncommon for the temporomandibular joint; however, these conditions do occur in clinical practice. These patients have intra-articular temporomandibular joint disorder that is localized to 1 joint, and is not caused by systemic disease or joint overload. The clinical presentation of this group of disorders is nonspecific, but ultimately the signs and symptoms (which occur with any internal derangement) include any combination of the following:

1. Joint pain
2. Joint noise: clicking and/or crepitus
3. Altered mandibular range of motion
4. Gross changes in the occlusion

SYSTEMIC ARTHROPATHY INVOLVING THE TEMPOROMANDIBULAR JOINT

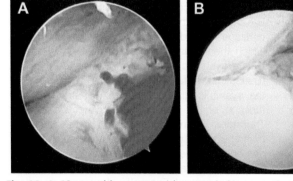
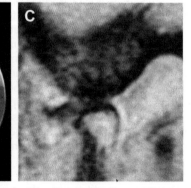

Fig. 11. A 46-year-old woman with systemic lupus erythematosus and synovitis, disc perforation, and severe degenerative changes involving the left temporomandibular joint. (*A*) Synovitis posterior recess. (*B*) Osteoarthritis and disc perforation. (*C*) MRI shows degenerative changes and anterior disc position.

SYSTEMIC ARTHROPATHY INVOLVING THE TEMPOROMANDIBULAR JOINT

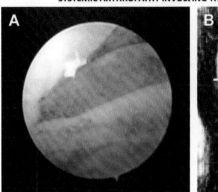 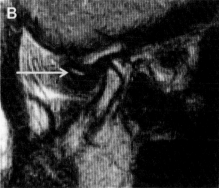

Fig. 12. A 41-year-old with psoriatic arthritis and severe synovitis left temporomandibular joint. (*A*) Severe inflammation of the synovial membrane. (*B*) MRI showing anterior disc position and small synovial effusion anterior recess (*arrow*).

Clinical findings that are suggestive of a localized atypical arthropathy include a gradual change in the occlusion, with the development of an ipsilateral posterior open bite, and shifting of the mandibular midline to the contralateral side. An osteochondroma of the condyle is the most common neoplasm affecting the temporomandibular joint and is in the category of an atypical (neoplastic) localized arthropathy (**Fig. 14**). Diagnostic images that show unusual findings, such as multiple loose dense bodies, calcifications, or very large synovial effusions are suggestive of atypical localized arthropathies such as synovial chondromatosis, crystal deposition joint disease, and a synovial cyst (**Fig. 15**). Some patients present with routine signs and symptoms

and the diagnosis is confirmed with arthroscopic examination and biopsy of pathologic tissue (**Fig. 16**). The algorithm for the diagnosis and management of patients with atypical localized arthropathies can be seen in **Fig. 17**. The importance of establishing the correct diagnosis cannot be overemphasized.

False Arthropathy

Some patients present with the signs and symptoms of temporomandibular joint internal derangement but the cause is not an intra-articular disorder. The most common example of this is the patients who develop trismus following an inferior alveolar nerve local anesthetic block. The

SYSTEMIC ARTHROPATHY INVOLVING THE TEMPOROMANDIBULAR JOINT

A   B

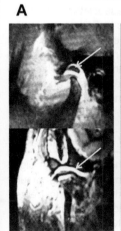 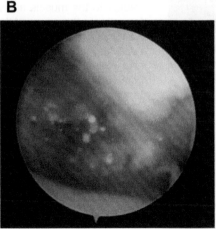 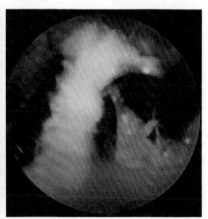

Fig. 13. A 61-year-old man with painful swelling of the right temporomandibular joint. Arthroscopic biopsy led to the diagnosis of chondrocalcinosis (pseudogout). The patient was referred to a rheumatologist for further work-up and management. (*A*) MRI images showing dense body (*Yellow arrow*) (*above*) and effusion (*Yellow arrow*) (*below*) in joint space. (*B*). Arthroscopic surgery identified the calcifications in the synovial membrane and biopsy of the tissue established the diagnosis of chondrocalcinosis.

LOCALIZED (NEOPLASTIC) ATYPICAL ARTHROPATHY INVOLVING THE TEMPOROMANDIBULAR JOINT

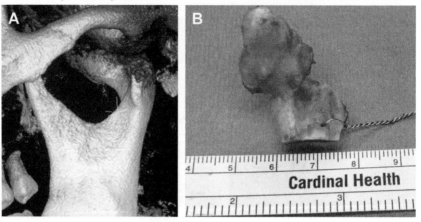

Fig. 14. A 45-year-old man with osteochondroma of the left mandibular condyle. (*A*). Cone beam scan three-dimensional reconstruction showing osteochondroma of the left condyle. (*B*) Surgical specimen following condylectomy.

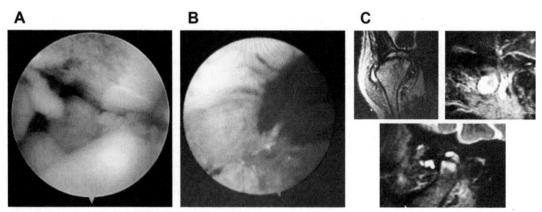

Fig. 15. Examples of atypical localized arthropathies affecting the temporomandibular joint. (*A*) Synovial chondromatosis. (*B*) Crystal deposition disease. (*C*) Synovial cyst.

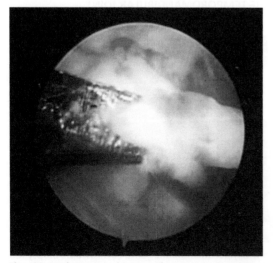

Fig. 16. Arthroscopic biopsy of synovial disorder is extremely valuable in establishing the correct diagnosis. Histopathology in this case was consistent with synovial chondromatosis.

trauma to the muscle and associated hematoma formation is the cause of the limitation of mandibular opening. Infection of the deep spaces of the head and neck, as well as radiation fibrosis, are also examples of a false arthropathy which are common and easy to diagnose based on the history and clinical presentation.

False Arthropathy Caused by Neoplasia

There are some patients who present with signs and symptoms of pain and limitation of mandibular range of motion, with a history of being treated as a routine temporomandibular joint internal derangement, who ultimately are diagnosed with a neoplastic process. It is essential for oral and maxillofacial surgeons to establish the diagnosis of false arthropathy caused by a neoplastic process as early as possible. Clinician should be suspicious of a neoplastic process in patients who

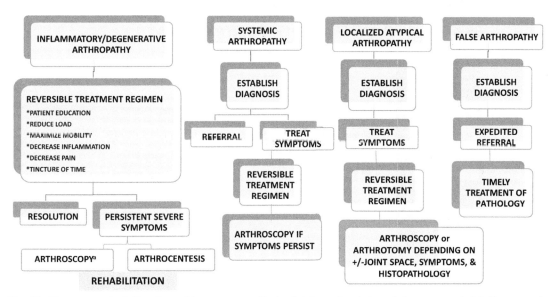

Fig. 17. Management of disorders of temporomandibular joint causing internal derangement. [a] Arthroscopy is minimally invasive treatment of choice.

present with temporomandibular joint symptoms with the following:

1. Recent rapid weight loss
2. Cranial nerve deficit
3. Prolonged nonsurgical therapy without a typical response to treatment in patients who have not had diagnostic imaging
4. Orofacial pain that is atypical and not well localized to the temporomandibular joint

Although each case presents differently, the essential component in making the diagnosis is for clinicians to be diligent in continually reevaluating the diagnosis and response to treatment. Diagnostic imaging of the head and neck (computed tomography [CT] and MRI) is critical in making the diagnosis (**Fig. 18**) and it is the responsibility of the treating clinician to review the images and not depend solely on the report by the radiologist. The algorithm for management of patients who are suspected of having a false arthropathy of the temporomandibular joint is shown in **Fig. 17**.

How Common Is Each Etiologic Category in the Classification of Arthropathies of the Temporomandibular Joint?

Because an etiologic classification of temporomandibular joint disorder has not been routinely used, there is a paucity of information on the prevalence of each category of arthropathy. Preliminary research on this classification based on cause has yielded surprising results. An unpublished review of 104 consecutive patients with signs and symptoms of internal derangement and failure of response to nonsurgical treatment, who underwent arthroscopic biopsies, has been conducted. The etiologic classification was based on the history,

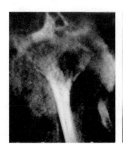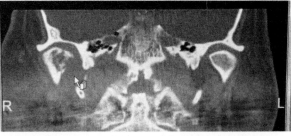

Fig. 18. A 79-year-old man referred to oral and maxillofacial surgery by ear, nose, and throat for treatment of severe right TMJ pain, limitation of opening, and mandibular dysfunction. Cone beam and CT scans showed lytic lesion of the right condyle. Simultaneously, the patient was diagnosed with pancreatic cancer. The lytic lesion of the condyle was caused by metastasis. This false arthropathy simulated routine TMJ symptoms.

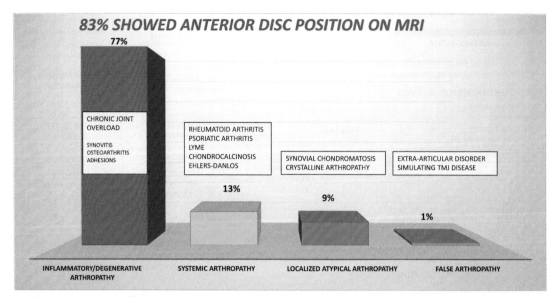

Fig. 19. Diagnostic classification based on cause in 104 consecutive patients undergoing arthroscopic diagnosis and biopsy.

diagnostic imaging, arthroscopic morphology, and histopathologic findings. The results revealed the following (**Fig. 19**):

Inflammatory/degenerative arthropathy caused by joint overload	77%
Systemic arthropathy	13%
Localized atypical arthropathy	9%
False arthropathy	1%

Further investigation using an etiologic classification system is required, but even in this small sample the results are surprising. Systemic arthropathies and localized atypical arthropathies affecting the temporomandibular joint were common. A total of 23% of the cases did not have the more common inflammatory/degenerative arthropathy, and thus treatment of these patient groups may be different from treatment of those with the more common inflammatory/degenerative arthropathy (Israel H. Etiologic classification of temporomandibular joint disease in 104 consecutive patients undergoing arthroscopic surgery. Manuscript in preparation, 2015).

SUMMARY: ETIOLOGIC CLASSIFICATION OF TEMPOROMANDIBULAR JOINT DISORDERS

A review of the current state of knowledge of internal derangement of the temporomandibular joint and synovial joint pathophysiology leads to the conclusion that internal derangement is not a disease. The signs and symptoms associated with internal derangement are caused by loss of the structure and function of the intra-articular tissues, ultimately leading to a failure in the biomechanics of the temporomandibular joint. The cause of this tissue failure is most often joint overload, leading to tissue failure and an inflammatory/degenerative arthropathy of the temporomandibular joint. However, the intra-articular changes associated with internal derangement of the temporomandibular joint can also be caused by a systemic arthropathy or a localized atypical arthropathy involving the temporomandibular joint. In addition, there is a group of disorders that simulates the signs and symptoms of internal derangement, but are caused by extra-articular disease, and thus are classified as a false arthropathy of the temporomandibular joint. Clinicians must be diligent in establishing the correct diagnosis and cause of the internal derangement, which ultimately leads to the appropriate management of patients with these disorders.

REFERENCES

1. Dworkin SF, LeResche L. Research diagnostic criteria for temporomandibular disorders: review, criteria, examinations and specifications, critique. J Craniomandib Disord 1992;6:301–55.
2. Schiffman E, Ohrbach R, Truelove E, et al. Diagnostic criteria for temporomandibular disorders (DC/TMD) for clinical and research applications:

recommendations of the international RDC/TMD consortium network and orofacial pain special interest group. J Oral Facial Pain Headache 2014; 28(1):6–27.

3. Peck CC, Goulet JP, Lobbezoo F, et al. Expanding the taxonomy of the diagnostic criteria for temporomandibular disorders. J Oral Rehabil 2014;41(1):2–23.

4. American Society of Temporomandibular Joint Surgeons. Guidelines for diagnosis and management of disorders involving the temporomandibular joint and related musculoskeletal structures. 2001.

5. Altman R, Alarcon G, Appelrouth D, et al. The American College of Rheumatology criteria for classification and reporting of osteoarthritis of the hip. Arthritis Rheum 1991;34(5):505–14.

6. Altman R, Asch E, Bloch D, et al. Development of criteria for classification and reporting of osteoarthritis: classification of osteoarthritis of the knee. Arthritis Rheum 1986;29:1039–49.

7. Mehta N. The Merck manual of diagnosis and therapy. In: Porter R, Kaplan J, editors. 19th edition. Whitehouse Station (New Jersey): Merck Sharp & Dohme; 2011.

8. Molinari F, Manicone PF, Raffaelli L, et al. Temporomandibular joint soft-tissue pathology, I: disc abnormalities. Semin Ultrasound CT MR 2007;28:192–204.

9. McCarty WL, Farrar WB. Surgery for internal derangements of the temporomandibular joint. J Prosthet Dent 1979;42(2):191–6.

10. Canale ST, Beaty JH. Campbell's operative orthopaedics. 12th edition. Elsevier; 2013.

11. Stegenga B. Nomenclature and classification of temporomandibular joint disorders. J Oral Rehabil 2010;37:760–5.

12. Kaplan PA, Ruskin JD, Tu HK, et al. Erosive arthritis of the temporomandibular joint caused by Teflon-Proplast implants: plain film features. Am J Roentgenol 1988;151(2):337–9.

13. Smith RM, Goldwasser MS, Sabol SR. Erosion of a Teflon-Proplast implant into the middle cranial fossa. J Oral Maxillofac Surg 1993;51(11):1268–71.

14. Lypka M, Yamashita DD. Exuberant foreign body giant cell reaction to a Teflon/Proplast temporomandibular joint implant: report of a case. J Oral Maxillofac Surg 2007;65(9):1680–4.

15. Trumpy IG, Lyberg T. Surgical treatment of internal derangement of the temporomandibular joint: Long-term evaluation of three techniques. J Oral Maxillofac Surg 1995;53:746–7.

16. Sanders B, Buoncristiani R. Diagnostic and surgical arthroscopy of the temporomandibular joint: Clinical experience with 136 procedures over a 2-year period. J Craniomandib Disord 1987;1:202.

17. Moses JJ, Poker ID. TMJ arthroscopic surgery: an analysis of 237 patients. J Oral Maxillofac Surg 1989; 47:790.

18. Indresano AT. Arthroscopic surgery of the temporomandibular joint: Report of 64 patients with long-term follow-up. J Oral Maxillofac Surg 1989; 47:439.

19. Israel H, Roser SM. Patient response to temporomandibular joint arthroscopy: Preliminary findings in 24 patients. J Oral Maxillofac Surg 1989;47:570.

20. Montgomery MT, Van Sickels J, Harms SE, et al. Arthroscopic TMJ surgery: Effects on signs, symptoms and disc position. J Oral Maxillofac Surg 1989; 47:1263.

21. McCain JP, Sanders B, Koslin M, et al. Temporomandibular joint arthroscopy: A 6-year multicenter retrospective study of 4,831 joints. J Oral Maxillofac Surg 1992;50:926.

22. Hoffman DC, Cubillos L. The effect of arthroscopic surgery on mandibular range of motion. Cranio 1994; 12(1):11.

23. Murakami K, Hosaka H, Moriya Y, et al. Short-term outcome study for the management of temporomandibular joint closed lock. Oral Surg Oral Med Oral Pathol 1995;80:253.

24. Murakami K, Moriya Y, Goto K, et al. Four-year follow-up study of temporomandibular joint arthroscopic surgery for advanced internal derangements. J Oral Maxillofac Surg 1996;54:285.

25. Reston JT, Turkelson CM. Meta-analysis of surgical treatments for temporomandibular articular disorders. J Oral Maxillofac Surg 2003;61:3–10.

26. Israel H, Behrman D, Friedman J, et al. Rationale for early versus late intervention with arthroscopy for treatment of inflammatory/degenerative temporomandibular joint disorders. J Oral Maxillofac Surg 2010;68(11):2661–7.

27. Al-Moraissi EA. Arthroscopy versus arthrocentesis in the management of internal derangement of the temporomandibular joint: a systematic review and meta-analysis. Int J Oral Maxillofac Surg 2015; 44(4):104–12.

28. Kircos LT, Douglas A, Mark AS, et al. Magnetic resonance imaging of the TMJ disc in asymptomatic volunteers. J Oral Maxillofac Surg 1987;45:852–4.

29. Katzberg RW, Westesson P, Tallents RH, et al. Anatomic disorders of the temporomandibular joint disc in asymptomatic subjects. J Oral Maxillofac Surg 1996;54:147–53.

30. Moore JB. Coronal and sagittal TMJ meniscus position in asymptomatic subjects by MRI. J Oral Maxillofac Surg 1989;47:75.

31. Larheim TA, Westesson P, Sano T. Temporomandibular joint disk displacement: comparison in asymptomatic volunteers and patients. Radiology 2001; 218(2):428–32.

32. Nitzan DW, Dolwick MF, Martinez GA. Temporomandibular joint arthrocentesis: a simplified treatment for severe limited mouth opening. J Oral Maxillofac Surg 1991;49(1):1163–7.

33. Nitzan DW. Arthrocentesis for management of severe closed lock of the temporomandibular joint. Oral Maxillofacial Surg Clin North Am 1994;6:245–57.

34. Dimitroulis G, Dolwick MF, Garza AM. Temporomandibular joint arthrocentesis and lavage for the treatment of closed lock: a follow-up study. Br J Oral Maxillofac Surg 1995;33:23–7.

35. Hosaka H, Murakami K, Goto K, et al. Outcome of arthrocentesis for temporomandibular joints with closed lock at 3 years follow-up. Oral Surg Oral Med Oral Pathol Oral Radiol Endod 1996;82:501–4.

36. Quinn JH, Bazan NG. Identification of prostaglandin E2 and leukotriene B4 in the synovial fluid of painful, dysfunctional temporomandibular joints. J Oral Maxillofac Surg 1990;48:968.

37. Shafer DM, Assael L, White LB, et al. Tumor necrosis factor alpha as a biochemical marker of pain and outcome in temporomandibular joints with internal derangements. J Oral Maxillofac Surg 1994;52:786.

38. Kopp S. Neuroendocrine, immune and local responses related to temporomandibular disorders. J Orofac Pain 2001;15:9.

39. Ratcliffe A, Israel HA. Proteoglycan components of articular cartilage in synovial fluids as potential markers of osteoarthritis of the temporomandibular joint. In: Sessle BJ, Bryant PS, Dionne RA, editors. Temporomandibular disorders and related pain conditions, progress in pain research and management, vol. 4. Seattle (WA): IASP Press; 1995. p. 141–50.

40. Israel H, Diamond B, Saed-Nejad F, et al. Correlation between arthroscopic diagnosis of osteoarthritis and synovitis of the human temporomandibular joint and keratan sulfate levels in the synovial fluid. J Oral Maxillofac Surg 1997;55:210.

41. Kubota E, Imamura H, Kubota T, et al. Interleukin 1 beta and stromelysin (MMP3) activity of synovial fluid as possible markers of osteoarthritis in the temporomandibular joint. J Oral Maxillofac Surg 1997;55:20.

42. Kubota E, Kubota T, Matsumoto J, et al. Synovial fluid cytokines and proteinases as markers of temporomandibular joint disease. J Oral Maxillofac Surg 1998;56:192.

43. Israel H, Diamond B, Saed-Nejad F, et al. Osteoarthritis and synovitis as major pathoses of the temporomandibular joint: comparison of clinical diagnosis and arthroscopic morphology. J Oral Maxillofac Surg 1998;56:1023–8.

44. Chang H, Israel H. Analysis of inflammatory mediators in TMJ synovial fluid lavage samples in symptomatic patients and asymptomatic controls. J Oral Maxillofac Surg 2005;63:761–5.

45. Shibata T, Murakami KI, Kubota E, et al. Glycosaminoglycan components in temporomandibular joint synovial fluid as markers of joint pathology. J Oral Maxillofac Surg 1998;56:209.

46. Israel H, Saed-Nejad F, Ratcliffe A. Early diagnosis of osteoarthrosis of the temporomandibular joint: correlation between arthroscopic diagnosis and keratan sulfate levels in the synovial fluid. J Oral Maxillofac Surg 1991;49:708–11.

47. Yoshida K, Takatsuka S, Tanaka A, et al. Aggrecanase analysis of synovial fluid of temporomandibular joint disorders. Oral Dis 2005;11(5):299–302.

48. Matsumoto K, Honda K, Ohshima M, et al. Cytokine profile in synovial fluid from patients with internal derangement of the temporomandibular joint: a preliminary study. Dentomaxillofac Radiol 2006;35(6):432–41.

49. Bouloux GF. Temporomandibular joint pain and synovial fluid analysis: a review of the literature. J Oral Maxillofac Surg 2009;67(11):2497–504.

50. Sato S, Goto S, Nasu F, et al. Natural course of disc displacement with reduction of the TMJ: changes in clinical signs and symptoms. J Oral Maxillofac Surg 2003;61:32–4.

51. Sato S, Goto S, Kawamura H, et al. The natural course of non-reducing disc displacement of the TMJ: relationship of clinical findings at initial visit to outcome after 12 months without treatment. J Orofac Pain 1997;11(4):315–20.

52. Kurita K, Westesson PL, Yuasa H, et al. Natural course of untreated symptomatic temporomandibular joint disc displacement without reduction. J Dent Res 1998;77(2):361–5.

53. Murakami K, Kaneshita S, Kanoh C, et al. Ten-year outcome of nonsurgical treatment for internal derangement of the temporomandibular joint with closed lock. Oral Surg Oral Med Oral Pathol Oral Radiol Endod 2002;94(5):572–5.

54. Minakuchi H, Kuboki T, Matsuka Y, et al. Randomized controlled evaluation of non-surgical treatments for temporomandibular joint anterior disk displacement without reduction. J Dent Res 2001;80(3):924–8.

55. Lundh H, Westesson PL, Eriksson L, et al. Temporomandibular joint disk displacement without reduction. Treatment with flat occlusal splint versus no treatment. Oral Surg Oral Med Oral Pathol 1992;73(6):655–8.

56. Truelove E, Huggins KH, Mancl L, et al. The efficacy of traditional, low-cost and non-splint therapies for temporomandibular disorders: a randomized controlled trial. J Am Dent Assoc 2006;137(8):1099–107.

57. Clark G, Minakuchi H. Oral appliances. In: Laskin DM, Greene CS, Hylander WL, editors. Temporomandibular disorders: an evidenced-based approach to diagnosis & treatment. Quintessence Publishing; 2006. p. 377–90.

58. Scrivani SJ, Keith DA, Kaban LB. Temporomandibular disorders. N Engl J Med 2008;359:2693–705.

59. Greene CS, Goddard G, Macaluso GM, et al. Topical review: placebo responses and therapeutic responses. How are they related? J Orofac Pain 2009; 23(2):93–107.

60. Laskin D. Surgical management of internal derangements. In: Laskin DM, Greene CS, Hylander WL, editors. Temporomandibular disorders: an evidenced-based approach to diagnosis & treatment. Quintessence Publishing; 2006. p. 469–81.

61. Kondoh T, Hamada Y, Kamei K, et al. Simple disc reshaping surgery for internal derangement of the temporomandibular joint: 5 year follow-up results. J Oral Maxillofac Surg 2003;61(1):41–8.

62. Abramowicz S, Dolwick F. 20-year follow-up study of disc repositioning surgery for temporomandibular joint internal derangement. J Oral Maxillofac Surg 2010;68(2):239–42.

63. Emshoff R, Rudisch A, Bosch R, et al. Effect of arthrocentesis and hydraulic distension on temporomandibular joint disk position. Oral Surg Oral Med Oral Pathol Oral Radiol Endod 2000;89(3): 271–7.

64. Moses J, Sartoris D, Glass R, et al. The effect of arthroscopic surgical lysis and lavage of the superior joint space on temporomandibular joint disc position and mobility. J Oral Maxillofac Surg 1989; 47(7):674–8.

65. Zhang S, Liu X, Yang, et al. Temporomandibular joint disc repositioning using bone anchors: an immediate post surgical evaluation by magnetic resonance imaging. BMC Musculoskelet Disord 2010;11:262.

66. Israel H, Langevin CJ, Singer M. The relationship between temporomandibular joint synovitis and adhesions: pathogenic mechanisms and clinical implications for surgical management. J Oral Maxillofac Surg 2006;64:1066–74.

67. Nakao Y, Konno-Nagasaka M, Toriya N, et al. Proteoglycan expression is influenced by mechanical load in temporomandibular joint discs. J Dent Res 2015; 94(1):93–100.

68. McCain J. TMJ Surgical Course. Miami OMS.

69. DiFabio V, Levin S, Moses J, et al. TMJ Surgery Mini Residency. Baltimore, U of Maryland.

70. Kaduk W. Endoscopy in Maxillofacial Surgery. TMJ Arthroscopy Course. Greifswald, Germany.

Temporomandibular Disorders and Headache

Steven B. Graff-Radford, DDS[a,b,c,*], Jeremy J. Abbott, DDS[d]

KEYWORDS

- Temporomandibular joint • Temporomandibular disorder • Treatment • Headache • Migraine

KEY POINTS

- In patients presenting with comorbid TMD and headache, each disorder should be separately identified and diagnosed using standardized diagnostic criteria.
- Once the disorders are identified, the predisposing, causative and perpetuating factors of each condition should be addressed and minimized.
- When necessary in headache patients, TMD treatment should involve patient education, self-care therapy, behavioral interventions, pharmacologic interventions, and physical therapies including occlusal splints.
- When considering appropriate headache treatment, physical, behavioral, and pharmacologic options should be evaluated for the potential benefit of both disorders without reducing headache treatment principles.

INTRODUCTION

Temporomandibular disorders (TMD) and primary headaches can be perpetual and debilitating musculoskeletal and neurological disorders. The presence of both can affect up to one-sixth of the population at any one time.[1–3] Initially, TMDs were thought to be predominantly musculoskeletal disorders, and migraine was thought to be solely a cerebrovascular disorder. The further understanding of their pathophysiology has helped to clarify their clinical presentation. This article focuses on the role of the trigeminal system in associating TMD and migraine. By discussing recent descriptions of prevalence, diagnosis, and treatment of headache and TMD, we will further elucidate this relationship. Historically, migraines were attributed to cerebrovascular change owing to arterial vasoconstriction producing aura, followed by vasodilation causing pain, mediated via the trigeminal

ophthalmic division afferent projections.[4,5] This theory has changed to a neurally mediated pain and aura and a secondary vascular role.[6] Migraine occurring outside of the ophthalmic division were reported in 1977 by Raskin,[7] who described recurring vascular neck pain with carotid tenderness that was reduced with prophylactic migraine medication. Subsequently, migraine has been associated with pain in the sinus, temporomandibular joint (TMJ),[8] teeth,[9] and cervical areas.[10] This association was clarified by Bartsch and Goadsby[11] when describing how central sensitization creates a neural pathway between trigeminal and central afferents. TMD has been described as a group of musculoskeletal and neuromuscular conditions that involve the TMJs, the masticatory muscles, and all associated tissues.[12] TMDs are functional disorders of the anatomic regions of the TMJ and associated musculature including arthritides and myogenous pains.[13] TMDs are thought to create

a The Pain Center, Cedars-Sinai Medical Center, 444 South San Vicente Boulevard #1101, Los Angeles, CA 90048, USA; b The Program for Headache and Orofacial Pain, Cedars-Sinai Medical Center, Los Angeles, CA, USA; c UCLA School of Dentistry, Los Angeles, CA, USA; d West Coast Ear, Nose & Throat Medical Group, 301 South Moorpark Road, Thousand Oaks, CA 91361, USA
* Corresponding author. The Pain Center, Cedars-Sinai Medical Center, 444 South San Vicente Boulevard #1101, Los Angeles, CA 90048.
E-mail address: graffs@cshs.org

Oral Maxillofacial Surg Clin N Am 28 (2016) 335–349
http://dx.doi.org/10.1016/j.coms.2016.03.004
1042-3699/16/$ – see front matter © 2016 Elsevier Inc. All rights reserved.

oralmaxsurgery.theclinics.com

Box 1
International Classification of Headache Disorders-3 (beta) criteria for headache attributed to TMD (11.7)

Description:

Headache caused by a disorder involving structures in the temporomandibular region

Diagnostic criteria:

A. Any headache fulfilling criterion C

B. Clinical and/or imaging evidence of a pathologic process affecting the TMJ, muscles of mastication, and/or associated structures

C. Evidence of causation shown by at least 2 of the following:

    1. Headache has developed in temporal relation to the onset of the TMD

    2. Either or both of the following:

        a. Headache has significantly worsened in parallel with progression of the TMD

        b. Headache has significantly improved or resolved in parallel with improvement in or resolution of the TMD

    3. The headache is produced or exacerbated by active jaw movements, passive movements through the range of motion of the jaw, and/or provocative maneuvers applied to temporomandibular structures such as pressure on the TMJ and surrounding muscles of mastication

    4. Headache, when unilateral, is ipsilateral to the side of the TMD

D. Not better accounted for by another International Classification of Headache Disorders-3 diagnosis

Abbreviations: TMD, temporomandibular disorder; TMJ, temporomandibular joint.
   From The Headache Classification Committee of the International Headache Society (IHS). The international classification of headache disorders, 3rd edition (beta version). Cephalgia 2013;33(9):765; with permission.

---

central sensitization and decrease in pain thresholds in migraine patients.[14] Also, parafunctional habits and associated painful TMD greatly increases the risk for chronic migraine.[15,16] Furthermore, genetic[17] and hormonal associations have also been made. Sex hormones, such as estrogen, may help to control trigeminal nerve sensitization by modulating nociceptive mediators such as calcitonin gene-related peptide (CGRP).[18]

EPIDEMIOLOGY OF HEADACHE AND TEMPOROMANDIBULAR DISORDERS COMORBIDITY

TMD epidemiology in nonpatient populations showed the prevalence of 1 joint dysfunction (clicking, limited range of motion) in 75% of patients. One symptom (pain or pain with palpation) occurred in 33% to 39% of patients. Painful TMD was present in 10% to 25% of the population, but fewer than 7% of patients required treatment. The presence of headache in TMD patients was 27.4% versus 15.2% in non-TMD patients.[1–3,12] Headache is more likely to be in myogenous TMD than arthrogenous TMD,[13] and chronic headache patients are more likely to meet Research Diagnostic Criteria/TMD criteria for myofascial pain[19,20] (**Box 1**).

Because TMD and headache occur frequently together in the young female population, assessing their relationship is difficult. There are, however, a number of studies suggesting the comorbidity is more than just coincidence. When assessing the prevalence of TMD in a headache population, it was described that 56.1% of headache patients had TMD. This percentage increased if the study population had both migraine and tension-type headache.[21] If the population is limited to females, 86.3% of migraine and 91.3% of chronic migraine patients had TMD. The TMD was more likely to be myogenous than arthrogenous.[22] Evaluating headache in a TMD population, the presence was 85.5%. Compared with a non-TMD control where the prevalence was 45.4%.[23]

Considering the presence of TMD in the various types of primary headaches, chronic migraine was most common (odds ratio, 95.9; P<.01; 95% CI, 12.5–734.64), followed by episodic migraine (7.0), then episodic tension-type headache (3.7). Painful TMD alone was associated with significant risk of chronic migraine (30.1) and episodic migraine (3.7), whereas the presence of sleep bruxism alone was not a significant risk factor for primary headaches. Compared with painful TMD and sleep bruxism individually, the combination of both significantly increased the risk for chronic migraine (87.1), episodic migraine (6.7), and episodic tension-type headache (3.8) with almost all chronic migraine subjects having TMD.[15]

A common symptom of migraines during (ictal) and in between (interictal) attacks is cutaneous allodynia. Cutaneous allodynia occurred between migraine attacks, in 86.9% of the patients with comorbid myofascial TMD and migraine, 84.0% of patients with mixed TMD (myofascial and arthrogenous) and migraine, but only 40% in migraine patients without TMD.[14]

Disability was assessed in a headache population with comorbid TMD compared with a non-TMD population using the Migraine Disability Assessment. The disability scores were significantly higher in the comorbid population than the non-TMD population. The severity of disability was strongly associated to the presence of musculoskeletal pain.[24]

In a double-blind, placebo-controlled study of treatment for comorbid migraine and TMD, patients were tested on the separate and combination effects of a migraine treatment and a TMD treatment in 4 groups of patients. No differences were seen among groups for the TMD treatment alone. The combination of TMD and migraine treatment was significantly greater to the other groups on all other headache endpoints and in disability.[25] Thus, efficient treatment requires a multidisciplinary approach by identifying, diagnosing, and addressing the comorbid disorders.[25,26]

THE PATHOPHYSIOLOGY RELATIONSHIP OF MIGRAINES AND TEMPOROMANDIBULAR DISORDERS

Understanding the mechanisms whereby facial pain (TMD) and head pain (migraine) may be linked physiologically may provide clues as to their clinical association and elucidate common targets for therapy. Whereas, in the face, maxillary and mandibular trigeminal nerve divisions are clearly separated from the ophthalmic division and cervical spine anatomically, it is clear that pain referral occurs between these sites. For this referral to occur, there must be proven anatomic links between these distant sites. It is thought that these referrals are facilitated by central sensitization, reducing activation thresholds, increasing the responsiveness to afferent stimuli, and expanding the receptive field. Bartsch and Goadsby[11] identified that, with peripheral sensitization in the facial region, there was an opening of silent connections between the trigeminal nucleus caudalis and the upper cervical segments. This finding clearly shows that pathways between trigeminal and central afferents exist.[8,11,27] Similarly, peripheral sensitization of the TMJ caused expansion of normal afferent pathways and increased muscle activity.[28]

TEMPOROMANDIBULAR JOINT STRUCTURE AND FUNCTION

The structure of the TMJ is formed by an inferior surface of the temporal bone and the mandibular condyle with a fibrocartilaginous disc inserted between with ligaments surrounding the joint forming a capsular structure and lined by fibrocartilage. The articular disc is absent of direct innervation or vascularization, and is not pain sensitive. The sensitive pain structures of the TMJ include the capsule, posterior disc attachment, which is highly vascularized and innervated, and discal ligaments. The fibrocartilage is unique in its increased ability for repair over hyaline cartilage, but when the TMJ is no longer able to repair itself,[29,30] joint deterioration begins. This deterioration can be identified as internal joint derangements, inflammatory or degenerative disorders, and muscular disorders. Although they can occur together, each may be a trigger for headache and is discussed separately.

Internal derangement is characterized by the articular disc being displaced. The displacement is described in coordination of the disc and condyle with the disc usually displaced in an anterior or anteromedial direction.[31,32] In nonpatient populations, disc displacement is the most common TMD with its subclinical signs existing more frequently than any awareness of symptoms.[30,33,34] Although the causes of disc displacement are not agreed on, macrotrauma, repeated microtrauma, insufficient lubrication, and adherences are possible etiologic factors.[35] No matter the cause, when disc displacement persists, the stretched or torn ligaments binding to the disc are elongated, allowing the disc to become permanently displaced.[36,37] Disc displacement can be subdivided into 2 categories, namely, disc displacement with reduction and disc displacement without reduction. Disc displacement with reduction is described as temporarily misaligned discs reducing or improving their structural relation with the condyle when mandibular translation occurs during opening, meaning that the condyle slides on to the anteriorly displaced disc. This can produce a joint noise (sound) described as clicking or popping. Disc displacement with reduction usually is characterized by what is termed reciprocal clicking, a reciprocal noise that is heard during the opening movement and again before the teeth occlude during the closing movement. Because disc displacement with reduction is so common, it may represent a physiologic accommodation without clinical significance.[38,39] In fact, clicking in reducing disc displacement is not pathologic because more than one-third of the asymptomatic population can have moderate to severe derangement, whereas as many as one-quarter of clicking joints show normal or only slightly displaced discs. Disc displacement may or may not be a painful condition. Correlation of pain and disc derangement disorders does not seem to be associated,[40] and no meaningful association was found between specific intraarticular disorders and the production of pain, functional limitations, or disability.[41–43] When a derangement becomes painful, inflammation of the retrodiscal tissue, synovial tissues, capsule, and ligaments, as well as pressure on the disc attachments, are likely causes of the pain.[44] TMJ disc displacement with reduction may persist for several years up to decades without pain, progression, or complication. Although, De Leeuw and colleagues[45] reported that if patients with disc displacement with reduction do not respond to treatment and it is present 2 to 4 years afterward, the condition will likely to persist for several decades.

Even though it is relatively uncommon, disc displacement with reduction can progress to disc displacement without reduction. This change is characterized by sudden cessation of clicking and a sudden onset of restricted mouth opening. It is frequently accompanied by pain. Disc displacement without reduction is described as having a permanently displaced disc, which does not improve with condylar position, meaning the condyle cannot slide or translate onto the disc. This condition may be owing to secondary adhesions, deformations, or dystrophy involving the disc. Often pain is present and especially present during attempts to open the mouth. The acute stage is exhibited clinically as a deflection to the affected side during opening, a marked limited laterotrusion to the contralateral side, and an absence of joint noise in the affected joint. As the condition becomes chronic, the pain is reduced significantly from the acute stage to the point of becoming nonpainful in a large percentage of patients,[46] with the opening range approaching normal dimensions over time.[47] If a patient presents with this condition in the chronic stage, a history of joint noise and/or limitation of mandibular opening is usually present.[48] It should be noted that most internal derangement disorders are not progressive. Even though symptoms may vary with time, few patients develop more serious disorders.[49]

INFLAMMATORY JOINT DISORDERS

Trauma or degenerative breakdown within the TMJ can result in an inflammatory joint disorder that affects the tissues that make up the joint. Unlike disc derangements, inflammatory TMDs have a constant dull aching pain that is worsened by joint movement. With the nonbony inflammatory disorders, it is difficult clinically to differentiate between these disorders, which include synovitis (inflammation of synovial membranes), capsulitis (inflammation of capsular ligaments), and retrodiscitis (inflammation of the retrodiscal attachment).[35] Inflammatory disorders affecting bony structures of the TMJ are destructive in nature. Osteoarthritis is the most common disorder affecting the TMJ, and is considered to be the result of excessive joint loading.[50] It occurs most commonly with disc displacement, and is thought to be the result of abnormal loading related to the displaced disc.[51] With this excessive loading, the articular surface experiences chrondromalacia (softening) and resorption of cortical layer, resulting in bone erosion and condylar changes that is evident radiographically. These radiographic changes are usually witnessed in the late stages of osteoarthritis, often with the patient being asymptomatic.[37] When the joint has a reduction in loading, the osteoarthritis can remit into its adaptive phase called osteoarthrosis. Osteoarthrosis is radiographically evident with the return of the cortical bony layer, often presenting with a flattened portion of the condyle. Clinically, osteoarthritis and osteoarthrosis can be observed with crepitation (grating sound on movement), occlusal changes, and pain.[50]

MUSCULAR PAIN

Considering the prevalence of internal derangements in the nonpatient population, the most prevalent diagnosis in the TMD patient population is myofascial pain. Myofascial pain is typically a chronic referring muscle pain, present when a muscle has been subjected to prolonged tension. Whereas myalgia or localized muscle pain is primarily owing to a strain or injury, and common in acute forms, with continued muscle tension it can present for a longer duration. Both muscle disorders can affect the movement and function of the TMJ; however, myofascial pain syndrome is more frequently involved with TMD and headache. Myofascial pain is described as regional muscle pain, with a dull and/or achy quality. Myofascial pain is a common cause of persistent regional pain such as neck pain, shoulder pain, headaches, and orofacial pain.[52] It is associated with the presence of trigger points in muscles, tendons, or fascia that can have similar pain referral patterns to areas outside of the muscle boundary.[53–55] Trigger points can be identified as localized spots of tenderness with a nodule in a palpable taut band of muscle, tendon, or ligament that produces a referred pain outside of the palpation area. These trigger points may be active or latent. An active trigger point is hypersensitive and displays a continuous and/or spontaneous pain in a referral zone consistent with palpation. The latent trigger point displays the characteristic referral with palpation, but does not have continuous or spontaneous pain. Latent trigger point pain is usually dull and deep in quality, diffuse in nature, and presents in subcutaneous tissues, including muscle and joints.[56]

The first correlation between muscle tenderness and pain were noted in experiments by Kellgren.[57] He injected patient muscles with hypertonic saline and asked the subjects where they perceived pain. The resulting mapped pain patterns were similar to those seen in tension-type headache. He then injected local anesthetic into these tender areas and was able to resolve the pain. These tender points became known as myofascial trigger points. Mense developed a hypothesis for muscle pain referral to other deep somatic tissues remote to the original muscle stimulation site. He hypothesized that the convergent connections from deep tissues (muscles) to dorsal horn neurons are only opened after nociceptive inputs from muscle are activated. He called them silent connections. According to this theory, the referral to muscle beyond the initially activated site is owing to central sensitization and spread to adjacent spinal segments, whereas the initiating stimulus requires a peripheral inflammatory process (neurogenic inflammation). In Mense's animal model, the noxious stimulus, bradykinin was injected into the muscle.[58–60] In work by Kellgren, a hypertonic saline solution was used to trigger the referred pain. This strategy seems to mimic what is seen in the animal model. It is unclear what triggers the muscle referral in the clinical setting, where there is usually no obvious inflammation producing incident. Mense's theory has been used by Simons to discuss a neurophysiological basis for trigger point pain. Simons hypothesized that, when the tender area in the muscle is palpated, there is a neurotransmitter release in the dorsal horn (trigeminal nucleus) resulting in previously silent nociceptive inputs becoming active. This in turn causes distant neurons to produce a retrograde referred pain.[61] This model accounts for most of the clinical presentation and therapeutic options seen in myofascial pain, but does not account for what initiates the peripheral tenderness that must be present to activate the silent connections.

Peripheral tenderness may be related to central nervous system–activated neurogenic inflammation, similar to migraine, except that stimulated nociceptors are in the muscle rather than around the blood vessel. Olesen was the first person to suggest a relationship between myofascial pain and tension type headache in 1991. He proposed a vascular–supraspinal–myogenic model for headache pain. This model hypothesizes that perceived pain (headache) intensity is modulated by the central nervous system.[62] Fields initially described a model where the central nervous system may switch on nociception. He describes the presence of "on" and "off" cells that, when stimulated, may produce or inhibit activation of trigeminal nucleus nociceptors that produce pain.[63] Similarly, Goadsby found that the stimulation of dural trigeminal afferents implicated in migraine increased pain in the greater occipital nerve (C2) through the trigeminal cervical complex with his studies.[11] Akerman and Goadsby further described that the brainstem and mid-brain are most likely to serve as a "migraine mediator," and their dysfunction may lead to activation of pathways that activate central structures, and may include mechanisms that involving the brainstem, higher centers, such as the thalamus and cortex. They described the signaling between these structures as bidirectional, which makes the symptoms of any associated disorder complex.[27]

When examining a neurochemical cause of myofascial pain, the neuroinflammatory peptides, such as CGRP and substance P, have been found to be increased in myofascial trigger points[64] and contribute to myofascial pain.[65] CGRP and substance P have also been implicated in migraine pathophysiology.[66] Recently, CGRP antagonist drugs have shown efficacy in the acute treatment of migraine in clinical trials,[67–69] and have also demonstrated pain reduction in various animal muscular pain models.[70,71] With these mechanisms, myofascial pain can be maintained, even after the initial eliciting factors are gone. This may contribute to transformation of episodic headache into its chronic form.

MANAGEMENT
Treating Headache by Targeting Temporomandibular Disorders

For successful treatment of comorbid TMDs and headaches, an accurate diagnosis of both disorders is needed. Primary headache disorders have the ability to cause pain in the TMJ and associated structures, whereas TMDs may have an associated headache or aggravate a primary headache. A common deficiency in TMD-related headache studies is the lack of a specific TMD diagnosis. This lack of proper diagnosis allows inaccurate correlation of headache improvement following TMD treatment. Nevertheless, treatment results could potentially be enhanced by managing both disorders, even though a causative association cannot be made. This relationship can be seen in the comparison of interventions that improve both TMD and primary headache.[24,26] When treating headache and TMD individually, the best results are often achieved by reducing as many predisposing, causative, and perpetuating factors as possible. For both groups of disorders, conservative treatments are recommended, which are inexpensive, modest, and reversible. A comparison of treatment for both disorders shows similarities in treatment that should be noted (**Box 2**).

Box 2
Management principles

Temporomandibular Joint Disorders[4,72]

- Patient education and self-care
- Pharmacotherapy:
  - NSAIDs, muscle relaxants, antidepressants, anesthetics, corticosteroids, antiepileptic drugs
- Physical therapies
  - Posture training, stretching exercises, mobilization, physical modalities, appliance therapy
- Cognitive behavioral interventions

Headaches (Migraine and Tension-type)[73,74]

- Patient education and self-care
- Trigger avoidance
  - Food, environmental
- Cognitive behavioral interventions
- Physical therapy
  - Posture training, mobilization, exercise, trigger point therapy
- Pharmacologic management
  - NSAIDs, muscle relaxants, antidepressants, antihypertensives, antiepileptic drugs, NMDA antagonist, corticosteroid, neurotoxins, serotonin antagonists, CGRP antagonists

Abbreviations: CGRP, calcitonin gene-related peptide; NMDA, N-methyl-D-aspartate; NSAIDs, nonsteroidal antiinflammatory drugs.
  Data from Refs.[4,72–74]

Nonsurgical Temporomandibular Disorder Treatment

Using treatment methods not explicitly directed toward TMJ noise or disc derangement disorders, Greene and Laskin[75] found that TMD-related symptoms improved overall by using conservative, nonsurgical methods. The outcomes they found support the concept that, if painful TMD can be treated successfully by conservative, nonsurgical modalities, it is generally not necessary to correct internal derangements with surgery.[75]

Patient Education

Because TMD symptoms are often being self-limiting, resolving in most patients within 7 years,[46,76] explanation alone is helpful in reducing fear leading to symptom improvement in the patient. An essential part of treatment is to educate the patient to rest the masticatory system, while avoiding perpetuating factors such as eating hard, chewy foods or chewing gum. Furthermore, patients should know how to avoid parafunctional habits like clenching and grinding.[77–81] In a long-term study, Randolph and associates[46] evaluated patients with myofascial pain, internal derangement, or both. Providing only conservative therapy with self-care advice versus advice only, they found that patients with acute conditions improved more than those with chronic problems, and 88% of all patients reported a substantial or total improvement in their symptoms of pain and dysfunction.[46]

Self-care

Among reversible therapies, physiotherapy is a common first choice treatment of TMD pain and dysfunction because it is simple, noninvasive, it is low in cost when compared with other treatments, it has an easy self-management style, it offers the opportunity for doctor and patients communication, and it can be managed by the general practitioner. For example, a home physiotherapeutic program of heat or ice to the painful areas, massage, and range of motion exercises have been shown to reduce pain and improve function.[82] Systematic have supported the effectiveness of self-care methods use in the reduction of TMD symptoms when compared with placebo.[82–85]

PHYSICAL THERAPY

Physical therapy can be used to control and manage causative and perpetuating factors while enhancing central inhibition. The use of active relaxation exercises, ethyl chloride spray and passive stretch, acupressure, ultrasound, deep massage, moist heat, laser therapy, electrical stimulation, transcutaneous electrical nerve stimulation, myofascial release, and orthopedic splints have been used with success.[86–88] In systematic reviews, postural exercises were found to increase range of motion and provide pain reduction. Additionally, the use of postural exercises in conjunction with other interventions has been effective.[89] Another study showed decreased pain and increased oral opening in patients using manual therapy in combination with active exercises.[84] Curricula involving relaxation techniques and biofeedback, electromyography training, and proprioceptive reeducation were found to be more effective than placebo. It should be recognized that the combination of multiple physical therapies including active exercises, manual therapy, postural correction, and relaxation techniques were more effective than the individual modality.[85]

ORTHOPEDIC JAW APPLIANCES (SPLINTS)

Splints, otherwise known as night guards, bite guards, stabilization appliances, orthotics, or orthopedic appliances, have often been the initial or only treatment that patients with TMD receive. These appliances are removable and either cover part or all of the teeth in 1 or both arches, which may or may not reposition the mandible anteriorly. Benefits of occlusal appliances include a stable temporary occlusal relationship, habit management assistance, alteration of TMJ structural relationships, prevention of dental and/or periodontal damage, and possible reduction of masticatory muscle activity during sleep.[90] When used inappropriately, occlusal appliances have potential complications, including dental caries, gingival irritation, odor, speech interferences, occlusal alterations, and psychological dependence on the appliance.[91,92]

Fricton and colleagues[93] performed a systematic review involving studies evaluating intraoral appliances. They found good evidence that single arch, hard, full-coverage stabilization appliances, when adjusted properly, had modest efficacy in the treatment of TMD pain compared with nonoccluding appliances or no treatment. Although other types of appliances, comprising soft appliances, anterior positioning appliances, and anterior bite appliances (nociceptive trigeminal inhibition, Lucia Jig) show evidence of effectiveness in reducing TMD pain, they showed no greater efficacy and with the potential for adverse events, the use of these appliances needs to be monitored more carefully. Furthermore, additional systematic reviews by Dao, Greene, Ekberg, Rubinoff, Jokstad, Wassell, and Conti and their many colleagues[88,94–101] studying the efficacy of splints have found similar results.

BEHAVIORAL INTERVENTIONS

The psychological aspect of TMD diagnosis and treatment is often overlooked. Psychological distress can initiate and perpetuate TMDs, which can result in chronic TMD pain.[102] Epidemiologic studies have shown that individuals who complained of pain had higher levels of anxiety, depression, nonpain somatic symptoms, poorer self-reported health status, and higher family stress than those who did not complain of pain.[103] Clinical studies have suggested that addressing the psychological aspects of pain early, improved pain outcomes,[104] whereas chronic pain increased the morbidity for psychological conditions.[105] In TMD-related psychological interventions, those receiving psychological interventions had significantly lower levels of self-reported pain and depression and were less likely to seek care for TMD related issues.[106] Those without psychological intervention were 12.5 times more likely to have a somatoform disorder, 7 times more likely to have an anxiety disorder, and 2.7 times more likely to have an affective disorder at 1 year compared with those with psychological intervention. When receiving cognitive–behavioral therapy, patients had reduced pain levels, improved coping abilities, and reduced emotional distress.[107] With chronic pain in other parts of the body, cognitive–behavioral therapy showed similar results.[108,109]

PHARMACOTHERAPY

Oral medication indicated for TMJ disorders include analgesics, nonsteroidal antiinflammatory drugs (NSAIDs), oral steroids, muscle relaxants, antiepileptic drugs, and antidepressants. Injectable pharmacotherapy includes local anesthetics, injectable corticosteroids, and botulinum toxin injections. Although analgesics and corticosteroids are indicated for treatment of acute pain, the use of NSAIDs, local anesthetics, and muscle relaxants may be used for both acute and chronic disorders. Tricyclic antidepressants are usually used for chronic TMD pain associated with tension-type headaches.[4,110,111]

Nonsteroidal Antiinflammatory Drugs and Corticosteroids

NSAIDs are often used for mild-to-moderate acute inflammatory conditions. Commonly used NSAIDs in orofacial pain include ibuprofen and naproxen. It is advised that NSAIDs not be used on the basis of pain, but use should be on a time-contingent basis to optimize reduction of inflammation.[112] The use of oral corticosteroids can be used for moderate inflammatory conditions and are particularly helpful in treatment of acute joint pain. The use of intracapsularly injected corticosteroid has been shown to significantly reduce TMJ pain.[113] It is indicated for painful intraarticular acute inflammation, unresponsive to other treatment,[114] such as polyarthritic disorders and acute disc displacements without reduction.[115–117] There is evidence that multiple frequent corticosteroid injections into the TMJ can cause damage osseous damage including condylysis. However, there is no evidence that individual steroid injections cause damage.[118]

Muscle Relaxants

Muscle relaxants may be prescribed for acute muscle tension associated with TMJ disorders, whereas tricyclic antidepressants like amitriptyline or nortriptyline may be used for chronic myofascial pain,[110,119] and there is a potential cross-benefit in headache prevention. Tricyclic antidepressants are used routinely as preventive medications in tension-type headache and migraine, but are used in doses that do not have significant antidepressant qualities, while retaining the antinociceptive effects and the potential for improved sleep.[120]

Local Anesthetics

The use of local anesthetics is primarily used in the presence of myofascial trigger points when physical therapy has not been effective in reducing dysfunction. In trigger point therapy, the use of 1% procaine is recommended owing to its low toxicity, but 1% lidocaine acceptable and commonly used; the use of epinephrine in trigger point injections is always contraindicated. Once the trigger point is identified, the needle is inserted and anesthetic is injected to a palpable taut band of muscle. Long-term success with trigger point injections remains in controlling perpetuating factors and providing a self-care and physical therapy programs to avoid recurrent pain.[110,121]

Botulinum Toxin

Initially used for muscle spasm and cosmetic purposes, botulinum toxin, specifically, onabotulinumtoxin A, is a peripherally acting neurotoxin that is injected into a muscle, preventing the release of acetylcholine into the neuromuscular junction, effectively paralyzing the muscle. Preceding the paralytic activity, it has an antinociceptive mechanism. Botulinum toxin is an approved treatment for chronic migraine and is also indicated in tension-type headache, but in respect to TMDs efficacy evidence is limited.[122,123] However, there are data to support the use of botulinum toxin as a treatment for some muscle-related TMDs.[124]

COMBINATION OF MULTIPLE THERAPIES

Use of combination therapies has been shown to be more advantageous than 1 single therapy. This combination of therapies does not seem depend on which specific therapy is provided; the therapies provided should attempt to address the causative and perpetuating factors.[89,125,126]

SURGICAL TREATMENT

TMJ surgery is considered to be a useful treatment for specific TMDs, but there is insufficient non-biased evidence to support or refute that arthrocentesis or orthognathic surgery is effective in initial treatment of common TMDs.[127] Türp and associates[126] found that quality of life ratings in patients who had multiple TMJ surgeries did not improve with multiple interventions. It should be noted that a significant amount of literature on surgical treatment of TMD is observational and is lacking test groups and controls. With respect to TMD and headache, there is minimal literature that examines headache response to TMJ surgery and the studies that do exist show conflicting outcomes. Therefore, TMJ surgery should be used only when conservative treatment options have been exhausted.[128]

TEMPOROMANDIBULAR DISORDER TREATMENTS NOT PROVEN HELPFUL OR EFFECTIVE

When considering appropriate treatment, a significant portion of the TMD literature consists of non-control observations, unsubstantiated views, and studies not adhering to modern scientific principal.[58,128] These approaches include occlusal adjustments, prosthetic reconstruction,[129–131] orthognathic surgery for TMD without dentofacial deformities,[127,132] and orthodontics.[133] These treatments did not show that they improved TMD outcomes or prevented TMD progression in the long term. The findings detailed herein support the concept that symptoms of pain and dysfunction can be treated successfully by conservative and nonsurgical modalities and irreversible treatments should only be considered if all conservative treatments have been exhausted.[75,134–139] The potential of comorbid TMDs and headaches to exacerbate each other is well-known. Because of this, each disorder should be treated concurrently, because they significantly escalate the prevalence of each other.[24] Most TMD treatments improve headache symptoms, although some TMD treatment methods are superior to others.

Occlusal Adjustment in Temporomandibular Disorders and Headache

The occlusal adjustment effects on headaches in TMD patients were studied by Vallon. Patients were assigned randomly to a treatment group or to a control group that received only counseling. All patients were evaluated periodically over a 2-year period. Over the 2 years, no differences were noted in the frequency of headaches between the group of patients who received occlusal adjustment treatment and the group of patients who just received counseling.[140–142] In the double-blind study, a group of patients seeking treatment for chronic headache, and neck and shoulder pain all received a preset physical therapy regimen. In addition, approximately one-half received occlusal adjustment, and the other one-half received a sham occlusal adjustment. Short-term responses to the physical therapy were good, but the improvement was not associated with any specific occlusal treatment. At 12 months, improvement was apparent in the real occlusal adjustment group. Compared with the sham group, the occlusal adjustment group showed a decrease in the occurrence of headache.[143] Forssell evaluated occlusal adjustment of teeth versus a sham adjustment in tension-type headache using a double-blind randomized controlled trial. All the patients had TMD and tension-type headache, but 36% of the patients also had migraine. Headache frequency decreased by 80% in the active group versus 50% in the placebo group. Headache intensity decreased 47% in the active group and 16% in the placebo group.[144] Patients in the placebo group with moderate to severe TMD symptoms, and were treated with occlusal therapy after the trial showed a significant reduction in headache frequency.[145] This study supports the value of TMD treatment for tension-type headache associated with TMD signs and symptoms.

Splint Therapy in Temporomandibular Disorders and Headache

When Forssell and colleagues[130] reevaluated the randomized controlled trials for occlusal adjustment, they concluded that there was insufficient evidence for its use, and suggested that there was evidence for splint therapy. This is similar to Koh and Robinson,[146] who found that occlusal adjustment did not treat or prevent TMDs, and recommended that occlusal adjustment not be used as a treatment for TMD.[146] Forssell also determined that there was no causal relationship between occlusion and headache, although they did find evidence suggesting that the management of TMD decreased the occurrence of comorbid migraine.[147] When looking at splint therapy in headache, an uncontrolled study found that 64% of patients had a decrease in headache frequency, and 30% showed a complete remission of headache at 4 weeks. Patients with higher starting headache frequency had more significant decrease than those with lower starting frequency.[148] In another uncontrolled study, TMD patients were followed for 1 year after the start of TMD treatment. Treatment consisted of occlusal splints, therapeutic exercises for masticatory muscles, occlusal adjustment, or a combination of these. Headaches were less frequent than 1 year earlier in 70% of patients, and 40% of patients reported a decrease in pain severity. At a 2.5-year follow-up, the results were relatively unchanged.[149,150] These studies, however, did not have a control for the placebo effect, nor was headache type defined.

Shankland[151] suggested an intraoral nociceptive trigeminal inhibition tension suppression system, a small commercially fabricated intraoral device. It is fitted over the 2 maxillary central incisors and is to be worn at night. A multicenter randomized trial was conducted to determine the effect of the nociceptive trigeminal inhibition tension suppression system on migraine compared with a full-coverage occlusal splint. Although this was labeled as a migraine study, the patients seemed diagnostically to have chronic tension-type headache. Also, no information was given on pretreatment days of headache, and the outcome was unclear by reporting the number of headaches reduced. It did show a decrease in headache, but the statistical analysis was not made clear. The evidence from the randomized, controlled trials suggests the nociceptive trigeminal inhibition may be beneficial in the management of bruxism and TMD. However, because of its potential unwanted effects, it should only be used if patients can be compliant with follow-up appointments. If not, a full-coverage appliance should be used.[152] Other authors found that care should be taken to avoid repositioning or partial coverage appliances because they may result in significant occlusal changes.[130,153,154]

Full-coverage splints in general headache patients with signs and symptoms of TMD were evaluated by Schokker and colleagues.[155,156] The patients were divided randomly into 2 groups.

One group was treated with conventional headache treatment by a neurologist, and the other group was treated with stabilization splints for 6 weeks with random patients receiving physical therapy. TMD treatment patients experienced a 56% decrease in headache frequency compared with a 32% decrease in headache frequency in patients receiving neurologic treatment. The headache intensity and abortive headache medication use also decreased in the TMD treatment group. Although the TMD treatment surpassed the neurologic treatment in patients, the TMD group did have more exposure to the treating clinician. Goncalves and colleagues,[25] performed a randomized placebo controlled clinical trial comparing migraine treatment and TMD treatment. Female patients with migraine with or without aura and myofascial TMD following the International Classification of Headache Disorders, second edition (ICHD-2) and the Research Diagnostic Criteria for TMD were studied. Patients were divided into 4 treatment groups that included propranolol and splint, propranolol placebo and splint, propranolol and nonocclusal splint, and propranolol placebo and nonocclusal splint. Migraine outcomes were determined by the change in headache days from baseline to 3 months and change in days with moderate or severe headache during the same period. TMD outcomes measured pain thresholds and mandibular vertical range of motion. The propranolol and stabilization group showed significant decrease in moderate to severe headaches days, and greater reduction in headache days and pain threshold with vertical opening compared with other groups. They found that migraine improved significantly only when both conditions were treated.

SUMMARY

In patients presenting with comorbid TMD and headache, each disorder should be separately identified and diagnosed using standardized diagnostic criteria. Once the disorders are identified, the predisposing, causative and perpetuating factors of each condition should be addressed and minimized. The inclusion of TMD treatment in headache patients is appropriate when 3 of the 4 following signs and symptoms are present:

- Pain in the preauricular and/or temporal region brought on by function (eg, chewing);
- Pain with palpation of the TMJ or associated structures;
- Joint noise (Clicking, popping, or crepitus); and
- Limited mandibular range of motion.

When necessary in headache patients, TMD treatment should involve a combination of patient education, self-care therapy, behavioral interventions, pharmacologic interventions, and physical therapies including occlusal splints. Also, during the consideration of appropriate headache treatment, physical, behavioral, and pharmacologic options should be evaluated for the potential benefit of both disorders without reducing headache treatment principles. Employment of both treatment regimens should be undertaken concurrently, which improves the overall outcome by reducing the frequency, intensity, and duration of both disorders.

REFERENCES

1. Goncalves DA, Dal Fabbro AL, Campos JA, et al. Symptoms of temporomandibular disorders in the population: an epidemiological study. J Orofac Pain 2010;24(3):270–8.
2. LeResche L. Epidemiology of temporomandibular disorders: implications for the investigation of etiologic factors. Crit Rev Oral Biol Med 1997;8(3):291–305.
3. Glass EG, McGlynn FD, Glaros AG, et al. Prevalence of temporomandibular disorder symptoms in a major metropolitan area. Cranio 1993;11(3):217–20.
4. Romero-Reyes M, Uyanik JM. Orofacial pain management: current perspectives. J Pain Res 2014;7:99–115.
5. Silberstein SD, Lipton RB, Dodick DW, et al. Wolff's headache and other head pain. 8th edition. New York: Oxford University Press; 2008. p. 95–104.
6. Bolay H, Moskowitz MA. The emerging importance of cortical spreading depression in migraine headache. Rev Neurol (Paris) 2005;161(6–7):655–7.
7. Raskin NH, Prusiner S. Carotidynia. Neurology 1977;27(1):43–6.
8. Cady R, Schreiber C, Farmer K, et al. Primary headaches: a convergence hypothesis. Headache 2002;42(3):204–16.
9. Graff-Radford SB. Headache problems that can present as toothache. Dent Clin North Am 1991;35(1):155–70.
10. Kaniecki RG. Migraine and tension-type headache: an assessment of challenges in diagnosis. Neurology 2002;58(9 Suppl 6):S15–20.
11. Bartsch T, Goadsby PJ. Increased responses in trigeminocervical nociceptive neurons to cervical input after stimulation of the dura mater. Brain 2003;126(Pt 8):1801–13.
12. Okeson JP. Diagnosis of temporomandibular disorders. Temporomandibular disorder and occlusion. 4th edition. Elsevier Mosby; 1998. p. 310–51.
13. Ciancaglini R, Radaelli G. The relationship between headache and symptoms of temporomandibular

disorder in the general population. J Dent 2001; 29(2):93–8.

14. Bevilaqua-Grossi D, Lipton RB, Napchan U, et al. Temporomandibular disorders and cutaneous allodynia are associated in individuals with migraine. Cephalalgia 2010;30(4):425–32.

15. Fernandes G, Franco AL, Gonçalves DA, et al. Temporomandibular disorders, sleep bruxism, and primary headaches are mutually associated. J Orofac Pain 2013;27(1):14–20.

16. Didier HA, Marchetti A, Marchetti C, et al. Study of parafunctions in patients with chronic migraine. Neurol Sci 2014;35(Suppl 1):199–202.

17. Plesh O, Noonan C, Buchwald DS, et al. Temporomandibular disorder-type pain and migraine headache in women: a preliminary twin study. J Orofac Pain 2012;26(2):91–8.

18. Gupta S, McCarson KE, Welch KM, et al. Mechanisms of pain modulation by sex hormones in migraine. Headache 2011;51(6):905–22.

19. Glaros AG, Urban D, Locke J. Headache and temporomandibular disorders: evidence for diagnostic and behavioural overlap. Cephalalgia 2007;27(6):542–9.

20. Dworkin SF, LeResche L. Research diagnostic criteria for temporomandibular disorders: review, criteria, examinations and specifications, critique. J Craniomandib Disord 1992;6(4):301–55.

21. Ballegaard V, Thede-Schmidt-Hansen P, Svensson P, et al. Are headache and temporomandibular disorders related? A blinded study. Cephalalgia 2008;28(8):832–41.

22. Goncalves MC, Florencio LL, Chaves TC, et al. Do women with migraine have higher prevalence of temporomandibular disorders? Braz J Phys Ther 2013;17(1):64–8.

23. Franco AL, Gonçalves DA, Castanharo SM, et al. Migraine is the most prevalent primary headache in individuals with temporomandibular disorders. J Orofac Pain 2010;24(3):287–92.

24. Mitrirattanakul S, Merrill RL. Headache impact in patients with orofacial pain. J Am Dent Assoc 2006;137(9):1267–74.

25. Goncalves DA, Camparis CM, Speciali JG, et al. Treatment of comorbid migraine and temporomandibular disorders: a factorial, double-blind, randomized, placebo-controlled study. J Orofac Pain 2013;27(4):325–35.

26. Goncalves DA, Camparis CM, Franco AL, et al. How to investigate and treat: migraine in patients with temporomandibular disorders. Curr Pain Headache Rep 2012;16(4):359–64.

27. Akerman S, Holland PR, Goadsby PJ. Diencephalic and brainstem mechanisms in migraine. Nat Rev Neurosci 2011;12(10):570–84.

28. Goncalves DA, Speciali JG, Jales LC, et al. Temporomandibular symptoms, migraine, and chronic daily headaches in the population. Neurology 2009;73(8):645–6.

29. Tanaka E, Detamore MS, Mercuri LG. Degenerative disorders of the temporomandibular joint: etiology, diagnosis, and treatment. J Dent Res 2008;87(4): 296–307.

30. Di Paolo C, Costanzo GD, Panti F, et al. Epidemiological analysis on 2375 patients with TMJ disorders: basic statistical aspects. Ann Stomatol (Roma) 2013;4(1):161–9.

31. Isberg-Holm AM, Westesson PL. Movement of the disc and condyle in temporomandibular joints with clicking: an arthrographic and cineradiographic study on autopsy specimens. Acta Odontol Scand 1982;40:151–64.

32. Farrar WB, MacCarty WL. A clinical outline of the temporomandibular joint diagnosis and treatment. Montgomery (AL): Walker Printing; 1983. p. 19.

33. Solberg WK, Woo MW, Houston JB. Prevalence of mandibular dysfunction in young adults. J Am Dent Assoc 1979;98(1):25–34.

34. Manfredini D, Guarda-Nardini L, Winocur E, et al. Research diagnostic criteria for temporomandibular disorders: a systematic review of axis I epidemiologic findings. Oral Surg Oral Med Oral Pathol Oral Radiol Endod 2011;112(4):453–62.

35. Okeson JP. Management of temporomandibular disorders and occlusion. 7th edition. Elsevier Mosby; 2013. p. 129–69.

36. Taskaya-Yylmaz N, Oğütcen-Toller M. Clinical correlation of MRI findings of internal derangements of the temporomandibular joints. Br J Oral Maxillofac Surg 2002;40(4):317–21.

37. Stegenga B, de Bont LG, Boering G, et al. Tissue responses to degenerative changes in the temporomandibular joint. J Oral Maxillofac Surg 1991; 49(10):1079–88.

38. Scapino RP. The posterior attachment: its structure, function, and appearance in TMJ imaging studies. Part 1. J Craniomandib Disord 1991;5(2):83–95.

39. Scapino R. The posterior attachment: its structure, function, and appearance in TMJ imaging studies. Part 2. J Craniomandib Disord 1991;5:155–66.

40. Tallents RH, Hatala M, Katzberg RW, et al. Temporomandibular joint sounds in asymptomatic volunteers. J Prosthet Dent 1993;69:298–304.

41. Chantaracherd P, John MT, Hodges JS, et al. Temporomandibular joint disorders' impact on pain, function, and disability. J Dent Res 2015; 94(3 Suppl):79s–86s.

42. Kozeniauskas JJ, Ralph WJ. Bilateral arthrographic evaluation of unilateral temporomandibular joint pain and dysfunction. J Prosthet Dent 1988;60: 98–105.

43. Davant TS, Greene CS, Perry HT, et al. A quantitative computer-assisted analysis of disc displacement in patients with internal derangement

using sagittal view magnetic resonance imaging. J Oral Maxillofac Surg 1993;51:974–9.

44. MF D. Intra-articular disc displacement. Part I: Its questionable role in temporomandibular joint pathology. J Oral Maxillofac Surg 1995;53:1069–72.

45. de Leeuw R, Boering G, Stegenga B, et al. Clinical signs of TMJ osteoarthrosis and internal derangement 30 years after nonsurgical treatment. J Orofac Pain 1994;8:18–24.

46. Randolph CS, Greene CS, Moretti R, et al. Conservative management of temporomandibular disorders: a posttreatment comparison between patients from a university clinic and from private practice. Am J Orthod Dentofacial Orthop 1990; 98(1):77–82.

47. Stegenga B, de Bont LG, Dijkstra PU, et al. Short-term outcome of arthroscopic surgery of temporomandibular joint osteoarthrosis and internal derangement: a randomized controlled clinical trial. Br J Oral Maxillofac Surg 1993;31:3–14.

48. Choi BH, Yoo JH, Lee WY. Comparison of magnetic resonance imaging before and after nonsurgical treatment of closed lock. Oral Surg Oral Med Oral Pathol 1994;78(3):301–5.

49. Magnusson T, Egermark I, Carlsson GE. A longitudinal epidemiologic study of signs and symptoms of temporomandibular disorders from 15 to 35 years of age. J Orofac Pain 2000;14(4): 310–9.

50. Stegenga B, de Bont LG, Boering G. Osteoarthrosis as the cause of craniomandibular pain and dysfunction: a unifying concept. J Oral Maxillofac Surg 1989;47(3):249–56.

51. DeBont LGM, Boering G, Liem RSB, et al. Osteoarthritis and internal derangement of the temporomandibular joint: a light microscopic study. J Oral Maxillofac Surg 1986;44:634–43.

52. Fricton J. Masticatory myofascial pain: an explanatory model integrating clinical, epidemiological and basic science research. Bull Group Int Rech Sci Stomatol Odontol 1999;41:14–25.

53. MH R. The neurophysiology of myofascial pain syndrome. Curr Pain Headache Rep 2001;5:432–40.

54. Gerwin RD. Classification, epidemiology, and natural history of myofascial pain syndrome. Curr Pain Headache Rep 2001;5:412–20.

55. Travell JG, Simons DG. Myofacial Pain and Dysfunction. The trigger point manual, vol. 1. Lippincott Williams and Wilkins; 1998. p. 1038.

56. Shah JP, Thaker N, Heimur J, et al. Myofascial trigger points then and now: a historical and scientific perspective. PM R 2015;7(7):746–61.

57. Kellgren JH. Referred pains from muscle. Br Med J 1938;1(4023):325–7.

58. Mense S. Considerations concerning the neurobiological basis of muscle pain. Can J Physiol Pharmacol 1991;69(5):610–6.

59. Mense S. Nociception from skeletal muscle in relation to clinical muscle pain. Pain 1993;54(3): 241–89.

60. Mense S. Referral of muscle pain new aspects. Pain Forum 1994;3(1):1–9.

61. Simons DG. Neurophysiological basis of pain caused by trigger points. APS Journal 1994;3(1): 17–9.

62. Olesen J, Jensen R. Getting away from simple muscle contraction as a mechanism of tension-type headache. Pain 1991;46(2):123–4.

63. Fields HL, Heinricher MM. Brainstem modulation of nociceptor-driven withdrawal reflexes. Ann N Y Acad Sci 1989;563:34–44.

64. Shah JP, Danoff JV, Desai MJ, et al. Biochemicals associated with pain and inflammation are elevated in sites near to and remote from active myofascial trigger points. Arch Phys Med Rehabil 2008; 89(1):16–23.

65. Pedersen-Bjergaard U, Nielsen LB, Jensen K, et al. Calcitonin gene-related peptide, neurokinin A and substance P: effects on nociception and neurogenic inflammation in human skin and temporal muscle. Peptides 1991;12(2):333–7.

66. Goadsby PJ, Edvinsson L. The trigeminovascular system and migraine: Studies characterizing cerebrovascular and neuropeptide changes seen in humans and cats. Ann Neurol 1993; 33(1):48–56.

67. Diener HC, Barbanti P, Dahlöf C, et al. BI 44370 TA, an oral CGRP antagonist for the treatment of acute migraine attacks: Results from a phase II study. Cephalalgia 2011;31(5):573–84.

68. Ho TW, Mannix LK, Fan X, et al. Randomized controlled trial of an oral CGRP receptor antagonist, MK-0974, in acute treatment of migraine. Neurology 2008;70(16):1304–12.

69. Olesen J, Mannix LK, Fan X, et al. Calcitonin gene-related peptide receptor antagonist BIBN 4096 BS for the acute treatment of migraine. N Engl J Med 2004;350(11):1104–10.

70. Romero-Reyes M, Pardi V, Akerman S. A potent and selective calcitonin gene-related peptide (CGRP) receptor antagonist, MK-8825, inhibits responses to nociceptive trigeminal activation: role of CGRP in orofacial pain. Exp Neurol 2015;271: 95–103.

71. Walsh DA, Mapp PI, Kelly S. Calcitonin gene-related peptide in the joint: contributions to pain and inflammation. Br J Clin Pharmacol 2015; 80(5):965–78.

72. Graff-Radford SB, Bassiur JP. Temporomandibular disorders and headaches. Neurol Clin 2014;32(2): 525–37.

73. Lipton RB, Bigal ME, Diamond M, et al. Migraine prevalence, disease burden, and the need for preventive therapy. Neurology 2007;68(5):343–9.

74. Estemalik E, Tepper S. Preventive treatment in migraine and the new US guidelines. Neuropsychiatr Dis Treat 2013;9:709–20.

75. Greene CS, Laskin DM. Long-term status of TMJ clicking in patients with myofascial pain and dysfunction. J Am Dent Assoc 1988;117(3):461–5.

76. de Bont LG, Dijkgraaf LC, Stegenga B. Epidemiology and natural progression of articular temporomandibular disorders. Oral Surg Oral Med Oral Pathol Oral Radiol Endod 1997;83(1):72–6.

77. de Leeuw R, Boering G, Stegenga B, et al. Temporomandibular joint osteoarthrosis: clinical and radiographic characteristics 30 years after nonsurgical treatment: a preliminary report. Cranio 1993; 11(1):15–24.

78. Kurita K, Westesson PL, Yuasa H, et al. Natural course of untreated symptomatic temporomandibular joint disc displacement without reduction. J Dent Res 1998;77(2):361–5.

79. Sato S, Sakamoto M, Kawamura H, et al. Long-term changes in clinical signs and symptoms and disc position and morphology in patients with nonreducing disc displacement in the temporomandibular joint. J Oral Maxillofac Surg 1999;57(1):23–9.

80. Minakuchi H, Kuboki T, Matsuka Y, et al. Randomized controlled evaluation of non-surgical treatments for temporomandibular joint anterior disk displacement without reduction. J Dent Res 2001; 80(3):924–8.

81. Sato S, Goto S, Nasu F, et al. Natural course of disc displacement with reduction of the temporomandibular joint: changes in clinical signs and symptoms. J Oral Maxillofac Surg 2003;61(1):32–4.

82. Michelotti A, de Wijer A, Steenks M, et al. Home-exercise regimes for the management of non-specific temporomandibular disorders. J Oral Rehabil 2005;32(11):779–85.

83. Feine JS, Lund JP. An assessment of the efficacy of physical therapy and physical modalities for the control of chronic musculoskeletal pain. Pain 1997;71(1):5–23.

84. McNeely ML, Armijo Olivo S, Magee DJ. A systematic review of the effectiveness of physical therapy interventions for temporomandibular disorders. Phys Ther 2006;86(5):710–25.

85. Medlicott MS, Harris SR. A systematic review of the effectiveness of exercise, manual therapy, electrotherapy, relaxation training, and biofeedback in the management of temporomandibular disorder. Phys Ther 2006;86(7):955–73.

86. Graff-Radford SB, Reeves JL, Jaeger B. Management of chronic head and neck pain: effectiveness of altering factors perpetuating myofascial pain. Headache 1987;27:186–90.

87. Solberg WK. Temporomandibular disorders: masticatory myalgia and its management. Br Dent J 1986;160:351–6.

88. Dao TT, Lavigne GJ, Charbonneau A, et al. The efficacy of oral splints in the treatment of myofascial pain of the jaw muscles: a controlled clinical trial. Pain 1994;56(1):85–94.

89. List T, Axelsson S. Management of TMD: evidence from systematic reviews and meta-analyses. J Oral Rehabil 2010;37(6):430–51.

90. Klasser GD, Greene CS, Lavigne GJ. Oral appliances and the management of sleep bruxism in adults: a century of clinical applications and search for mechanisms. Int J Prosthodont 2010; 23(5):453–62.

91. Abbott DM, Bush FM. Occlusions altered by removable appliances. J Am Dent Assoc 1991; 122(2):79–81.

92. Brown DT, Gaudet EL Jr, Phillips C. Changes in vertical tooth position and face height related to long term anterior repositioning splint therapy. Cranio 1994;12(1):19–22.

93. Fricton J, Look JO, Wright E, et al. Systematic review and meta-analysis of randomized controlled trials evaluating intraoral orthopedic appliances for temporomandibular disorders. J Orofac Pain 2010;24(3):237–54.

94. Greene CS, Laskin DM. Splint therapy for the myofascial pain–dysfunction (MPD) syndrome: a comparative study. J Am Dent Assoc 1972;84(3): 624–8.

95. Rubinoff MS, Gross A, McCall WD Jr. Conventional and nonoccluding splint therapy compared for patients with myofascial pain dysfunction syndrome. Gen Dent 1987;35(6):502–6.

96. Ekberg EC, Vallon D, Nilner M. Occlusal appliance therapy in patients with temporomandibular disorders. A double-blind controlled study in a short-term perspective. Acta Odontol Scand 1998; 56(2):122–8.

97. Ekberg E, Vallon D, Nilner M. The efficacy of appliance therapy in patients with temporomandibular disorders of mainly myogenous origin. A randomized, controlled, short-term trial. J Orofac Pain 2003;17(2):133–9.

98. Ekberg E, Nilner M. Treatment outcome of appliance therapy in temporomandibular disorder patients with myofascial pain after 6 and 12 months. Acta Odontol Scand 2004;62(6):343–9.

99. Jokstad A, Mo A, Krogstad BS. Clinical comparison between two different splint designs for temporomandibular disorder therapy. Acta Odontol Scand 2005;63(4):218–26.

100. Wassell RW, Adams N, Kelly PJ. The treatment of temporomandibular disorders with stabilizing splints in general dental practice: one-year follow-up. J Am Dent Assoc 2006;137(8):1089–98 [quiz: 1168–9].

101. Conti PC, dos Santos CN, Kogawa EM, et al. The treatment of painful temporomandibular joint

clicking with oral splints: a randomized clinical trial. J Am Dent Assoc 2006;137(8):1108–14.

102. Carlson CR. Psychological factors associated with orofacial pains. Dent Clin North Am 2007;51(1): 145–60.

103. Von Korff M, Dworkin SF, Le Resche L, et al. An epidemiologic comparison of pain complaints. Pain 1988;32(2):173–83.

104. Boersma K, Linton SJ. Psychological processes underlying the development of a chronic pain problem: a prospective study of the relationship between profiles of psychological variables in the fear-avoidance model and disability. Clin J Pain 2006;22(2):160–6.

105. Vlaeyen JW, Linton SJ. Fear-avoidance and its consequences in chronic musculoskeletal pain: a state of the art. Pain 2000;85(3):317–32.

106. Stowell AW, Gatchel RJ, Wildenstein L. Cost-effectiveness of treatments for temporomandibular disorders: biopsychosocial intervention versus treatment as usual. J Am Dent Assoc 2007; 138(2):202–8.

107. Gatchel RJ, Stowell AW, Wildenstein L, et al. Efficacy of an early intervention for patients with acute temporomandibular disorder-related pain: a one-year outcome study. J Am Dent Assoc 2006; 137(3):339–47.

108. Turk DC, Okifuji A, Scharff L. Chronic pain and depression: role of perceived impact and perceived control in different age cohorts. Pain 1995;61(1):93–101.

109. Malow FM, Olson RE. Changes in pain perception after treatment for chronic pain. Pain 1981;11(1): 65–72.

110. Graff-Radford SB. Regional myofascial pain syndrome and headache: principles of diagnosis and management. Curr Pain Headache Rep 2001; 5(4):376–81.

111. List T, Axelsson S, Leijon G. Pharmacologic interventions in the treatment of temporomandibular disorders, atypical facial pain, and burning mouth syndrome. A qualitative systematic review. J Orofac Pain 2003;17(4):301–10.

112. Gregg JM, RJ. Pharmacological therapy. In: Mohl ND, Zarb GA, Carlsson GE, et al, editors. A textbook of occlusion. Chicago: Quintessence; 1983. p. 351–75.

113. Wenneberg B, Kopp S, Grondahl HG. Long-term effect of intra-articular injections of a glucocorticosteroid into the TMJ: a clinical and radiographic 8-year follow-up. J Craniomandib Disord 1991; 5(1):11–8.

114. de Leeuw R, Klasser GD. Orofacial pain: guidelines for assessment, diagnosis, and management. Chicago: Quintessence Books; 2013.

115. Kopp S, Akerman S, Nilner M. Short-term effects of intra-articular sodium hyaluronate, glucocorticoid, and saline injections on rheumatoid arthritis of the temporomandibular joint. J Craniomandib Disord 1991;5(4):231–8.

116. Samiee A, Sabzerou D, Edalatpajouh F, et al. Temporomandibular joint injection with corticosteroid and local anesthetic for limited mouth opening. J Oral Sci 2011;53(3):321–5.

117. Stoll ML, Good J, Sharpe T, et al. Intra-articular corticosteroid injections to the temporomandibular joints are safe and appear to be effective therapy in children with juvenile idiopathic arthritis. J Oral Maxillofac Surg 2012;70(8):1802–7.

118. Toller PA. Use and misuse of intra-articular corticosteroids in treatment of temporomandibular joint pain. Proc R Soc Med 1977;70(7):461–3.

119. Graff-Radford SB. Myofascial pain: diagnosis and management. Curr Pain Headache Rep 2004; 8(6):463–7.

120. Silberstein SD. Preventive migraine treatment. Neurol Clin 2009;27(2):429–43.

121. Hong CZ. Treatment of myofascial pain syndrome. Curr Pain Headache Rep 2006;10(5):345–9.

122. Ernberg M, Hedenberg-Magnusson B, List T, et al. Efficacy of botulinum toxin type A for treatment of persistent myofascial TMD pain: a randomized, controlled, double-blind multicenter study. Pain 2011;152(9):1988–96.

123. Guarda-Nardini L, Stecco A, Stecco C, et al. Myofascial pain of the jaw muscles: comparison of short-term effectiveness of botulinum toxin injections and fascial manipulation technique. Cranio 2012;30(2):95–102.

124. Song PC, Schwartz J, Blitzer A. The emerging role of botulinum toxin in the treatment of temporomandibular disorders. Oral Dis 2007;13(3):253–60.

125. Türp JC, Jokstad A, Motschall E, et al. Is there a superiority of multimodal as opposed to simple therapy in patients with temporomandibular disorders? A qualitative systematic review of the literature. Clin Oral Implants Res 2007;18:138–50.

126. Türp JC, Motschall E, Schindler HJ, et al. In patients with temporomandibular disorders, do particular interventions influence oral health-related quality of life? A qualitative systematic review of the literature. Clin Oral Implants Res 2007;18:127–37.

127. Abrahamsson C, Ekberg E, Henrikson T, et al. Alterations of temporomandibular disorders before and after orthognathic surgery: a systematic review. Angle Orthod 2007;77(4):729–34.

128. Reid KI, Greene CS. Diagnosis and treatment of temporomandibular disorders: an ethical analysis of current practices. J Oral Rehabil 2013;40(7): 546–61.

129. Koh H, Robinson PG. Occlusal adjustment for treating and preventing temporomandibular joint disorders. Cochrane Database Syst Rev 2003;(1):CD003812.

130. Forssell H, Kalso E, Koskela P, et al. Occlusal treatments in temporomandibular disorders: a qualitative systematic review of randomized controlled trials. Pain 1999;83(3):549–60.

131. Tsukiyama Y, Baba K, Clark GT. An evidence-based assessment of occlusal adjustment as a treatment for temporomandibular disorders. J Prosthet Dent 2001;86(1):57–66.

132. Al-Riyami S, Cunningham SJ, Moles DR. Orthognathic treatment and temporomandibular disorders: a systematic review. Part 2. Signs and symptoms and meta-analyses. Am J Orthod Dentofacial Orthop 2009;136(5):626.e1–16.

133. Macfarlane TV, Kenealy P, Kingdon HA, et al. Twenty-year cohort study of health gain from orthodontic treatment: temporomandibular disorders. Am J Orthod Dentofacial Orthop 2009;135(6):692.e1–8 [discussion: 692–3].

134. Greene CS, Laskin DM. Long-term evaluation of treatment for myofascial pain-dysfunction syndrome: a comparative analysis. J Am Dent Assoc 1983;107(2):235–8.

135. Okeson JP, Hayes DK. Long-term results of treatment for temporomandibular disorders: an evaluation by patients. J Am Dent Assoc 1986;112(4):473–8.

136. Okeson JP. Long-term treatment of disk-interference disorders of the temporomandibular joint with anterior repositioning occlusal splints. J Prosthet Dent 1988;60(5):611–6.

137. Mejersjö C, Carlsson GE. Long-term results of treatment for temporomandibular joint pain-dysfunction. J Prosthet Dent 1983;49(6):809–15.

138. Garefis P, Grigoriadou E, Zarifi A, et al. Effectiveness of conservative treatment for craniomandibular disorders: a 2-year longitudinal study. J Orofac Pain 1994;8(3):309–14.

139. de Leeuw R, Boering G, Stegenga B, et al. Radiographic signs of temporomandibular joint osteoarthrosis and internal derangement 30 years after nonsurgical treatment. Oral Surg Oral Med Oral Pathol Oral Radiol Endod 1995;79(3):382–92.

140. Vallon D, Ekberg EC, Nilner M, et al. Short-term effect of occlusal adjustment on craniomandibular disorders including headaches. Acta Odontol Scand 1991;49(2):89–96.

141. Vallon D, Ekberg E, Nilner M, et al. Occlusal adjustment in patients with craniomandibular disorders including headaches. A 3- and 6-month follow-up. Acta Odontol Scand 1995;53(1):55–9.

142. Vallon D, Nilner M. A longitudinal follow-up of the effect of occlusal adjustment in patients with craniomandibular disorders. Swed Dent J 1997;21(3):85–91.

143. Karppinen K. Purennan hoito osana kroonisten pää-, niska- ja hartiakipujen hoitoa [dissertation]. Turkey: Annales Universitatis Turkuensis; 1995. Ser C,114.

144. Forssell H, Kirveskari P, Kangasniemi P. Changes in headache after treatment of mandibular dysfunction. Cephalalgia 1985;5(4):229–36.

145. Forssell H, Kirveskari P, Kangasniemi P. Response to occlusal treatment in headache patients previously treated by mock occlusal adjustment. Acta Odontol Scand 1987;45(2):77–80.

146. Koh H, Robinson PG. Occlusal adjustment for treating and preventing temporomandibular joint disorders. J Oral Rehabil 2004;31(4):287–92.

147. Forssell H, Kalso E. Application of principles of evidence-based medicine to occlusal treatment for temporomandibular disorders: are there lessons to be learned? J Orofac Pain 2004;18(1):9–22 [discussion: 23–32].

148. Kemper JT Jr, Okeson JP. Craniomandibular disorders and headaches. J Prosthet Dent 1983;49(5):702–5.

149. Magnusson T, Carlsson GE. Changes in recurrent headaches and mandibular dysfunction after various types of dental treatment. Acta Odontol Scand 1980;38(5):311–20.

150. Magnusson T, Carlsson GE. A 21/2-year follow-up of changes in headache and mandibular dysfunction after stomatognathic treatment. J Prosthet Dent 1983;49(3):398–402.

151. Shankland WE. Nociceptive trigeminal inhibition-tension suppression system: a method of preventing migraine and tension headaches. Compend Contin Educ Dent 2002;23(2):105–8, 110, 112–3; [quiz: 114].

152. Stapelmann H, Turp JC. The NTI-tss device for the therapy of bruxism, temporomandibular disorders, and headache - where do we stand? A qualitative systematic review of the literature. BMC Oral Health 2008;8:22.

153. Kreiner M, Betancor E, Clark GT. Occlusal stabilization appliances. Evidence of their efficacy. J Am Dent Assoc 2001;132(6):770–7.

154. Al-Ani MZ, Davies SJ, Gray RJ, et al. Stabilisation splint therapy for temporomandibular pain dysfunction syndrome. Cochrane Database Syst Rev 2004;(1):CD002778.

155. Schokker RP, Hansson TL, Ansink BJ. Craniomandibular disorders in headache patients. J Craniomandib Disord 1989;3(2):71–4.

156. Schokker RP, Hansson TL, Ansink BJ. The result of treatment of the masticatory system of chronic headache patients. J Craniomandib Disord 1990;4(2):126–30.

Cranial Neuralgias

Zahid H. Bajwa, MD[a],*, Sarah S. Smith, ANP-BC, GNP-BC[b],
Shehryar N. Khawaja, BDS, MS[c], Steven J. Scrivani, DDS, DMSc[d]

KEYWORDS

- Cranial neuralgias • Trigeminal neuralgia • Compression

KEY POINTS

- Cranial neuralgia is defined as a paroxysmal pain along a specific cranial nerve.
- Neuralgias are diagnosed by clinical exam, no objective test exists currently.
- Cranial neuralgias are treatable; treatment of these neuralgias typically start with antiepileptic medications.

INTRODUCTION

Advances in diagnostic modalities have improved the understanding of the pathophysiology of neuropathic pain involving head and face. Recent updates in nomenclature of cranial neuralgias and facial pain have rationalized accurate diagnosis. Clear diagnosis and localization of pain generators are paramount, leading to better use of medical and targeted surgical treatments.[1–5]

Cranial neuralgia is defined as paroxysmal pain along a specific cranial nerve. Old classification system categorized pain into "typical," "atypical," and "secondary" neuralgias. New nomenclature divided pain into "classical" and "symptomatic"[2] (**Boxes 1–3**). The term classical, for example, refers to trigeminal neuralgia (TN) of unknown cause. The term secondary or symptomatic defines cranial neuralgias that are due to another source such as a tumor or infection. Atypical facial pain was previously an umbrella term for less definitive facial pain symptoms. However, this term has been replaced with painful posttraumatic trigeminal neuropathy or persistent idiopathic facial pain; this better describes the lack of known mechanism of action and factors that contribute to the pain[6–9] (**Table 1**).

CLASSICAL TRIGEMINAL NEURALGIA
History

TN was first documented in the first century AD and was described in the writings of Aretaeus. At that time, treatments were primitive, including bloodletting and the administration of arsenic-, cobra-, hemlock-, and mercury-soaked bandages.[10] Centuries later, Johannes Bausch and John Locke documented clinical descriptions of TN in 1672 and 1677, respectively. French physician Nicolaus Andre, who in 1765 outlined 5 cases of "unbearable painful twitch," is credited with first recognizing the condition as a unique medical entity. Andre also coined the term *tic douloureux* ("painful spasm"). Other names for TN include prosopalgia and neuralgia of the fifth.[10–12]

In the nineteenth century, susceptibility to TN was thought to be secondary to hereditary factors, in addition to other factors such as disease, intemperance, or insufficient diet. Medical treatment was unsuccessful until the introduction of trichloroethylene inhalation in the 1920s. Before this, treatments included focusing on a nutritious diet, improved sleep, exercise, and things in moderation. Moderation was recommended because extremes in stress (including work) and toxins such as alcohol and tobacco use were thought to be

a Clinical Research, Boston Pain Care, Boston Headache Institute, Tufts University School of Medicine, Waltham, MA, USA; b Boston Pain Care, Boston Headache Institute, Waltham, MA, USA; c Orofacial Pain Training Program, Department of Oral and Maxillofacial Surgery, Massachusetts General Hospital, Boston, MA, USA; d Orofacial Pain Residency Training Program, Division of Oral and Maxillofacial Pain, Department of Oral and Maxillofacial Surgery, Massachusetts General Hospital, Boston, MA, USA
* Corresponding author.
E-mail address: zbajwa@bostonpaincare.com

Oral Maxillofacial Surg Clin N Am 28 (2016) 351–370
http://dx.doi.org/10.1016/j.coms.2016.04.001
1042-3699/16/$ – see front matter © 2016 Elsevier Inc. All rights reserved.

Box 1
International Headache Society's International Classification of Headache Disorders III

14 Categories

- Primary headaches: 1 to 4
- Secondary headaches: 5 to 12
- Painful cranial neuropathies, other facial pains and other headaches: 13 to 14
- Appendix

From Headache Classification Committee of the International Headache Society (IHS). The International Classification of Headache Disorders, 3rd edition (beta version). Cephalalgia 2013;33:629–808.

the impetus for pain attacks.[12,13] Early attempts at surgical treatments of TN were conducted by Mareschal, the surgeon to King Louis XIV of France, around 1750, and by Veillard and Dussans in 1768, but were unsuccessful. In the early nineteenth century, Bell and Megendie's description of the anatomy and function of the trigeminal and the facial nerve is thought to have been the start of subsequent effective surgical treatments. There are several different surgical approaches including middle fossa approach, demonstrated by Horsley, Taylor, and Coleman in 1981, and the subtemporal approach by Hartley and Krause in 1892. In 1925, Dandy reported a novel lateral suboccipital or cerebellar approach. He was able to observe vascular loops that were pinching on the root entry

Box 2
Painful cranial neuropathies and other facial pains

1. Trigeminal neuralgia
   a. Classical trigeminal neuralgia
      i. Classical trigeminal neuralgia, purely paroxysmal
      ii. Classical trigeminal neuralgia with concomitant persistent facial pain
   b. Painful trigeminal neuropathy
      i. Painful trigeminal neuropathy attributed to acute Herpes zoster
      ii. Postherpetic trigeminal neuropathy
      iii. Painful posttraumatic trigeminal neuropathy
      iv. Painful trigeminal neuropathy attributed to multiple sclerosis plaque
      v. Painful trigeminal neuropathy attributed to space-occupying lesion
      vi. Painful trigeminal neuropathy attributed to other disorder
2. Glossopharyngeal neuralgia
3. Nervus intermedius (facial nerve) neuralgia
4. Occipital neuralgia
5. Optic neuritis
6. Headache attributed to ischemic ocular motor nerve palsy
7. Tolosa-Hunt syndrome
8. Paratrigeminal oculosympathetic (Raeder) syndrome
9. Recurrent painful ophthalmoplegic neuropathy
10. Burning mouth syndrome
11. Persistent idiopathic facial pain
12. Central neuropathic pain
    a. Central neuropathic pain attributed to multiple sclerosis
    b. Central poststroke pain

From Headache Classification Committee of the International Headache Society (IHS). The International Classification of Headache Disorders. 3rd edition (beta version). Cephalalgia 2013;33:629–808.

> **Box 3**
> **Classification of trigeminal neuralgia**
>
> - "Classical" or primary TN: idiopathic
>   - TN type 1
>   - TN type 2 (Burchiel K: 2005)
> - "Symptomatic" or STN: associated with another disease process

zone (REZ). REZ was hypothesized to be the cause of TN.[12,13] In 1967, Peter Jannetta used an operating microscope with the posterior fossa approach confirming the vascular loop compression of the REZ that was documented by Dandy, leading to the development of the microvascular decompression (MVD) surgery.[14,15]

Epidemiology

A UK study by Brewis and colleagues[16] published in 1966 reported an incidence of 2 per 100,000. More recent studies have published an incidence of 26 per 100,000 per year between January 1992 and April 2002. TN continues to be considered a rare neurologic disorder. The incidence of TN has consistently been found to be higher in women with a 1.74:1 female:male ratio. Onset is typically after age 40 with peak occurrence

between ages 50 and 80. It is much more common in the second and third divisions of the trigeminal system and rare solely in the first division, unlike shingles (varicella zoster) (**Box 4**, **Fig. 1**, **Table 2**). If patients are younger than 40, then suspicion should be raised for a secondary cause.[17,18]

Cause and Pathophysiology

The various pathologic findings reported and complex theories advanced in the TN literature attempt to explain the combination of unique clinical features of the TN, such as

- Stereotyped paroxysms of lancinating pain, which occur in a limited part of the trigeminal territory
- Separation of the trigger area from the painful region
- Nonnoxious triggers
- Absence of sensory or motor deficit
- Characteristic response of TN to antiepileptic medications

Observation of surgical techniques and outcomes led to the twentieth century vascular compression therapy of TN; this was hypothesized by Dandy, Gardner, and Miklos as well as Jannetta. Jannetta's review of more than 4000 operative procedures ranging from 1969 to 1999 showed a

Table 1
Characteristics of cranial neuralgias

Feature	Typical Neuralgia	Atypical Neuralgia Unilateral Facial Pain	Persistent Idiopathic Facial Pain
Frequency	Intermittent	Constant, can fluctuate	Constant, less fluctuation
Pain freedom	Exists	Rare	Never
Symptom description	Electric shock, stabbing, shooting	Burning, aching	Burning, aching
Location	Unilateral, usually trigeminal	Unilateral, usually trigeminal or upper cervical	No specific cranial nerve, starts unilateral and can progress to bilateral
Sensory changes	None to mild hypesthesia	Mild to moderate hypesthesia	Hypesthesia, dysthesia, paresthesia
Precipitating factors	Trigger by nonnoxious stimuli	Rarely triggered	Not triggered
Autonomic changes	None	Rare	None
Causative factors	Vascular compression of nerve in subarachnoid space, rarely MS	Tumor, infection, trauma, or mechanical impingement of nerve, MS	None known
Common age of onset (y)	>50	30	Variable
Gender	60% female	75% female	90% female

Box 4
Key facts about trigeminal neuralgia

- Not very common (5 per 100,000 population annually)
- Typically in persons around age 60
- More often in women
- More often on the right side of the face
- More often in the region around the mouth and jaws (see **Fig. 1**)

Table 2
Characteristics of patients

	Scrivani	Combined[a]
Average age	61.5 (range: 41–95)	65
Sex	69% Female	62% Female
Side of face	58% Right	60% Right
Division involved (%)		
V-1	0	1
V-2	13	16
V-3	38	15
V-1, V-2	8	15
V-2, V-3	33	40
V-1, V-2, V-3	4	13

[a] Tew JM, van Loveren H, 1995.
Data from Scrivani SJ, Keith DA, Mathews ES, et al. Percutaneous stereotactic differential radiofrequency thermal rhizotomy for the treatment of trigeminal neuralgia. J Oral Maxillofac Surg 1999;57(2):104–11; [discussion: 111–2]; and Mathews ES, Scrivani SJ. Percutaneous stereotactic radiofrequency thermal rhizotomy for the treatment of trigeminal neuralgia. Mt Sinai J Med 2000;67(4):288–99.

rostroventral superior cerebellar artery loop compressing the trigeminal nerve either at the brainstem or distally to be the most common cause of vascular compression.[19] Compression by the posterior inferior cerebellar, vertebral, and anterior inferior cerebellar arteries has also been found. Other reported causes of compression of the nerve include meningioma, epidermoid cysts, arachnoid cysts, and schwannomas.[20] Kerr[21] proposed a peripheral versus central mechanism for TN. Kerr's peripheral hypothesis suggested that the paroxysmal neuralgic pain with TN with associated trigger zones is consistent with minor mechanical or pulsatile compression superimposed on predisposing axonal degenerative changes due to hypertension, atherosclerosis, or other diseases such as multiple sclerosis (MS).[21] King[18] argued a central cause for TN based on injections into the spinal nucleus of the fifth nerve, which resulted in a syndrome of dysesthesia of the face with hypersensitivity to tactile stimulation. The compression theory postulates that the mechanism of action involves degenerative changes to the central peripheral myelin of the trigeminal nerve, whether directly or indirectly, from the pons to the entry of Meckel cave.[22]

THE COMPRESSION THEORY

How does mild compression of the trigeminal nerve result in TN? Cutting or compressing the trunk of an undamaged nerve elicits, at most, only a brief discharge in sensory axons.[23,24] However, following a partial nerve injury, a cascade of changes takes place over time in the sensory neurons as part of the repair process.[18,23–27] It seems likely that several of these changes contribute to the signs and symptoms observed in clinical neurogenic pain disorders, including TN. Focal areas of axonal demyelination due to nerve compression generate spontaneous action potentials that travel in either direction along the nerve. In some cases, single-action potentials may evoke sustained after-discharges.[28–30] Spontaneous activity, evoked after-discharges, and abnormal coupling between primary afferents may all be important mechanisms in TN.

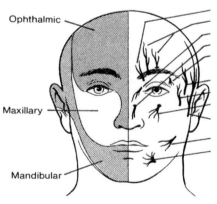

Fig. 1. Facial diagram of TN.

Devor and colleagues[31] analyzed trigeminal root surgical biopsy specimens taken from the site of presumed vascular compression. Their cases again showed evidence of demyelination and close apposition of axons in the area of compression. These anatomic findings demonstrate the right anatomic substrate for ephaptic transmission[32]: a substantial loss of myelin as well as abnormal close apposition of trigeminal axons in the area of injury. Love and colleagues[23] examined trigeminal nerve specimens from 6 patients with MS undergoing rhizotomy for intractable TN, obtaining data that strongly support the above view. In all of Love's MS cases, the trigeminal roots revealed areas of demyelination and axons in close apposition. These findings are similar to the changes seen in TN cases with vascular compression, even though the cause of nerve injury in MS is quite different. It should also be noted that ephaptic cross-talk provides a plausible mechanism to explain the "trigger zone" phenomenon. In TN, often a minimal intensity cutaneous stimulus (such as hair-bending, drinking a cool liquid, or air blowing over a small area of skin) will reliably evoke typical TN pain attacks. The trigger phenomenon is strongly consistent with interaction between large, rapidly conducting cutaneous afferents, and the smaller-caliber A-δ and C fibers that carry pain information. Ephaptic interaction between low-threshold, large-caliber sensory afferents and nociceptive sensory axons could account for this observation. Experimental studies also indicate that this anatomic arrangement favors the ectopic generation of spontaneous nerve impulses and their ephaptic conduction to adjacent fibers, and that spontaneous nerve activity is likely to be increased by deformity of the nerve and frequently associated pulsatile vasculature.[18,23,31,33]

Based on these morphologic and physiologic changes following partial nerve injury, Devor and colleagues[34] proposed an "ignition hypothesis" to explain the principal signs and symptoms in TN. In this model, a partial injury to the trigeminal roots or ganglion results in a group of hyperexcitable and functionally linked primary sensory neurons. The spontaneous or evoked discharge of individual neurons can quickly spread by ephaptic and other means to excite an entire population of adjacent sensory neurons, resulting in the sudden jolt of pain characteristic of TN. This model is attractive, not only because it explains many of the key features of TN listed at the beginning of this section but also because it encourages specific, testable hypotheses that should stimulate advances in both basic science and clinical investigation related to TN.

More conclusive evidence of the peripheral versus central cause of TN can be found in recent electrophysiological studies. One such recent study

has revealed evidence of peripheral damage to small fibers of the trigeminal nerve near the REZ in the brainstem due to demyelination and axonal degeneration or isolated advanced axonal damage on the symptomatic side in patients with classical trigeminal neuralgia (CTN). In patients with CTN and concomitant chronic facial pain, facilitation of central trigeminal processing at the supraspinal level was found, consistent with divergent results of MVD in these 2 groups of patients. Outcome data from MVD in patients with CTN show excellent or good pain relief in 97% immediately postoperatively and in 80% of those with 5-year follow-up. In patients with TN and concomitant persistent facial pain (previously defined as "atypical"), only 51% show good or excellent pain relief at 5 years.[24,25] Preoperative and postoperative electrophysiological recording sessions revealed that relief of pain correlates with normalization of previously prolonged trigeminal reflex responses. Electrophysiological testing has also been able to differentiate CTN from secondary trigeminal neuralgia (STN) with a high degree of sensitivity and specificity (92% and 95%).[26,27] Although not practical for routine patient diagnostic purposes, this research is helpful in understanding the decreased response rates in these distinct groups of patients.

Although substantial advances have been made in the understanding of the pathophysiology of TN over the past 2 decades, it is important to emphasize that many basic questions and problems remain and to re-emphasize that the cause and pathophysiological mechanism for TN is still unknown.

PROBLEMS WITH CURRENT THEORIES

Although substantial advances have been made in the understanding of the pathophysiology of TN over the past 2 decades, it is important to emphasize that many basic questions and problems remain. A few of these include the following.

THERE IS NO OBJECTIVE TEST FOR TRIGEMINAL NEURALGIA

The diagnosis of CTN is based on a history of characteristic symptoms, in the absence of any objective abnormality or clinical examination findings. The lack of an objective test to confirm the diagnosis is a significant stumbling block for research and therapy. In other common painful compression neuropathies (such as carpal tunnel syndrome or lumbar disc herniation), clinical electrophysiological studies (including nerve conduction, electromyogram, and evoked responses) demonstrate physiologic changes that at least partially correlate with clinical findings. These tests have substantial value for diagnosis, clinical correlation, and research. However, at the present time, there are no physiologic tests that sufficiently correlate with TN symptoms to make them helpful in the diagnosis or investigation of TN.

Recent studies demonstrate functional MRI abnormalities in patients with TN. These findings are encouraging, and the present authors think this line of investigation may prove useful in the near future.

TRIGEMINAL NEURALGIA PATIENTS HAVE NO CLINICAL SENSORY ABNORMALITY

Many forms of clinical or experimental nerve compression commonly result in a sensory deficit. If nerve compression is an important factor in the pathophysiology of TN, why is not a trigeminal sensory loss more commonly found in the disorder?

This question is an obvious, significant concern. However, for unclear reasons, a nerve compression injury producing facial pain does not appear to produce a sensory deficit in the trigeminal system as readily as it does at spinal levels.[35] Vos and colleagues[36] found very few patients who exhibited an associated sensory deficit. The infraorbital nerve compression model discussed earlier is also notable for an absence of any sensory loss, despite major evidence that the nerve injury results in a neurogenic pain disorder.[36]

These observations are particularly interesting because the physiologic changes following experimental nerve compression (ectopic impulse generation and after-discharges) are most prominent in large, myelinated sensory fibers rather than the small-diameter fibers that code for pain. Large myelinated sensory afferents convey light touch, joint position, and muscles spindle information. It is surprising that nerve compression would result in a painful disorder without evidence of large-fiber damage, such as paraesthesia or sensory loss. The lack of sensory deficit in patients with TN remains a puzzling and very interesting feature of the disorder.

TRIGEMINAL COMPRESSION DOES NOT PRODUCE TRIGEMINAL NEURALGIA IN ANIMALS

The animal model discussed earlier[36] provides strong experimental evidence that chronic, mild compression of the infraorbital nerve results in a trigeminal neuropathic pain disorder. However, the experimental model also shows that localized allodynia and hyperalgesia are consistent findings following infraorbital nerve (ION) compression; these sensory abnormalities are virtually never found in human clinical TN. The Vos animal model is potentially more consistent with the clinical findings of human painful trigeminal traumatic neuropathy.[36]

It is appropriate to emphasize that much of the earlier stated criticism regarding TN is based on a comparison with other neuropathic pain disorders. However, most of these other disorders result from nerve injuries that are peripheral to the sensory ganglion; TN seems to result from injuries to the segment proximal to the brain (the central segment and dorsal REZ). The biology of the peripheral and central trigeminal sensory axons segments is quite different. It is possible that the unique features of TN may, in some fashion, result from selective chronic compression of the central trigeminal axon segments.

SYMPTOMS AND SIGNS

Clear classification of TN is essential in establishing a diagnosis and conducting research. Clear classification is particularly important because there is no objective laboratory test to confirm the clinical diagnosis of TN. White and Sweet developed their own criteria to help facilitate early and accurate clinical recognition of TN.[37,38] This criterion also helped to facilitate research (**Box 5**).

The International Headache Society (IHS) recently developed new clinical diagnostic criteria for TN as part of the International Classification of Headache Disorders, 3rd edition (ICHD-III Beta)[5] (see **Boxes 1** and **2**, **Table 3**).

CTN has pathognomonic features, which differentiate from other facial pains. It is characterized by severe paroxysmal, electrical pain, which may include muscle spasms on the affected side of the face. The attacks typically last from fractions of a second to 2 minutes at a time. The pain is then followed by a refractory period during which

---

Box 5
Sweet criteria

1. The pain in TN is paroxysmal

2. The pain in TN may be provoked by light touch to the face

3. The pain in TN is confined to the trigeminal zone

4. The pain in TN is unilateral

5. In the patient with TN, the clinical sensory examination is normal

From White JC, Sweet WH. Pain: its mechanisms and neurosurgical control. Thomas; 1955.

Table 3
International Classification of Headache Disorders III beta diagnostic criteria

ICHD-III Beta Diagnostic Criteria for CTN	ICHD-III Beta Diagnostic Criteria for Painful Trigeminal Neuropathy (PTN) Head and/or facial pain in the distribution of one or more branches of the trigeminal nerve caused by another disorder and indicative of neural damage

A. At least 3 attacks of unilateral facial pain fulfilling criteria B and C
 B. Occurring in one or more divisions of the trigeminal nerve, with no radiation beyond the trigeminal distribution
 C. Pain has at least 3 of the following 4 characteristics:
   I. Recurring in paroxysmal attacks lasting from a fraction of a second to 2 min
   II. Severe in intensity
   III. Electric shocklike, shooting, stabbing, or sharp in quality
   IV. Precipitated by innocuous stimuli to the affected side of the face (note 1)
 D. No clinically evident neurologic deficit (note 2)
 E. Not better accounted for by another ICHD-3 diagnosis
	A. Unilateral head and/or facial pain persisting or recurring for 3 mo and fulfilling criterion C
	 B. Presence or history of herpetic lesions along distribution of TN, identifiable traumatic event, diagnosis of MS, a presence of space-occupying lesion, or another disorder capable of causing PTN
	 C. Evidence of causation of PTN demonstrable
	 D. Not better accounted for by another ICHD-3 diagnosis

From Headache Classification Committee of the International Headache Society. The International Classification of Headache Disorders, 3rd edition (beta version). Cephalalgia 2013;33:629–808.

the pain cannot be elicited. The pain starts and stops in an abrupt manner.[24] Spontaneous remission from pain can occur for weeks, months, or years. This feature is welcome by the patient but can also complicate accurate evaluation of treatments.[25]

The pain occurs along one or more divisions of the trigeminal nerve. It most often occurs in division 2 (V2) or division 3 (V3), or a combination of both. The first division (V1) is rare with TN.[26] Trigger zones, or areas of the face or head that on nonnoxious stimulation elicit a TN episode, are also a characteristic feature of TN. In 2 large series of patients with TN, trigger zones were reported to be present in 91% of patients.[37,39] Most often, the central part of the face near the nose and lips is a trigger zone. Touch and vibration are found to be the most noxious stimuli.[40] Attacks have been reported to be set off by washing the face, shaving, talking, chewing, brushing the hair/scalp, or a light breeze on the face. Because of the high number of stimuli that elicit the pain, patients may have poor hygiene, weight loss, dehydration, and social withdrawal in order to avoid the pain.

Over time, patients with CTN can develop persistent background pain in addition to the paroxysmal pain; this is defined as atypical TN in past literature. These patients are significantly less responsive to therapies, pharmacologic and interventional. It is hypothesized that this is due to central facilitation of trigeminal nociceptive processing in these patients in accordance with recent electrophysiological findings.[25]

Pre-TN is a syndrome that was initially documented in 1949 by Symonds.[41] In these patients, a dull aching pain involving a part of the upper or lower jaw develops. Patients may experience remission for weeks, months, or years, but these are followed by sudden onset of the paroxysmal pain of CTN. Unfortunately, some patients undergo multiple dental procedures before the syndrome is recognized and diagnosed as the early signs of TN.[41–43]

COMMENTS ON THE SWEET CRITERIA

Despite the wide acceptance of the Sweet criteria, however, few studies have actually critically analyzed the scientific foundations of this or any other TN diagnostic scheme. In most cases, diagnostic criteria for clinical syndromes develop gradually, based on the shared knowledge of experienced practitioners. The Sweet criteria are an example of this type of consensus, empirical approach.

THE PAIN IN TRIGEMINAL NEURALGIA IS PAROXYSMAL

Paroxysmal attacks of pain are the key feature, and invariably the presenting complaint of patients with TN. The pain has an electrical shocklike quality. It is sudden in onset and often severe in intensity, usually resulting in a facial grimace.

Most published descriptions of TN report a pain duration between 1 second and 2 minutes for each attack. However, this duration probably includes both the patient's initial pain and the immediate response to the attack. On more careful questioning, essentially all of the patients report an instantaneous electric shock sensation that is over in much less than a second. The pain is frequently described as a "lightning strike," an instantaneous electric jolt sensation.

Patients who describe pain that lasts for 1 or 2 minutes, particularly those who report a gradual buildup and decrement of pain symptoms, are very atypical in TN. Even though such patients may meet the other diagnostic criteria listed earlier, such patients deserve a very thorough evaluation.

It is important to emphasize another diagnostic feature of the pain in TN: between the paroxysmal attacks of pain, patients are pain free. Some patients with CTN develop a persistent background pain in addition to their paroxysmal pain. This presentation is referred to as atypical TN in much of the past and current literature. Many studies report that these patients are significantly less responsive to pharmacologic and interventional therapies than those with CTN; this may be due to central facilitation of trigeminal nociceptive processing in these patients in accordance with recent electrophysiological findings.[24] Patients with significant dull pain as part of their clinical presentation do not cleanly fit the diagnostic criteria for TN. On further evaluation, such patients often have a different syndrome, or more than one pain diagnosis.

An additional syndrome reported initially in 1949 by Symonds[41] is pre-TN. In these patients, a dull aching or burning pain involving a part of the upper or lower jaw develops for hours, days, or weeks and may be triggered by jaw movements or liquids. Patients may have several bouts of this pain with remissions for weeks, months, or years followed by sudden onset of the paroxysmal pain of CTN, which is responsive to carbamazepine and/or baclofen in most cases. Unfortunately, some patients undergo multiple dental procedures before the syndrome is recognized as an early sign of TN.[42,43]

It is worth commenting on the intensity of pain associated with attacks of TN. Many descriptions of the syndrome emphasize the severe intensity of pain associated with the disorder, to the point where "excruciating" pain becomes part of the diagnostic criteria.

Pain is a personal, subjective experience. It is difficult to meaningfully gauge and compare pain intensity between patients and across diagnoses. The clinical report of pain severity reflects not only the sensory symptom, but also the patient's psychological state and their cumulative past experience. Depression and "learned pain behavior" can amplify the subjective pain complaints of any patient with legitimate pain symptoms, including those of TN.

THE PAIN IN TRIGEMINAL NEURALGIA MAY BE PROVOKED BY LIGHT TOUCH TO THE FACE

A TN trigger zone is a localized trigeminal sensory area (facial skin or oral cavity), often only a few millimeters in size, where low-intensity mechanical stimulation (such as light touch, an air puff, or even bending a facial hair) can trigger a typical pain attack. Trigger zones are commonly present in TN,[44] but are not essential for the diagnosis. However, if present, a trigger zone is virtually pathognomonic of TN. In 2 large series of patients with TN, trigger zones were reported to be present in 91%.[37,39]

TN trigger zones are nearly exclusively found in the perioral region or nasolabial fold and can be located in either the second or the third trigeminal division. In occasional cases, a second division trigger zone can elicit pain that occurs exclusively in the third division. First-division trigger zones are rare.

The detailed studies of Kugelberg and Lindblom[40] demonstrated several additional interesting features that are typical of TN trigger zones:

1. A low threshold stimulus provokes an attack more effectively than a noxious stimulus.
2. There is a short delay between the trigger point stimulus and the evoked pain response.
3. Low-threshold trigger point stimulation demonstrates temporal summation.

After a pain attack, the trigger zone becomes relatively refractory for several seconds. During the refractory period, trigger zone stimulation is ineffective.

The trigger zone in TN is occasionally confused with the diagnostic "trigger point" frequently described in so-called myofascial pain disorders. The 2 findings are very different and should be easily distinguished by most, if not all, clinicians.

THE PAIN IN TRIGEMINAL NEURALGIA IS CONFINED TO THE TRIGEMINAL ZONE

Pain paroxysms in TN are confined to the sensory distribution of the trigeminal nerve on one side. Patients who report significant pain that extends outside the trigeminal distribution do not have TN.

Even within the trigeminal distribution, the location of pain attacks is circumscribed. The lancinating attacks of pain typical of TN most frequently occur in the third trigeminal division, radiating along the mandible. Less frequently, pain occurs in the second division or includes both divisions. First-division pain is rare in TN. In individual patients, the pain attacks are "stereotyped." In other words, they share similar features, with the same quality, location, and intensity. In some patients, the location of typical paroxysmal pain can "drift" over time within the second or third trigeminal division. However, it is rare for individual patients to experience paroxysms of pain in different trigeminal locations.

THE PAIN IN TRIGEMINAL NEURALGIA IS UNILATERAL

Paroxysmal pain attacks in TN are exclusively unilateral. Pain occurs on the right side of the face more often than on the left with predominance ranging from 59% to 66%. Reviews have reported a 3% to 5% occurrence of bilateral pain. Pain rarely occurs on both sides simultaneously. Rather, the painful paroxysms occur on one side for weeks or months and then, following a period of remission, occur on the opposite side.[28,30,45,46] Pain occurring on both sides simultaneously or in the presence of an abnormal neurologic examination should raise concerns of a secondary cause such as tumor or MS.[47,48] Occurrence of spontaneous remission of pain for weeks, months, or years is another feature of TN, which may complicate accurate assessment of therapies.[29]

THE CLINICAL SENSORY EXAMINATION IS NORMAL IN TRIGEMINAL NEURALGIA

Several clinical series describe subtle impairment of facial sensation in a minority of patients with TN.[33,43,44,49,50] However, this deficit is not usually apparent at the bedside or on a standard clinical examination. A patient who demonstrates a trigeminal sensory deficit combined with pain reminiscent of TN should raise strong clinical suspicions of another underlying disease process affecting the trigeminal system.

DIFFERENTIAL DIAGNOSIS

As mentioned earlier, there is no objective laboratory test to confirm TN. The diagnosis is made from clinical information such as the patient's history and clinical presentation. A thorough history is required, including defining characteristics, frequency, duration of pain, exacerbating factors, presence or absence of triggers, and associated symptoms to make the diagnosis. A complete neurologic examination is necessary to confirm the presence or absence of neurologic deficits. The examination can help the clinician determine if there is suspicion of a secondary cause. Secondary causes are often evaluated by more advanced testing with computed tomography or MRI/angiography (MRA). Differentiation between CTN and STN is essential because treatment of the underlying cause of STN can limit patient morbidity and mortality.

MS is a common cause for STN and should be considered in patients who are younger than 50 and present with TN. In addition to MRI testing, brainstem auditory-evoked potential and blink reflex testing are sensitive methods for evaluating for MS.[26,51–54]

Expedient treatment of the underlying disease process or lesion in these cases may limit patient morbidity and mortality and improve overall patient outcome. Although most patients with malignant and benign tumors present with sensory deficit or persistent idiopathic facial pain, the literature does contain reports of patients with tumors initially presenting with TN and no neurologic deficits. Nguyen and colleagues[55] at the Massachusetts General Hospital evaluated patients with facial pain and atypical findings and found cerebellopontine angle tumors in 4%. They reported 3 tumors: meningioma, with variable pattern of cranial nerve V, VII, VIII deficits; acoustic neuroma, with primarily cranial nerve VII deficits; and epidermoid tumor, with few signs or symptoms other than facial pain. Cheng and colleagues[56] at the Mayo Clinic reported a "Comprehensive Study of Diagnosis and Treatment of Trigeminal Neuralgia Secondary to Tumors." They evaluated 5058 patients from 1976 to 1990 with the diagnosis of TN in 2972 patients. Tumors were found in 296 of 2972 (9.95%), consisting of meningioma, schwannoma, pituitary tumor, and others, such as glioma, lymphoma, arachnoid cyst, and squamous cell carcinoma. Neurologic deficits were seen in 47%. Mathews and Scrivani,[57] at the Massachusetts General Hospital, reported on 575 patients from 1992 to 1996 with chronic neurogenic facial pain They also noted structural abnormality in many patients that fit the diagnosis of TN.

The cranial neuralgias that are covered in further depth later in this article must also be differentiated from TN. Neuralgias such as glossopharyngeal neuralgia are similar in presentation related to symptoms and duration; however, they differ in location. Glossopharyngeal neuralgia pain typically occurs in the ear, tonsils, larynx, and tongue and can radiate to the neck and shoulder. This type of neuralgia is rarely associated with patients with MS or CTN. Other neuralgias that are often mistaken for TN include tic convulsif and hemifacial spasm. Pain with tic convulsif is associated with severe otalgia in addition to the unilateral facial pain. Hemifacial spasm involves the facial nerve and is characterized by intermittent, involuntary, irregular, unilateral contractions of muscles supplied by the ipsilateral facial nerve.[58–60]

Trigeminal autonomic cephalalgias (TACs) include cluster headaches, chronic paroxysmal hemicrania, hemicrania continua, and short-lasting unilateral neuralgiform headaches either with conjunctival injection and tearing or with autonomic symptoms can sometimes be confused as TN due to the unilateral prevention of pain.[5,61] The main differentiating characteristic is that the severe and stabbing pain is associated with autonomic symptoms such as ptosis, mitosis, tearing, and rhinorrhea. The TACs are typically defined by duration of pain.

Painful ophthalmoplegia, such as seen in Tolosa-Hunt syndrome, ocular diabetic neuropathy, ophthalmic herpes zoster (HZ), and ophthalmoplegic migraine, must also be differentiated from TN. Tolosa-Hunt syndrome is a painful ophthalmoplegia due to a granulomatous inflammation in the cavernous sinus. It is characterized by episodic unilateral or bilateral orbital pain associated with paralysis of one or more of the third, fourth, or sixth cranial nerves. Involvement of the V2 and V3 divisions of the trigeminal nerve, the optic nerve, and the facial nerve has been reported. The pain is typically described as steady gnawing or boring. Spontaneous resolution may be followed by remissions and relapses of symptoms. Involvement of the optic, facial, acoustic, or trigeminal nerves has been reported. Treatment with corticosteroids results in resolution of pain and paresis in most cases within 72 hours. Failure of response to steroids or recurrence of symptoms should prompt further workup.

Ocular diabetic neuropathy may present as eye and forehead pain associated with ocular cranial nerve paresis (usually cranial nerve III). As in other diabetic neuropathies, pain improves with glucose control, treatment with tricyclics, and anticonvulsant medications.

HZ involving the trigeminal ganglion affects the ophthalmic division in most cases. Ophthalmic herpes may be accompanied by palsies of the third, fourth, and/or sixth cranial nerves or with facial palsy. Burning pain, sometimes accompanied by neuralgic pain, is followed by vesicular eruption typically within 7 days. Pain may resolve or persist as postherpetic neuralgia (PHN).

Ophthalmoplegic migraine is a rare clinical entity presenting as recurrent migrainelike headaches accompanied by paresis of one or more of the ocular cranial nerves in the absence of other intracranial lesion. There may be a latent period of up to 4 days from onset of headache to onset of ocular cranial nerve paresis. Demonstration on MRI of thickening and enhancement of the cisternal part of the occulomotor nerve in these patients suggests the cause of recurrent demyelinating neuropathy.

TREATMENT
Medication Treatment

Medical treatments include the use of antiepileptics. The use of this class of medication was first suggested by Bergouignan in 1942.[62] He trialed phenytoin in patients based on Trousseau's therapy that the paroxysmal pain of TN was similar to the paroxysmal brain activity in patients with epilepsy.[63] Surgical consultation should be sought in patients with structural lesions and in patients who are refractory to medical treatments. Patients who are unresponsive to medical therapy and those deemed to not be surgical candidates can look into treatments with radiation or percutaneous therapies. These therapies are described in later discussion.

The European Federation of Neurological Societies and the Quality Standards Subcommittee of the American Academy of Neurology currently support the use of carbamazepine as the drug of choice for treatment of TN.[64] However, more and more studies are supporting the use of oxcarbazepine as first-line treatment. Oxcarbazepine has a lesser side-effect profile and requires less laboratory monitoring compared with carbamazepine.[65]

Carbamazepine is metabolized in the cytochrome P450 isoenzyme center. The medication slows the recovery rate of the voltage-gated sodium channels, modulates activated calcium channel activity, and activates the ascending inhibitory modulation system.[66–70] The recommended starting dose is 100 to 200 mg twice daily with gradual titration until pain relief or side effects develop. The average maintenance dose of carbamazepine is 600 to 1200 mg daily in divided doses.[71] Side effects with carbamazepine include drowsiness, dizziness, constipation, nausea, and ataxia. Less common but more severe side effects include rashes, leucopenia, abnormal liver function, aplastic anemia, and hyponatremia due to inappropriate secretion of antidiuretic hormone. Monitoring of complete blood count, liver function, and sodium is recommended when using carbamazepine.[72–74]

Oxcarbazepine is the 10-keto analogue of carbamazepine. A large double-blind, crossover trial compared oxcarbapezine with carbamazepine, and 3 multicenter, double-blind randomized trials revealed oxcarbazepine to have equal efficacy with fewer side effects. Tolerability was reported as "good" to "excellent" by 62% of patients receiving oxcarbazepine compared with 48% of patients receiving carbamazepine.[73,75]

Lamotrigine also decreases repetitive firing of sodium channels by slowing the recovery rate of voltage-gated channels. In a small, double-blind, crossover, randomized controlled trial evaluating patients on carbamazepine or phenytoin who were refractory to treatment with these medications, lamotrigine (400 mg) versus placebo increased the number of patients who improved after 4 weeks of treatment.[76] Side effects include dizziness, constipation, nausea, and drowsiness. Stevens-Johnson syndrome has been reported in 1 in 10,000 patients on lamotrigine.

Phenytoin is one of the oldest anticonvulsants. It acts by blocking sodium channels in rapidly discharging neurons and inhibiting presynaptic glutamate release. There are no controlled trials supporting its efficacy despite being one of the longer used antiepileptics in the treatment of TN. Phenytoin interacts with several medications, including digoxin and warfarin. Side effects include hyperglycemia, hepatotoxicity, gingival hyperplasia, and megaloblastic anemia.[77–79]

Baclofen is an analogue of the neurotransmitter γ-aminobutyric acid. Baclofen is used in the treatment of TN because it depresses the excitatory synaptic transmission in the spinal trigeminal nucleus.[80] The starting dose is 5 mg 3 times a day with gradual titration to 50 to 60 mg per day in divided doses. Side effects include sedation, dizziness, and dyspepsia. Other medications that have shown efficacy in recent trials include subcutaneous sumatriptan and intranasal lidocaine.

In summary, the current literature supports carbamazepine as first-line therapy for TN; however, recent data also support the use of oxcarbazepine as first-line therapy. Patients who do not improve with monotherapy may benefit from adjunctive therapy with lamotrigine, baclofen, gabapentin, or a different antiepileptic drug.

Treatment of Acute Attacks

Occasionally, patients may present in acute attacks, with frequent spontaneous, or easily triggered, high-intensity jolts of pain. In this situation, some form of acute intervention is warranted because the patient's functioning is generally severely affected by the pain attacks, and if it continues, may alter their ability to be able to properly eat or drink. In such cases, the present authors have had some success with local anesthetic trigeminal division nerve blocks typically with a long-acting local anesthetic (bupivacaine). Occasionally, the application of a topical amide local anesthetic preparation (lidocaine 2%–5%) may be effective. However, there are modest amounts of good data that show that local anesthetic applications are consistently effective in stopping acute attacks and/or eliminating recurrence of pain after the duration of the applied anesthetic. Furthermore, some patients may benefit from intravenous administration of fosphenytoin (Cerebyx), valproic acid (Depacon), or lidocaine. These infusions need to be conducted in a carefully monitored setting with appropriate medical attention and emergency equipment available (outpatient surgical center or in hospital).

Nerve and Neurolytic Blockade Treatment

Local anesthetic injection or transfusion has been used for diagnostic purposes. They can also be used to temporarily reduce or eliminate TN that is refractory to medical therapy or for patients who are waiting for MVD surgery.[81] No controlled studies of nerve blockade for relief for TN have been reported. Controlled studies are needed to validate this approach. Different combinations of 4% tetracaine and 0.5% bupivacaine have provided pain relief when injected along the infraorbital nerve in patients with TN along V2. A combination of ketamine, morphine, and bupivacaine produced similar pain relief and duration as reported following a series of symptomatic peripheral trigeminal nerve branches in patients with TN.[82–84]

Careful aspiration, fluoroscopic guidance when available, using contrast (when no contraindication exists) and digital subtraction can decrease the risk of intravascular or intrathecal injection. As with intravenous injection, injections should be performed in a monitored setting with appropriate medical attention. Alcohol, phenol, or glycerol injections have long been reported in the treatment of TN. Percutaneous gangliolysis-using glycerol is discussed later. A retrospective study of patients who received peripheral alcohol injections for TN from 1994 to 1999 found a mean duration of effect of 11 months.[85] Peripheral alcohol injections are thought to be comparable in efficacy to peripheral cryotherapy. Glycerol injections provided a mean of 7 months of pain relief.[86] A retrospective analysis of 157 cases of intractable CTN treated with peripheral glycerol injections reported an initial 98% success rate with 60 patients having recurrent pain between 25 and 36 months. The study reports complete, or near complete, pain relief in 154 patients at 4 years, with inclusion of patients with recurrent pain who were reinjected.[87] No serious complications or dysesthetic pain was reported with the above described injections. In patients who did experience some facial sensory loss, sensation returned within 6 months.[88]

Surgical Treatment

Surgical treatments are meant to either damage or destroy the pain transmitting nerve fibers or relieve the pressure on the nerve at the REZ. Radiation therapy may relieve pain in patients who are not surgical candidates. Surgery should be reserved for patients who are refractory to medical management of TN.

MVD is performed under general anesthesia using a microscope to visualize the trigeminal nerve as it leaves the pons and is done by way of a suboccipital craniotomy. Repositioning of the offending artery or vein relieves compression of the nerve. Despite being invasive, MVD is associated with the best long-term outcome. Mortality and complication rates are low.[89] Barker and colleauges[90] recently reported results of 1185 patients who underwent MVD over a 20-year period. It was shown that the rates of complications were reduced and no deaths occurred after 1980 when intraoperative monitoring of brainstem-evoked response was used. Of note, female gender, symptoms lasting more than 8 years, venous compression of the terminal REZ, and lack of immediate postoperative cessation of pain were significant predictors of eventual recurrence.

Percutaneous stereotactic radiofrequency rhizotomy or gangliolysis is a better option for the elderly or debilitated patients who are not surgical candidates due to increased risk factors. Gangliolysis is performed under fluoroscopic guidance by placing a needle percutaneously through the foramen ovale and advancing it to the trigeminal cistern. The 3 techniques for gangliolysis are percutaneous radiofrequency ablation/thermocoagulation, trigeminal ganglion compression, and retrogasserian glycerol rhizolysis. Percutaneous radiofrequency ablation involves the use of radiofrequency to create lesions every 45 to 90 seconds at 60°C to 90°C. These lesions reduce the brain's ability to interpret pain signals from the trigeminal nerve. The trigeminal ganglion compression is performed by placing a catheter into the trigeminal cistern and inflating it with radiocontrast dye to compress the gasserian ganglion. This particular technique requires close monitoring because of the possibility of severe bradycardia and hypotension that may result.

Mathews and Scrivani[57] presented results of 258 patients (1991–1997) treated with radiofrequency thermal rhizotomy (RTR). Early pain relief (0–6 months) was excellent or good (successful) in 224 of 258 (87%), fair (unsuccessful) in 21 of 258 (8%), and poor (failures) in 3 of 258 (5%). There were 11% recurrences that underwent reoperation and 16% with recurrence that did not undergo reoperation. Long-term overall pain relief (12 months to 80 months) was 83%. Side effects included dysesthesia (13%), corneal anesthesia (2%), and keratitis in only 2 patients that were adequately treated.

Finally, glycerol rhizolysis occurs when anhydrous glycerol is injected into the cistern of Meckel cave.[91] The radiofrequency ablation technique provided pain relief without medication in a median of 88% of patients at 6-month follow-up; this percentage dropped to 61% at 3-year follow-up. The glycerol rhizolysis provided complete pain relief without medication in 84% at 6-month follow-up; this percentage dropped to 54% at 3-year follow-up. There are insufficient data to compare pain relief from the trigeminal ganglion compression with the other techniques. Dysesthetic changes can occur as a complication of the procedures above in 4% to 10% of patients. Other complications include corneal numbness and keratitis, anesthesia dolorous, transient masseter weakness, cranial nerve deficits, and vascular injuries.[91]

Ablative procedures are less invasive than MVD and are associated with a high initial response rate. Recurrence of pain is common, and the incidence of facial numbness is higher than that with MVD. Patients who have recurrence of pain after an ablative procedure can successfully undergo MVD surgery.[90]

Peripheral neurectomy is the surgical destruction of the peripheral branches of the trigeminal nerve and is indicated for patients who have failed medical therapy, who have failed gangliolysis, or who have severe cardiopulmonary disease and are unable to tolerate a suboccipital craniotomy with MVD. A more recent analysis of 40 patients reported good to excellent results in all 40 patients from 2 to 5 years.[92,93] The procedure can be repeated if necessary; however, the risks of developing a neuroma as well as less successful results are possible. Cryoablation of the peripheral branches of the trigeminal nerve produces a disruption of the nerve structure. This technique has been described as providing analgesia for 6 to 13 months. There are a few reports of development of atypical facial pain as a result of the procedure.[94–96]

Professor Lars Leksell first developed stereotactic radiosurgery in the 1950s. Stereotactic radiosurgery led to the invention of the gamma knife, which can precisely irradiate small intracranial targets with gamma ray photons. This technique delivers energy to the proximal trigeminal root with minimal injury to the surrounding structures.[97,98] Gamma knife surgery (GKS) is now used in conjunction with MRI to improve targeting and outcome results. Pain improvement was reported in 65% to 88% of patients; pain relief occurs a month after the procedure.[99] Complications include sensory disturbances.[100] Although radiosurgery is less effective than MVD, it is a good option for patients who are refractory to medical treatments and are not surgical candidates.[101,102] In recent years, CyberKnife radiosurgery has been developed and is an improvement on linear accelerator radiosurgery, which uses x-ray beans. GKS has the most years of clinical data. However, recent observational studies using CyberKnife radiosurgery show promising results. Long-term response rate at 11 months was 78% with CyberKnife radiosurgery.[103] Larger studies with long-term research are required to further evaluate this technique against GKS.

SECONDARY TRIGEMINAL NEURALGIA (PAINFUL TRIGEMINAL NEUROPATHY)

STN differs from CTN because there is another cause for the development of the TN pain. TN pain can be due to a lesion or a tumor. MS and benign or malignant neoplasms are the most common causes of STN, although fungal infection and bacterial infection are sometimes causes.[103–108]

MS is an inflammatory autoimmune disease that involves the development of demyelinating lesions and plaques in the central nervous system. The disease often fluctuates with periods of remyelination/remission. MS affects more women more than men, 1.77:1. The typical age of onset is the early 20s.[109] TN occurs in about 2% of patients with MS. This population of patients who have MS and TN represents only about 0.2% of patients with TN. These patients often present with unique bilateral symptoms and persistent background facial pain.[110] The pathophysiology of TN in

patients with MS is debated. Demyelinating lesions affecting the trigeminal REZ have been seen on autopsy; however, some patients have had lesions in that zone, which were clinically silent.[111,112] MVD surgery was previously contraindicated in patients with MS; however, there is a small subset of 35 patients who received 22% fair and 39% excellent long-term pain relief.[113] In general, patients with STN due to MS respond less to medical and interventional treatments. These patients may require more aggressive treatments compared with patients with CTN.

Neoplasm should be a suspicion for patients who present with CTN. Some practitioners advocate for advanced imaging with all patients presenting with CTN due to the delayed neurologic symptoms in patients with space-occupying lesions.[107] The most common posterior fossa tumors associated with STN are meningioma, epidermoid tumor, and acoustic neuroma.[114,115] Cranial nerve dysfunction, intracranial hypertension, and gait disturbance are frequent presenting symptoms with the above-mentioned tumors. Twenty cases of TN caused by contralateral tumors of the posterior fossa have been reported. Only 4 of the cases presented as CTN. The mechanism of contralateral tumor causing TN is thought to be due to displacement of the brainstem and compression of the contralateral Meckel cave.[116,117] Pain in all 3 nerve distributions of the trigeminal nerve is the first sign of a tumor in Meckel cave in 65% of patients.[118]

HZ and resulting PHN originate from the reactivation of the varicella zoster virus, which is commonly called "chicken pox" in children and "shingles" in adults. The virus remains dormant in the dorsal root ganglia of cranial and spinal nerves. The virus can reactivate along peripheral nerves if immunity is decreased due to disease, chemotherapy, and age. The virus replicates and results in direct nerve sheath and neuronal injury. Inflammation causes excitation of nociceptors and dorsal horn sensitization.[119] HZ and complications associated with HZ increase with age. HZ can involve the trigeminal nerve. Neuronal spread of the virus first occurs along the ophthalmic and less commonly the maxillary division of the trigeminal nerve. Pain occurs when the vesicular eruptions occur at the terminal points of sensory innervation. Inflammation of the eye can lead to impairment of vision or even temporary blindness. HZ involving the eye is considered a medical emergency requiring immediate treatment to avoid long-term vision loss. Acute HZ presents with a prodrome of hyperesthesia, paraesthesia, burning dysesthesia, or pruritis along the affected dermatome. Fever and general malaise often present with the prodrome phase. The prodrome precedes vesicular skin lesions by up to 3 weeks. The vesicles will leak fluid and eventually scab over in a week. During this vesicular/inflammatory stage, pain is severe. Pain that persists after the healing of the rash but resolves within 4 months is called subacute herpetic neuralgia. PHN is defined by pain persisting longer than 4 months after onset of the rash.[120] Patients with PHN often describe constant severe burning along the affected nerve in addition to allodynia. Diagnosis of acute HZ is clinical based on the distribution of the rash along a dermatome. Treatment of NZ includes treatment of the acute HZ viral infection, management of the acute pain symptoms, and prevention of PHN. Acute HZ infection is treated with antiviral medications within 72 hours of the appearance of the rash. Oral steroids are sometimes used to reduce the acute pain associated with HZ.[121] Neuropathic analgesics such as anticonvulsants and tricyclic antidepressants can be used to help reduce pain within 48 hours of the development of the rash.[122–124] Opioids are often provided to help reduce the severe pain associated with the acute phase of HZ. Patients with ocular involvement require immediate evaluation and treatment of their symptoms by a specialist.

The US Food and Drug Administration approved the varicella vaccine in May 2006. This vaccine was found to reduce the incidence of shingles by 51%. Pain was reduced by 61% in those patients who received the vaccine but still developed the viral infection. PHN was reduced compared with placebo in patients who received the vaccine.[125]

OTHER CRANIAL NEURALGIAS

Nervus intermedius neuralgia is an uncommon disorder affecting the sensory branch of the facial nerve. This disorder is often attributed to a vascular compression. The pain associated with this neuralgia is described as sharp, lancinating, and paroxysmal. The pain occurs unilaterally and deep inside the ear. It may be triggered by cold, noise, swallowing, or touch. On occasion, patients with this neuralgia may also have pain along the trigeminal nerve due to cross-compression.[126] Diagnosis is made after a thorough history and full examination to determine the distribution of the pain. Examination of the entire HEENT (head, eye, ear, nose, and throat) system is appropriate. MRI with gadolinium of the brain, cerebellopontine angle, and facial nerve should be completed in addition to an MRA. Of note, nervous intermedius neuralgia can be caused by an acute HZ infection. Treatment is similar to that with TN. When medical management is not effective, local anesthetic blocks can sometimes be helpful. If the pain does not respond to conservative measures, surgical management involves MVD or sectioning of the nervous intermedius.[127]

Glossopharyngeal neuralgia is a rare disease; this neuralgia occurs in 1% compared with TN.[128,129] Paroxysmal pain occurs in areas supplied by cranial nerves IX and X. The glossopharyngeal nerve or ninth cranial nerve exits the upper medulla. Sensory fibers supply the posterior aspect of the tongue, tonsils, pharynx, middle ear, and carotid body. Similar to TN, classical or secondary forms of this neuralgia exist. Secondary causes include tumors, abscess, aneurysm, Chiari I type malformation, and Eagle syndrome. Patients with glossopharyngeal neuralgia describe intolerable, electrical pain that is unilateral.[130–132] The pain is typically located in the ear, larynx, tonsillar fossa, or base of the tongue and occurs from seconds to minutes at a time. The attacks can occur up to a dozen times per day. Triggers include swallowing, yawning, coughing, and talking. Diagnosis is made after a thorough history and physical examination. MRI/MRA studies are typically completed to rule out secondary causes such as a mass lesion. Treatment is again similar to that with TN through medical and surgical options.[82,133]

Vagal neuralgia can be classical or secondary in nature. The 2 sensory branches of the vagus nerve are involved in this type of neuralgia. This pain is described as severe paroxysmal pain in the submandibular region, throat, and/or under the ear. Triggers include swelling, talking, yawning, coughing, and turning the head. Compression of the vagal nerve is also associated with intractable hiccups, coughing, spontaneous gagging, and dysphagia.[83,84] Similar to the other neuralgias mentioned earlier, diagnosis is made from the clinical history, examination, and oftentimes, advanced imaging. Treatment is the same as with TN. Vagal neuralgia can respond well to high-concentration lidocaine injection nerve blocks if the pain is refractory to typical conservative medications such as carbamazepine.[134] Surgical interventions such as MVD can be considered when other conservative treatments fail.[135]

OTHER TRIGEMINAL BRANCH NEURALGIAS

Even less frequent neuralgias involving the trigeminal nerve have been reported. These neuralgias include supraorbital neuralgia, nasociliary neuralgia, infraorbital neuralgia, and nummular headache. Supraorbital neuralgia typically presents as paroxysmal or even constant pain at the supraorbital notch. Small-volume local anesthetic nerve blocks can provide long-term pain relief. Medical treatment is often less effective if entrapment of the nerve is present. In that case, cryoablation or surgical release would be considered.[136,137] Nasociliary neuralgia is a localized stabbing pain lasting seconds to hours on one side of the nose. Nerve blocks are considered diagnostic with this type of neuralgia. Surgical release and section of the nasociliary nerve are often suggested.[138] Intraorbital neuralgia is often reported as a result of post-traumatic entrapment syndrome.[139] Treatment is often reduction of the zygomatic fracture and mobilization of the surrounding soft tissue. Nummular headache is considered a TN that affects a 2- to 6-cm area on the head. Nummular headache is a primary headache disorder that often goes undiagnosed. Local anesthetic nerve blocks can be diagnostic, and treatment can include botulinum toxin A injections.[140]

ANESTHESIA DOLOROSA

Anesthesia dolorosa is the perception of pain in an area that has been anesthetized; it is a complication of trigeminal nerve surgery, nerve resections, MVD, percutaneous gangliolysis, neurolytic injections, and even stereotactic radiosurgery.[141] The pain is typically described as burning, pulling, or stabbing. Patients also report an electrical element to the pain. The pain fluctuates with changes in weather and temperature. This diagnosis is made by excluding other factors. Empiric treatment with anticonvulsants, tricyclic antidepressants, and serotonin norepinephrine reuptake inhibitors can help. In some instances, intravenous lidocaine and ketamine infusions can be a second line of treatment if conservative treatments are not effective.[142,143]

Motor cortex stimulation was the recommended surgical treatment of choice for facial anesthesia dolorosa according to authors of a recent review of literature on central and neuropathic pain over the last 15 years. Motor cortex stimulation may act by replacing nociceptive with nonnociceptive sensory input at the cortical, thalamic, brainstem, and spinal level. It may also interfere with the emotional component of nociceptive perception.[144] In a prospective study of 10 patients undergoing trial and treatment with motor cortex stimulation, patients with facial weakness and sensory loss regained both strength and discriminative sensation during stimulation.[145] Multicenter randomized studies are now in progress to further evaluate this modality of treatment. Anesthesia dolorosa did not appear to respond to deep brain stimulation according to one 15-year series of 141 patients.[146]

SUMMARY

It is essential to have an understanding of neuropathic pain and the associated disorders that can affect the trigeminal nerve and other nerves in the face. Understanding the presentation, anatomy, and treatment options can lead a clinician to more accurate diagnoses and treatment options for the patient.

REFERENCES

1. Burchiel KJ. A new classification for facial pain. Neurosurgery 2003;53:1164–6 [discussion: 1166–7].
2. Headache Classification Subcommittee of the International Headache Society. The International Classification of Headache Disorders. Cephalalgia 2004;24:9.
3. Nurmikko TJ, Eldridge PR. Trigeminal neuralgia–pathophysiology, diagnosis and current treatment. Br J Anaesth 2001;87:117–32.
4. Zebenholzer K, Wober C, Vigl M, et al. Facial pain and the second edition of the International Classification of Headache Disorders. Headache 2006;46:259–63.
5. Headache Classification Committee of the International Headache Society. The International Classification of Headache Disorders, 3rd edition (beta version). Cephalalgia 2013;33:629–808.
6. Jaaskelainen SK, Forssell H, Tenovuo O. Electrophysiological testing of the trigeminofacial system: aid in the diagnosis of atypical facial pain. Pain 1999;80:191–200.
7. Nielsen LA, Henriksson KG. Pathophysiological mechanisms in chronic musculoskeletal pain (fibromyalgia): the role of central and peripheral sensitization and pain disinhibition. Best Pract Res Clin Rheumatol 2007;21:465–80.
8. Burchiel KJ. Trigeminal neuropathic pain. Acta Neurochir Suppl (Wien) 1993;58:145–9.
9. Merskey H, Bogduk N. Task Force on Taxonomy of the International Association for the Study of Pain. Classification of chronic pain: descriptions of chronic pain syndromes and definition of pain terms. 1994.
10. Cowan J, Brahma B, Sagher O. Surgical treatment of trigeminal neuralgia: comparison of microvascular decompression, percutaneous ablation, and stereotactic radiosurgery. Tech Neurosurg 2003;8:157–67.
11. Block AR, Fernandez E, Kremer E. Handbook of pain syndromes: biopsychosocial perspectives. Psychology Press; 2013.
12. Cole CD, Liu JK, Apfelbaum RI. Historical perspectives on the diagnosis and treatment of trigeminal neuralgia. Neurosurg Focus 2005;18:E4.

13. Hurd EP, Davis GS. A treatise on neuralgia. 1890.

14. Jannetta PJ. Neurovascular compression in cranial nerve and systemic disease. Ann Surg 1980;192:518–25.

15. Jannetta PJ. Arterial compression of the trigeminal nerve at the pons in patients with trigeminal neuralgia. J Neurosurg 1967;26(Suppl):159–62.

16. Brewis M, Poskanzer DC, Rolland C, et al. Neurological disease in an English city. Acta Neurol Scand 1966;42(Suppl 24):21–89.

17. Lopes PG, Castro ES Jr, Lopes LH. Trigeminal neuralgia in children: two case reports. Pediatr Neurol 2002;26:309–10.

18. Ramanathan M, Parameshwaran AA, Jayakumar N, et al. Reactivation of trigeminal neuralgia following distraction osteogenesis in an 8-year-old child: report of a unique case. J Indian Soc Pedod Prev Dent 2007;25:49–51.

19. Love S, Barber R. Expression of P-selectin and intercellular adhesion molecule-1 in human brain after focal infarction or cardiac arrest. Neuropathol Appl Neurobiol 2001;27:465–73.

20. McLaughlin MR, Jannetta PJ, Clyde BL, et al. Microvascular decompression of cranial nerves: lessons learned after 4400 operations. J Neurosurg 1999;90:1–8.

21. Kerr F. Evidence for a peripheral etiology of trigeminal neuralgia. 1967. J Neurosurg 2007;107:225.

22. Peker S, Kurtkaya Ö, Üzün I, et al. Microanatomy of the central myelin-peripheral myelin transition zone of the trigeminal nerve. Neurosurgery 2006;59:354–9.

23. Love S, Gradidge T, Coakham HB. Trigeminal neuralgia due to multiple sclerosis: ultrastructural findings in trigeminal rhizotomy specimens. Neuropathol Appl Neurobiol 2001;27:238–44.

24. Obermann M, Yoon MS, Ese D, et al. Impaired trigeminal nociceptive processing in patients with trigeminal neuralgia. Neurology 2007;69:835–41.

25. Watson JC. From paroxysmal to chronic pain in trigeminal neuralgia: implications of central sensitization. Neurology 2007;69:817–8.

26. Cruccu G, Biasiotta A, Galeotti F, et al. Diagnostic accuracy of trigeminal reflex testing in trigeminal neuralgia. Neurology 2006;66:139–41.

27. Leandri M, Parodi CI, Favale E. Early trigeminal evoked potentials in tumours of the base of the skull and trigeminal neuralgia. Electroencephalogr Clin Neurophysiol 1988;71:114–24.

28. Davis EW, Naffziger HC. Major trigeminal neuralgia: an analysis of two hundred and forty-five cases. Calif Med 1948;68:130.

29. Rushton JG, MacDonald HN. Trigeminal neuralgia: special considerations of nonsurgical treatment. J Am Med Assoc 1957;165:437–40.

30. Peet MM, Schneider RC. Trigeminal neuralgia: a review of six hundred and eighty-nine cases with a follow-up study on sixty-five percent of the group. J Neurosurg 1952;9:367–77.

31. Devor M, Govrin-Lippmann R, Rappaport ZH. Mechanism of trigeminal neuralgia: an ultrastructural analysis of trigeminal root specimens obtained during microvascular decompression surgery. J Neurosurg 2002;96:532–43.

32. Devor M. Neuropathic pain: what do we do with all these theories? Acta Anaesthesiol Scand 2001;45:1121–7.

33. Rappaport ZH, Govrin-Lippmann R, Devor M. An electron-microscopic analysis of biopsy samples of the trigeminal root taken during microvascular decompressive surgery. Stereotact Funct Neurosurg 1997;68:182–6.

34. Devor M, Amir R, Rappaport ZH. Pathophysiology of trigeminal neuralgia: the ignition hypothesis. Clin J Pain 2002;18:4–13.

35. Starke RM, Williams BJ, Hiles C, et al. Gamma knife surgery for skull base meningiomas: clinical article. J Neurosurg 2012;116:588–97.

36. Vos BP, Strassman AM, Maciewicz RJ. Behavioral evidence of trigeminal neuropathic pain following chronic constriction injury to the rat's infraorbital nerve. J Neurosci 1994;14:2708–23.

37. White JC, Sweet WH. Pain and the neurosurgeon: a forty-year experience. C. C. Thomas; 1969.

38. White JC, Sweet WH. Pain: its mechanisms and neurosurgical control. Thomas; 1955.

39. Albrecht K, Krump J. Diagnosis, differential diagnosis and possibilities for treatment of trigeminal neuralgia: with special reference to the conservative treatment with hydantoin drugs and vitamin B12. Munch Med Wochenschr 1954;96:985–7.

40. Kugelberg E, Lindblom U. The mechanism of the pain in trigeminal neuralgia. J Neurol Neurosurg Psychiatr 1959;22:36–43.

41. Symonds C. Facial pain. Ann R Coll Surg Engl 1949;4:206–12.

42. Mitchell RG. Pre-trigeminal neuralgia. Br Dent J 1980;149:167–70.

43. Fromm GH, Graff-Radford SB, Terrence CF, et al. Pre-trigeminal neuralgia. Neurology 1990;40:1493–5.

44. MacDonald BK, Cockerell OC, Sander JW, et al. The incidence and lifetime prevalence of neurological disorders in a prospective community-based study in the UK. Brain 2000;123(Pt 4):665–76.

45. Harris W. An analysis of 1,433 cases of paroxysmal trigeminal neuralgia (trigeminal-tic) and the end-results of gasserian alcohol injection. Brain 1940;63:209–24.

46. Ruge D, Brochner R, Davis L. A study of the treatment of 637 patients with trigeminal neuralgia. J Neurosurg 1958;15:528–36.

47. Jackson EM, Bussard GM, Hoard MA, et al. Trigeminal neuralgia: a diagnostic challenge. Am J Emerg Med 1999;17:597–600.

48. Gass A, Kitchen N, MacManus DG, et al. Trigeminal neuralgia in patients with multiple sclerosis: lesion localization with magnetic resonance imaging. Neurology 1997;49:1142–4.

49. Lin YW, Lin SK, Weng IH. Fatal paranasal sinusitis presenting as trigeminal neuralgia. Headache 2006;46:174–8.

50. Sawaya RA. Trigeminal neuralgia associated with sinusitis. OHL J Otorhinolaryngol Rolat Spec 2000;62:160–3.

51. Metzer WS. Trigeminal neuralgia secondary to tumor with normal exam, responsive to carbamazepine. Headache 1991;31:164–6.

52. Jamjoom AB, Jamjoom ZA, al-Fehaily M, et al. Trigeminal neuralgia related to cerebellopontine angle tumors. Neurosurg Rev 1996;19:237–41.

53. Meng L, Yuguang L, Feng L, et al. Cerebellopontine angle epidermoids presenting with trigeminal neuralgia. J Clin Neurosci 2005;12:784–6.

54. Tanaka T, Morimoto Y, Shiiba S, et al. Utility of magnetic resonance cisternography using three-dimensional fast asymmetric spin-echo sequences with multiplanar reconstruction: the evaluation of sites of neurovascular compression of the trigeminal nerve. Oral Surg Oral Med Oral Pathol Oral Radiol Endod 2005;100:215–25.

55. Nguyen M, Maciewicz R, Bouckoms A, et al. Facial pain symptoms in patients with cerebellopontine angle tumors: a report of 44 cases of cerebellopontine angle meningioma and a review of the literature. Clin J Pain 1986;2:3–9.

56. Cheng TM, Cascino TL, Onofrio BM. Comprehensive study of diagnosis and treatment of trigeminal neuralgia secondary to tumors. Neurology 1993;43:2298.

57. Mathews ES, Scrivani SJ. Percutaneous stereotactic radiofrequency thermal rhizotomy for the treatment of trigeminal neuralgia. Mt Sinai J Med 2000;67:288–99.

58. Yentür EA, Yegül I. Nervus intermedius neuralgia: an uncommon pain syndrome with an uncommon etiology. J Pain Symptom Manage 2000;19:407–8.

59. Yeh HS, Tew JM. Tic convulsif, the combination of geniculate neuralgia and hemifacial spasm relieved by vascular decompression. Neurology 1984;34:682–3.

60. Samii M, Günther T, Iaconetta G, et al. Microvascular decompression to treat hemifacial spasm: long-term results for a consecutive series of 143 patients. Neurosurgery 2002;50:712–9.

61. Bussone G, Usai S. Trigeminal autonomic cephalalgias: from pathophysiology to clinical aspects. Neurol Sci 2004;25:s74–6.

62. Bergouignan M. Cures heureuses de nevralgies faciales essentielles par le diphenylhydantoinate de soude. Rev Laryngol Otol Rhinol 1942;63: 34–41.

63. Trousseau A. De la névralgie épileptiforme. Arch Gen Med 1853;1:33–44.

64. Jorns T, Zakrzewska J. Evidence-based approach to the medical management of trigeminal neuralgia. Br J Neurosurg 2007;21:253–61.

65. Cruccu G, Gronseth G, Alksne J, et al. AAN-EFNS guidelines on trigeminal neuralgia management. Eur J Neurol 2008;15:1013–28.

66. Campbell F, Graham J, Zilkha K. Clinical trial of carbazepine (tegretol) in trigeminal neuralgia. J Neurol Neurosurg Psychiatr 1966;29:265.

67. Rockliff BW, Davis EH. Controlled sequential trials of carbamazepine in trigeminal neuralgia. Arch Neurol 1966;15:129.

68. Killian JM, Fromm GH. Carbamazepine in the treatment of neuralgia: use and side effects. Arch Neurol 1968;19:129.

69. Nicol CF. A four year double-blind study of tegretol (r) in facial pain. Headache 1969;9:54–7.

70. Wiffen P, Collins S, McQuay H, et al. Anticonvulsant drugs for acute and chronic pain. Cochrane Database Syst Rev 2005;(3):CD001133.

71. Tomson T, Ekbom K. Trigeminal neuralgia: time course of pain in relation to carbamazepine dosing. Cephalalgia 1981;1:91–7.

72. Hart RG, Easton JD. Carbamazepine and hematological monitoring. Ann Neurol 1982;11: 309–12.

73. Liebel JT, Menger N, Langohn H. Oxcarbazepin in der Behandlung der idiopathischen Trigeminusneuralgie. Nervenheikunde 2001;20:461–5.

74. Gronseth G, Cruccu G, Alksne J, et al. Practice parameter: the diagnostic evaluation and treatment of trigeminal neuralgia (an evidence-based review) report of the Quality Standards Subcommittee of the American Academy of Neurology and the European Federation of Neurological Societies. Neurology 2008;71:1183–90.

75. Beydoun A, Schmidt D, D'souza J. Oxcarbazepine versus carbamazepine in trigeminal neuralgia: a meta-analysis of three double-blind comparative trials. In: Neurology, vol. 7. Philadelphia: Lippincott Williams & Wilkins; 2002. p. A131.

76. Zakrzewska JM, Chaudhry Z, Nurmikko TJ, et al. Lamotrigine (lamictal) in refractory trigeminal neuralgia: results from a double-blind placebo controlled crossover trial. Pain 1997;73:223–30.

77. Iannone A, Baker A, Morrell F. Dilantin in the treatment of trigeminal neuralgia. Neurology 1958;8:126.

78. Braham J, Saia A. Phenytoin in the treatment of trigeminal and other neuralgias. Lancet 1960;276: 892–3.

79. McCleane GJ. Intravenous infusion of phenytoin relieves neuropathic pain: a randomized, double-blinded, placebo-controlled, crossover study. Anesth Analg 1999;89:985.

80. Fromm GH, Terrence CF, Chattha AS, et al. Baclofen in trigeminal neuralgia its effect on the spinal trigeminal nucleus: a pilot study. Arch Neurol 1980; 37:768.

81. Umino M, Kohase H, Ideguchi S, et al. Long-term pain control in trigeminal neuralgia with local anesthetics using an indwelling catheter in the mandibular nerve. Clin J Pain 2002;18:196–9.

82. Zhao K, Zuo H, Zhang L, et al. Long-term follow-up results of microsurgical treatment for glossopharyngeal neuralgia. Zhonghua Wai Ke Za Zhi 2000; 38:598–600 [in Chinese].

83. Johnson DL. Intractable hiccups: treatment by microvascular decompression of the vagus nerve: case report. J Neurosurg 1993;78:813–6.

84. Resnick DK, Jannetta PJ. Hyperactive rhizopathy of the vagus nerve and microvascular decompression: case report. J Neurosurg 1999;90: 580–2.

85. McLeod NM, Patton D. Peripheral alcohol injections in the management of trigeminal neuralgia. Oral Surg Oral Med Oral Pathol Oral Radiol Endod 2007;104:12–7.

86. Fardy M, Zakrzewska J, Patton D. Peripheral surgical techniques for the management of trigeminal neuralgia—alcohol and glycerol injections. Acta Neurochir 1994;129:181–4.

87. Erdem E, Alkan A. Peripheral glycerol injections in the treatment of idiopathic trigeminal neuralgia: retrospective analysis of 157 cases. J Oral Maxillofac Surg 2001;59:1176–9.

88. Wilkinson HA. Trigeminal nerve peripheral branch phenol/glycerol injections for tic douloureux. J Neurosurg 1999;90:828–32.

89. Kondo A. Microvascular decompression surgery for trigeminal neuralgia. Stereotact Funct Neurosurg 2001;77:187–9.

90. Barker FG, Jannetta PJ, Bissonette DJ, et al. The long-term outcome of microvascular decompression for trigeminal neuralgia. N Engl J Med 1996; 334:1077–84.

91. Lopez BC, Hamlyn PJ, Zakrzewska JM. Systematic review of ablative neurosurgical techniques for the treatment of trigeminal neuralgia. Neurosurgery 2004;54:973–83.

92. Quinn J, Weil T. Trigeminal neuralgia: treatment by repetitive peripheral neurectomy. Supplemental report. J Oral Surg 1975;33:591–5.

93. Murali R, Rovit RL. Are peripheral neurectomies of value in the treatment of trigeminal neuralgia? An analysis of new cases and cases involving previous radiofrequency gasserian thermocoagulation. J Neurosurg 1996;85:435–7.

94. Zakrzewska JM, Nally FF, Flint SR. Cryotherapy in the management of paroxysmal trigeminal neuralgia: four year follow up of 39 patients. J Maxillofac Surg 1986;14:5–7.

95. Pradel W, Hlawitschka M, Eckelt U, et al. Cryosurgical treatment of genuine trigeminal neuralgia. Br J Oral Maxillofac Surg 2002;40:244–7.

96. Zakrzewska JM, Nally F. The role of cryotherapy (cryoanalgesia) in the management of paroxysmal trigeminal neuralgia: a six year experience. Br J Oral Maxillofac Surg 1988;26:18–25.

97. Hoh DJ, Liu CY, Pagnini PG, et al. Chained lightning, part I: exploitation of energy and radiobiological principles for therapeutic purposes. Neurosurgery 2007;61:14–28.

98. Hoh DJ, Liu CY, Chen JC, et al. Chained lightning, part II: neurosurgical principles, radiosurgical technology, and the manipulation of energy beam delivery. Neurosurgery 2007;61:433–46.

99. Young R, Vermeulen S, Grimm P, et al. Gamma Knife radiosurgery for treatment of trigeminal neuralgia: idiopathic and tumor related. Neurology 1997;48:608–14.

100. Sheehan J, Pan H-C, Stroila M, et al. Gamma knife surgery for trigeminal neuralgia: outcomes and prognostic factors. J Neurosurg 2005;102: 434–41.

101. Shetter AG, Rogers CL, Ponce F, et al. Gamma knife radiosurgery for recurrent trigeminal neuralgia. J Neurosurg 2002;97:536–8.

102. Pollock BE, Foote RL, Link MJ, et al. Repeat radiosurgery for idiopathic trigeminal neuralgia. Int J Radiat Oncol Biol Phys 2005;61:192–5.

103. Lim M, Villavicencio AT, Burneikiene S, et al. CyberKnife radiosurgery for idiopathic trigeminal neuralgia. Neurosurg Focus 2005;18:1–7.

104. Kiya K, Sakoda K, Gen M, et al. A case of aspergillotic meningoencephalitis associated with trigeminal neuralgia. No Shinkei Geka 1982;10:861–6 [in Japanese].

105. Suzuki K, Iwabuchi N, Kuramochi S, et al. Aspergillus aneurysm of the middle cerebral artery causing a fatal subarachnoid hemorrhage. Intern Med 1995;34:550–3.

106. Arai M, Nakamura A, Shichi D. Case of tsutsugamushi disease (scrub typhus) presenting with fever and pain indistinguishable from trigeminal neuralgia. Rinsho Shinkeigaku 2007;47:362–4 [in Japanese].

107. Vitali A, Sayer F, Honey C. Recurrent trigeminal neuralgia secondary to Teflon felt. Acta Neurochir 2007;149:719–22.

108. Hojaili B, Barland P. Trigeminal neuralgia as the first manifestation of mixed connective tissue disorder. J Clin Rheumatol 2006;12:145–7.

109. Irizarry MC. Neurologic disorders in women. In: Cudkowicz ME, Irizarry MC, editors. Neurologic disorders in women, vol. 491. Boston: Butterworth-Heinemann; 1997.

110. Rovit RL. Trigeminal neuralgia. Baltimore (MD): Williams & Wilkins; 1990.

111. Da Silva C, Da Rocha A, Mendes M, et al. Trigeminal involvement in multiple sclerosis: magnetic resonance imaging findings with clinical correlation in a series of patients. Mult Scler 2005;11:282–5.

112. Van der Meijs A, Tan I, Barkhof F. Incidence of enhancement of the trigeminal nerve on MRI in patients with multiple sclerosis. Mult Scler 2002; 8:64–7.

113. Broggi G, Ferroli P, Franzini A, et al. Operative findings and outcomes of microvascular decompression for trigeminal neuralgia in 35 patients affected by multiple sclerosis. Neurosurgery 2004;55:830–9.

114. Roberti F, Sekhar LN, Kalavakonda C, et al. Posterior fossa meningiomas: surgical experience in 161 cases. Surg Neurol 2001;56:8–20.

115. Lobato R, Gonzalez P, Alday R, et al. Meningiomas of the basal posterior fossa. Surgical experience in 80 cases. Neurocirugia 2004;15:525–42.

116. Haddad FS, Taha JM. An unusual cause for trigeminal neuralgia: contralateral meningioma of the posterior fossa. Neurosurgery 1990;26:1033–8.

117. Florensa R, Llovet J, Pou A, et al. Contralateral trigeminal neuralgia as a false localizing sign in intracranial tumors. Neurosurgery 1987;20:1–3.

118. Mewes H, Schroth I, Deinsberger W, et al. Pain of the trigeminal nerve as the first symptom of a metastasis from an oesohaguscarcinoma in Meckel's cave—case report. Zentralbl Neurochir 2000; 62:65–8 [in German].

119. Wu CL, Marsh A, Dworkin RH. The role of sympathetic nerve blocks in herpes zoster and postherpetic neuralgia. Pain 2000;87:121–9.

120. Dworkin RH, Portenoy RK. Pain and its persistence in herpes zoster. Pain 1996;67:241–51.

121. Schmader K. Management of herpes zoster in elderly patients. Infect Dis Clin Pract 1995;4:293–9.

122. Crooks RJ, Jones DA, Fiddian AP. Zoster-associated chronic pain: an overview of clinical trials with acyclovir. Scand J Infect Dis Suppl 1991;80: 62–8.

123. Whitley RJ, Weiss H, Gnann JW Jr, et al. Acyclovir with and without prednisone for the treatment of herpes zoster: a randomized, placebo-controlled trial. Ann Intern Med 1996;125:376–83.

124. Kuraishi Y, Takasaki I, Nojima H, et al. Effects of the suppression of acute herpetic pain by gabapentin and amitriptyline on the incidence of delayed postherpetic pain in mice. Life Sci 2004; 74:2619–26.

125. Oxman M, Levin M, Johnson G, et al. A vaccine to prevent herpes zoster and postherpetic neuralgia in older adults. N Engl J Med 2005;352: 2271–84.

126. Pulec JL. Geniculate neuralgia: long-term results of surgical treatment. Ear Nose Throat J 2002; 81:30.

127. Rupa V, Saunders RL, Weider DJ. Geniculate neuralgia: the surgical management of primary otalgia. J Neurosurg 1991;75:505–11.

128. Laha RK, Jannetta PJ. Glossopharyngeal neuralgia. J Neurosurg 1977;47:316–20.

129. Chawla JC, Falconer MA. Glossopharyngeal and vagal neuralgia. Br Med J 1967;3:529–31.

130. Bryun GW. Glossopharyngeal neuralgia. In: Vinkin PJ, Gruyn GW, Klawans HL, editors. Handbook of clinical neurology. Amsterdam: Elsevier; 1985.

131. Fini G, Gasparini G, Filippini F, et al. The long styloid process syndrome or Eagle's syndrome. J Craniomaxillofac Surg 2000;28:123–7.

132. Soh K. The glossopharyngeal nerve, glossopharyngeal neuralgia and the Eagle's syndrome—current concepts and management. Singapore Med J 1999;40:659–65.

133. Sampson JH, Grossi PM, Asaoka K, et al. Microvascular decompression for glossopharyngeal neuralgia: long-term effectiveness and complication avoidance. Neurosurgery 2004;54:884–90.

134. Sato KT, Suzuki M, Izuha A, et al. Two cases of idiopathic superior laryngeal neuralgia treated by superior laryngeal nerve block with a high concentration of lidocaine. J Clin Anesth 2007;19: 237–8.

135. Kunc Z. Treatment of essential neuralgia of the 9th nerve by selective tractotomy. J Neurosurg 1965; 23:494–500.

136. Trescot AM, Helm S, Hansen H, et al. Opioids in the management of chronic non-cancer pain: an update of American Society of the Interventional Pain Physicians' (ASIPP) Guidelines. Pain Physician 2008;11:S5–62.

137. Sjaastad O, Stolt-Nielsen A, Pareja J, et al. Supraorbital neuralgia. On the clinical manifestations and a possible therapeutic approach. Headache 1999; 39:204–12.

138. Zhao Y, Li H, Cai Q, et al. Partial middle turbinatectomy and folded for nasonsociliary neuralgia by transnasal endoscopic surgery. Lin Chuang Er Bi Yan Hou Ke Za Zhi 2004;18:91–2 [in Chinese].

139. Rath E. Surgical treatment of maxillary nerve injuries. The infraorbital nerve. Atlas Oral Maxillofac Surg Clin North Am 2001;9:31–41.

140. Mathew NT, Kailasam J, Meadors L. Botulinum toxin type A for the treatment of nummular headache: four case studies. Headache 2008;48: 442–7.

141. Tatli M, Keklikci U, Aluclu U, et al. Anesthesia dolorosa caused by penetrating cranial injury. Eur Neurol 2006;56:162–5.

142. Stillman M. Clinical approach to patients with neuropathic pain. Cleve Clin J Med 2006;73:726.

143. Wallace MS. Emerging drugs for neuropathic pain. Expert Opin Emerg Drugs 2001;6:249–59.

144. Lazorthes Y, Sol J, Fowo S, et al. Motor cortex stimulation for neuropathic pain. In: Operative neuromodulation. Springer; 2007. p. 37–44.

145. Brown JA, Pilitsis JG. Motor cortex stimulation for central and neuropathic facial pain: a prospective study of 10 patients and observations of enhanced sensory and motor function during stimulation. Neurosurgery 2005;56:290–7.

146. Levy RM, Lamb S, Adams JE. Treatment of chronic pain by deep brain stimulation: long term follow-up and review of the literature. Neurosurgery 1987;21: 885–93.

Painful Traumatic Trigeminal Neuropathy

Benoliel Rafael, BDS (Hons)[a],*, Teich Sorin, DMD, MBA[b], Eliav Eli, DMD, PhD[c]

KEYWORDS

- Neuropathic pain • Trauma • Implants • Root canal therapy • Extractions

KEY POINTS

- Painful traumatic trigeminal neuropathy (PTTN) may result from a wide variety of nerve injuries, ranging from mild to severe.
- These include external trauma (altercations, road traffic accidents) and iatrogenic injuries, such as root canal therapies, extractions, dental implants, orthognathic surgery, and other invasive procedures.
- Early diagnosis and treatment are essential, because once chronic pain is established the condition is hard to treat.

INTRODUCTION

Neuropathic pain (NP) has been recently redefined as "pain arising as a direct consequence of any lesion or disease affecting the somatosensory system."[1] NP may result from active or past systemic or local diseases.[2] Neuropathic orofacial (or craniofacial) pain[3] is an umbrella term that includes a group of entities that are included in the article (see Edens MH, Khaled Y, Napeñas JJ: Intraoral Pain Disorders, in this issue) the most recent classification of the International Headache Society.[4] This excellent resource details inclusion criteria for all painful head and neck neuropathies, and is essential for all clinicians treating painful neuropathies and indeed any craniofacial pain (freely available at http://www.ihs-headache.org). There are, however, some very important nonpainful neuropathies, beyond the scope of this article, but interested readers should consult.[5]

This article presents the clinical features and pathophysiology of painful traumatic trigeminal neuropathy (PTTN). Use of the International Headache Society's classification[4] for details on inclusion criteria for all head and neck neuropathies is essential (freely available at http://www.ihs-headache.org). Description of nonpainful neuropathies is also available.[5]

PAINFUL TRAUMATIC TRIGEMINAL NEUROPATHY

PTTN may occur following major craniofacial or oral trauma[6,7] but may also be induced by relatively minor dental interventions.[8] This entity has been termed phantom tooth pain, atypical odontalgia or atypical facial pain, anesthesia dolorosa, and orofacial complex regional pain syndrome.

Neural damage can induce pain originating in a peripheral nerve (peripheral neuropathy), in a ganglion (ganglionopathy), in a dorsal root (radiculopathy), or from the central nervous system (central NP). The focus here is on pain resulting from injury to the peripheral branch of the trigeminal neuron. Pain arising as a consequence of damage to the cell soma at the level of the trigeminal ganglion or the dorsal root is usually a result of

[a] Department of Diagnostic Sciences, Center for Orofacial Pain and Temporomandibular Disorders, Rutgers School of Dental Medicine, Rutgers, The State University of New Jersey, Room D741, 110 Bergen Street, Newark, NJ 07101, USA; [b] Department of Comprehensive Care, CWRU School of Dental Medicine, 2124 Cornell Road, Cleveland, OH 44106, USA; [c] Eastman Institute for Oral Health, University of Rochester Medical Center, 625 Elmwood Avenue, Box 683, Rochester, NY 14620, USA
* Corresponding author.
E-mail address: rafael.benoliel@rutgers.edu

Oral Maxillofacial Surg Clin N Am 28 (2016) 371–380
http://dx.doi.org/10.1016/j.coms.2016.03.002

neurosurgery. Although injury at the level of the peripheral branch of the neuron may leave the cell soma and its central branch (nerve root) intact, damage at the level of the trigeminal ganglion may potentially kill the afferent completely thus deafferenting the area. Injury to the dorsal root is also different, potentially cutting all peripheral input to the central nervous system. Clearly each of these injuries needs to be examined individually, but is beyond the scope of this article.

HOW COMMON IS PAINFUL TRAUMATIC TRIGEMINAL NEUROPATHY?

It is important to stress that traumatic injuries to the trigeminal nerve largely result in either no residual deficit or in a nonpainful neuropathy. A minority, as discussed later, develop a painful neuropathy. Following identical injuries, the onset of PTTN and its characteristics vary from patient to patient. Such variability is probably caused by a combination of environmental, psychosocial, and genetic factors. A further consideration is that, relative to spinal nerves, the trigeminal nerve may show subtle differences in the pathophysiologic events that may lead to pain.[9,10]

MACROTRAUMA

In patients with zygomatic complex fractures residual, mild hypoesthesia of the infraorbital nerve is common but chronic NP developed in only 1 out of 30 patients (3.3%) followed up for 6 months.[6] This compares with about 5% to 17% in other body regions.[11,12]

IMPLANTS

Dental implants pose the risk of neuropathy secondary to direct or indirect neuronal trauma. A common neuronal complication following implant insertion is damage to adjacent nerves, altered sensory perception, and possibly pain.[13–15]

The incidence of nonpainful neurosensory disturbance ranges from 0.6% to 36%.[16–21] This large range suggests that both transient and permanent changes were included. The incidence of postimplant PTTN is unclear, but some studies suggest around 8%.

Postimplant PTTN is divided into four interrelated groups. (1) Clear and documented injury to a nerve, usually the inferior alveolar nerve, during the osteotomy or implant placement. These patients usually complain of immediate postoperative and significant sensory dysfunction in the target organ of innervation (eg, the lower lip). (2) Persistent pain associated with implants not in the vicinity of a large nerve trunk, as in most implants placed in the maxilla. In these cases there is often no clinical complaint of sensory dysfunction. Theoretically these cases may be caused by direct injury to small nerve branches and, as in all traumatic neuropathies, inflammation is involved. (3) In patients with no history of intraoperative injury and no evidence of the implant itself causing damage, but where there is proximity between the implant and a large nerve trunk. (4) Patients with apparent, implant-related complications and characterized by a good postoperative course. However, on implant-loading the patients complain of ongoing pain and "sensitivity" to mechanical (chewing, brushing) and often thermal stimuli. Radiographs usually show good osseointegration. In some of these patients, pain appears on implant loading and disappears when unloaded, or a temporary restoration is in place. In others, loading seems to trigger pain that then continues regardless of loading or type of restoration.

MANDIBULAR THIRD MOLARS

Mandibular third molar extractions are often associated with transient hypoesthesia.[22] Disturbed sensation may persist in the lingual or inferior alveolar nerve for varying episodes and has been found in 0.3% to 1% of cases.[23] Inferior alveolar nerve injuries are more common than lingual nerve damage[24–26] but the latter may commonly occur in certain extraction techniques, involving nerve retraction (up to 4%).[10] Large case series have failed to identify any NP cases.[27,28] However, complaints of tongue dysesthesia after injury may remain in a small group of patients (0.5%).

ROOT CANAL THERAPY

Nonpainful sensory changes related to endodontics are probably common and underreported. Nerve injury may be a result of apical infection or inflammation,[29,30] accidental injection of hypochlorite,[31–33] and extrusion of filling materials[34,35] that may cause chemical injury in addition to the physical insult.

Persistent pain after successful endodontics was found to occur in 3% to 13% of cases.[8,36,37] In surgical endodontics chronic NP may reach 5% of cases.[38]

Factors significantly associated with persistent pain were long duration of preoperative pain, marked symptomatology from the tooth, previous chronic pain problems or a history of painful treatment in the orofacial region, and female gender.[39,40] Recently we have found that these patients have a reduced endogenous ability to inhibit pain,[41] but it is still unclear if this is a risk factor for, or a response to, chronic pain.

LOCAL ANESTHETIC INJECTIONS

Local anesthetic injections may induce nerve injury secondary to physical trauma by the needle or by chemical insult from the anesthetic solution.[42–44] These injuries are more common in delivery of blocks to the inferior alveolar and lingual nerves. They are probably caused by the anatomic features.Findings suggest that lingual nerve injuries are more permanent than inferior alveolar nerves.[45] Lingual nerve injury is more common following repeated injections and when the injection was reported as painful.[45] The presenting features are, however, similar to other PTTNs: burning pain accompanied by paresthesia, allodynia, or hyperalgesia.

There has been discussion on the possibility that different local anesthetic agents in use (eg, lidocaine, prilocaine, mepivicaine, artocaine) may induce varying degrees of nerve toxicity,[46,47] but results had been equivocal. A paper published in 2011 showed that articaine 4% was significantly associated with nerve injury and clinical symptoms,[48] particularly when given as an inferior alveolar nerve block.[48] Based on this it would seem prudent to limit the use of 4% articaine, particularly for blocks.

CLINICAL FEATURES OF POSTTRAUMATIC TRIGEMINAL PAIN

Following identical injuries onset of NP and its characteristics vary. Such variability is probably caused by a combination of environmental, psychosocial, and genetic factors. A further consideration is that the trigeminal nerve may show subtle differences in the pathophysiologic events that may lead to pain[9,10] when compared with spinal nerves.

The considerable complexity of the sensory processing in the scenario of nerve damage or neuritis (nerve inflammation) results in altered activity by different nerve fibers and hence clinical presentation. Painful neuropathies may present with a clinical phenotype involving combinations of spontaneous and evoked pain and of positive (eg, dysesthesia) and negative symptomatology (eg, numbness).

MAJOR FEATURES OF PAINFUL TRAUMATIC TRIGEMINAL NEUROPATHY

Pain occurs in the area of injury, or at the distal dermatome of an injured nerve, and is accompanied by demonstrable sensory dysfunction, particularly if a major nerve branch has been injured.[49] The pain is unilateral.[49] It may be precisely located to the dermatome of the affected nerve, and may become diffuse and spread across dermatomes. It rarely if ever crosses the midline. Pain is of moderate to severe intensity (VAS 5–8) and usually burning or shooting.[50–53]

PTTN cases with a clear "triggering-like" mechanism have been seen but are rare.[49] These are not accompanied by a latency or refractory period (trigeminal neuralgia). More often there is severe allodynia or a positive Tinel sign.[53]

The pain is usually continuous, lasting most of the day and on most days.[49] Paroxysmal pain may be spontaneous or initiated by touch or function.[53]

Painful neuropathies present with a clinical phenotype involving positive (eg, dysesthesia) and negative neurologic symptoms (eg, numbness).[49,51,54] Hyperalgesia and other sensory changes may be found in extratrigeminal sites suggesting more extensive changes in central somatosensory processing.[55–57] Thermal modalities are usually preserved.[57,58] There are complaints of swelling (not always verifiable clinically), foreign body, hot or cold, local redness, or flushing.[49,53]

Age at onset is typically around 45 to 50 years, and patients are usually female.[49,51,58,59] It is characterized by multiple treatment modalities aimed at eliminating pain, often including pharmacotherapy, occlusal adjustments, and surgery.[51]

PTTN is associated with a substantial psychosocial burden.[51] Patients with PTTN with more severe pain demonstrate elevated levels of depression and pain catastrophizing, and substantially reduced quality of life and coping efficacy levels.[60] Pain intensity is a good predictor for quality of life measures and emotional problems, such as depression.

Theprognosis is poor. Long-term follow-up indicates that only about one-third of patients report improvement.[51,61] Only 10% to 20% report significant improvement. About half reported the same or worsened pain. Most experience some degree of pain even at an average of 13 years after onset.[51]

ASSESSING AND DIAGNOSING PAINFUL TRAUMATIC TRIGEMINAL NEUROPATHY

The symptomatology of PTTN includes sensory symptoms that may be positive (eg, hyperalgesia) and/or negative (eg, numbness) and these should be assessed and recorded using accepted terminology.[62] Some of these, such as thermal and mechanical allodynia, are frequently associated with PTTN.[63]

Many techniques are available to assess and quantify sensory changes in the affected. Advanced electrophysiologic techniques show distinct abnormalities but are not usually available in primary care.[64,65] Sensory testing should therefore be performed, preferably with quantitative and dynamic assessment.[54,55] Advanced quantitative sensory testing apparatus is not usually available in dental clinics, so dental instruments may be adapted to test gross changes. For example, a dental probe to test pin-prick sensation, warm/cool instruments for thermal sensation, and cotton wool for mechanosensation may be used. Areas affected should be carefully mapped, marked, and photographed so as to form part of the patient's documentation, evaluation, and follow-up.

Thorough clinical and imaging evaluation of orofacial structures is needed. Imaging may be needed to assess the degree of injury from a dental implant, detect foreign bodies, sequestra, and so forth. The choice of plain radiography or cone beam computerized tomography depends entirely on the case. In select cases previous (preoperative) radiographs may be of use. Trauma cases should be carefully assessed to detect fractures and other injuries.

PATHOPHYSIOLOGY OF PAINFUL TRAUMATIC TRIGEMINAL NEUROPATHY

The pathophysiology of painful inflammatory or traumatic neuropathies involves a cascade of events in nervous system function. Generally events are time dependent, progressing from the peripheral to the central nervous system. These events include alterations in functional, biochemical, and physical characteristics of neurons and glia on a background of genetic sensitivity.[66–73]

Peripheral Sensitization

This is commonly the result of tissue inflammation and initiated by inflammatory molecules produced in response to tissue injury. It develops rapidly, resulting in the activation or sensitization of nociceptors, but is reversible.

Inflammation around a nerve with no axonal nerve damage elevates spontaneous activity and induces mechanosensitivity.[74] Data show that inflammation anywhere along a nerve can be a source of pain in the organ supplied by the nerve.[75,76] If inflammation is allowed to persist, secondary nerve damage may ensue.

Peripheral sensitization is characterized by hyperalgesia (increased pain to a normally painful stimulus) and/or allodynia (ordinarily nonpainful stimuli induce pain). Common examples include irreversible pulpitis where application of cold, normally mildly painful, now induces extreme pain (hyperalgesia) and periapical periodontitis where tooth sensitivity to percussion represents allodynia.

Nerve Injury and Ectopic Activity

Nerve injury may induce cell death of involved neurons. It is often the case that the proximal stump survives and healing ensues. However, healing may involve disorganized sprouting of nerve fibers that form a neuroma.

Neuroma formation is dependent on the degree and type of nerve damage. This usually occurs when the perineurium is cut. Milder injuries, such as nerve constriction or compression, may also cause regions of neuroma formation and focal demyelination. These regions are characterized by ectopic neuronal discharge. Ectopic activity is also seen in the cell bodies of injured nerves in the trigeminal ganglia. These phenomena partly explain spontaneous NP.

Phenotypic Changes

Neuropeptide expression is altered in trigeminal ganglion following nerve injury indicating functional modification. For example, Aß fibers usually transmit innocuous stimuli, but catalyzed by inflammation or injury a phenotypic change results in the expression of substance-P.[69] Aß fibers acquire the ability to induce painful sensations in response to peripheral stimulation and may underlie the phenomenon of allodynia.

Novel Sensitivity to Catecholamines

Patients may report increased pain during periods of stress or anxiety, characterized by increased sympathetic activity. This is possibly caused by upregulation of α-adrenoreceptors in the dorsal root ganglion and the site of injury that induce sensitivity to circulating catecholamines. Basket-like sprouting of sympathetic fibers occurs around the neuronal cell bodies within the dorsal root ganglion, augmenting sensory-sympathetic interactions. This phenomenon has not, however, been experimentally detected in the trigeminal ganglion and may explain the relative rarity of sympathetically maintained craniofacial pain.[9]

Central Sensitization

Central changes are induced by ongoing activity from primary afferents transmitted to the central nervous system. Repeated primary nociceptive afferent input increasingly sensitizes the central nervous system resulting in amplified responses, a phenomenon termed "wind up." Hypersensitivity may induce activation of adjacent areas in the central nervous system. This condition is termed "central sensitization" and accounts for increased pain and spread to adjacent structures in patients with severe facial pain.

Of importance is the increasing evidence that unmanaged, ongoing pain leads to sensitization and changes in the peripheral and central nervous systems that may help establish chronic pain. Therefore, the inescapable progression of events after nerve or extensive tissue damage suggests that intervention is most effective within an early time frame. Prevention is clearly a primary objective but is not always attainable, so early treatment is essential.

CAN PAINFUL TRAUMATIC TRIGEMINAL NEUROPATHY BE PREVENTED?

Preventive analgesia, previously referred to as pre-emptive analgesia, aims to avert persistent post-surgical pain. The current term shifts the focus of possible strategies from solely before the surgery to all stages. However, reduced acute postsurgical pain has been demonstrated with such techniques; there are no reliable data indicating that the incidence of chronic pain can be reduced.[77] Notwithstanding, it is sensible in selected procedures and patients to provide a preventive strategy. This strategy could include the following:

- Minimize tissue damage and nerve involvement.
  - Consider alternative surgical approaches to avoid nerve stretching, crushing, or cutting.
- Adequate dosing and duration of preoperative anti-inflammatories and analgesics.
- Deep local or regional anesthesia to ensure no intraoperative pain.
  - Blocking regional nerve activity may also be useful in patients under general anesthetic.
- Suitable postoperative analgesic cover.

MANAGEMENT OF PAINFUL TRAUMATIC TRIGEMINAL NEUROPATHY
Pharmacotherapy

Our clinical experience in the management of PTTN suggests that this is extremely difficult to manage.[78] The mainstays of pharmacologic treatment of PTTN remain antiepileptic drugs and tricyclic antidepressants.[79–81] In contrast to the traditional 50% pain reduction for clinical significance, research has shown that about a 30% reduction represents meaningful pain relief for patients with NP.[82]

Based on current evidence pharmacotherapy of PTTN should progress as follows.[79–81] Begin with an antidepressant possessing mixed serotonin/noradrenaline (eg, amitriptyline and nortriptyline) or serotonin and noradrenaline reuptake inhibition (eg, venlaflaxine and duloxetine).[83,84] The more novel antidepressants drugs, such as duloxetine, are effective and because they have fewer side effects than the tricyclic antidepressants, are attractive aternatives.[81] If the patient's medical history precludes the use of an antidepressant, anticonvulsants are good alternatives, although they are generally inferior to antidepressants. Based on the efficacy of pregabalin and gabapentin in other peripheral neuropathies these are the recommended drugs.[81]

Failure of either of the previous strategies is an indication to begin a trial of the alternate drug, if the medical status of the patient allows (ie, move patients on antidepressants to the anticonvulsants and vice versa). Failure of this second phase is an indication to try combined therapy, if the medical status of the patient allows.Duloxetine or amitriptyline may be combined with one of the anticonvulsants, such as gabapentin or pregabalin.[85,86]

If the previous strategy fails opioids and opioid combinations may be a viable alternative. Opioids have been shown to improve painful polyneuropathies, but are less efficacious in traumatic neuropathies.[81] Opioid combinations may be advantageous, particularly gabapentin and opioid combinations,[87] such as gabapentin-oxycodone[88] or gabapentin-morphine.[89] It is important to bear in mind that opioid prescription practices have been under intense scrutiny because of their addictive and abuse potential. Strategies to prevent these must be in place in all clinics prescribing opioid drugs.

We have tested this protocol in an open study on a cohort of patients with PTTN.[78] Only 11% of patients with PTTN achieved a greater than or equal to 50% reduction in pain intensity and higher pain intensity scores were associated with a significantly reduced response to therapy. This is in line with response rates of other, similar painful neuropathies[81] and underpins the need for new drugs and other treatment options targeting chronic NP.

Topical treatments carry the benefit of minimal side effects but affected areas are not always amenable to treatment.[90] Evidence-based topicals include lidocaine or capsaicin (low and high concentrations) patches and locally injected botulin toxin A.

Cognitive Behavioral Therapy

NP, like many other chronic pains, is associated with comorbid anxiety and depression. This would suggest that psychosocial therapy (eg, cognitive behavioral therapy) might be beneficial. However, a meta-analysis did not show a significant effect of cognitive behavioral therapy on pain intensity and quality of life measures in NP.[91] Notwithstanding, psychotherapeutic support should be offered to distressed patients.

Surgery

The role of surgery in the management of nonpainful neuropathies is well established and nerve repair may improve the level of sensation in injured patients.[92–94] Surgery is marginally more successful in inferior alveolar than in lingual nerve injuries.[95,96] The presence of a neuroma is a negative prognostic factor.[97,98] Repair within 1 year of injury shows good success rates, as measured by sensory recovery.[93,98–101] About 50% of repaired cases recover with complete sensory function by 7 months.[97]

The efficacy of surgery for painful trigeminal neuropathies is unclear. Further peripheral surgical procedures (exploration, further apicoectomies) for PTTN may result in more pain. Unless there are specific indications we advise patients with painful traumatic neuropathies not to undergo further surgery.

Carefully considered surgical interventions for patients with PTTN may be justified and include exploration, release of scar tissue, decompression, and neuroma excision. All may lead to good success rates.[102] In cases where surgery is aimed at nerve repair and restoration of sensation in larger nerve branches (eg, lingual nerve), some improvement in pain may also be attained. No rigorous trials have been published.

Offending Implants: Remove or Leave?

By decompressing an injured nerve, healing may be encouraged avoiding neuropathy and pain. This may be achieved by removing the implant completely or alternatively by shortening it so there is no nerve-to-implant contact. Additionally, anti-inflammatory drugs may achieve indirect decompression by reducing edema.

There are no prospective studies that indicate whether removing is better than leaving the implant as is. Each situation needs to be weighed according to the degree of nerve injury, type of injury, and time elapsed since insertion. Clinical experience and published case reports suggest that if the implants are removed or replaced early after placement (<24–48 hours) there is a reduced incidence of neuropathy and pain.[102,103] Iatrogenic and accidental resections of nerve bundles (eg, inferior alveolar) should have an oral surgery consultation to discuss the possibility of microsurgical repair.

Management of early nerve injury beyond the previously discussed modalities should be aimed at controlling associated inflammation. If there are no contraindications, we use steroids at suitable doses (discussed next). The situation is different for offending implants that have osseintegrated; the collateral damage in removing these can be significant. We have not seen any such cases improve and the removal of implants must be weighed against the potential tissue damage and dental handicap of removing the implants. Use of anti-inflammatory drugs at a late stage does not seem to be indicated. In patients with NP pharmacotherapy should be offered as discussed previously.

Controlling Injury-Associated Inflammation

In the orofacial region, dental and other invasive procedures can generate temporary perineural inflammation, termed neuritis, which is usually asymptomatic. However, misplaced implants or periapical inflammation can induce sensory changes. The involvement of inflammation in a clinical painful neuropathy is a clear indication for anti-inflammatory therapy.

In mild cases or in cases where surgical or endodontic therapy is planned to further relieve inflammation consider the use of standard nonsteroidal anti-inflammatory drugs (eg, naproxen, 500 mg twice a day; ibuprofen, 400 mg three times a day). In severe cases with marked pain and/or sensory changes, or in milder cases where adjuvant therapy is impractical, steroids may be warranted (prednisone, 40–60 mg initially then tapered over 7–10 days; dexamethasone, 12–16 mg initially then similarly tapered). Tapering is aimed at reducing side effects from consistently high dosages. Preclinical data show that early dexamethasone relieves NP,[104] but there is no evidence from clinical studies. Common side effects include facial flushing, dyspepsia, and sleeplessness, so treatment should be as short as possible. Antacids may be coprescribed. If treatment is successful we transfer patients to a nonsteroidal anti-inflammatory drug with an antacid and continue treatment for a further 7 to 10 days.

Central Surgery

Anecdotal evidence suggests that central procedures may be useful for recalcitrant PTTN cases.[105,106] The primary choice of operation should be minimally invasive, such as computed tomography–guided percutaneous trigeminal tractotomy-nucleotomy (surgical division of the descending fibers of the trigeminal tract in the medulla), effectively ablating pathways that carry sensation from the face. Trigeminal dorsal root entry zone operation (surgical damage to a portion of neurons in the trigeminal nerve root at the brainstem level) may subsequently be performed for failures.[106]

REFERENCES

1. Haanpaa M, Attal N, Backonja M, et al. NeuPSIG guidelines on neuropathic pain assessment. Pain 2011;152:14–27.

2. Elad S, Sroussi H, Klasser GD, et al. Secondary orofacial pain and headache: systemic diseases, tumors, and trauma. In: Sharav Y, Benoliel R, editors. Orofacial pain & headache. 2nd edition. Quintessence International; 2015. p. 487–540.

3. Benoliel R, Heir G, Eliav E. Neuropathic orofacial pain. In: Sharav Y, Benoliel R, editors. Orofacial pain & headache. 2nd edition. Chicago: Quintessence International; 2015. p. 407–74.

4. Headache Classification Subcommittee of the International Headache Society (IHS). The International Classification of Headache Disorders, 3rd edition (beta version). Cephalalgia: Chicago 2013;33: 629–808.

5. Smith JH, Cutrer FM. Numbness matters: a clinical review of trigeminal neuropathy. Cephalalgia 2011; 31:1131–44.

6. Benoliel R, Birenboim R, Regev E, et al. Neurosensory changes in the infraorbital nerve following zygomatic fractures. Oral Surg Oral Med Oral Pathol Oral Radiol Endod 2005;99:657–65.

7. Benoliel R, Eliav E, Elishoov H, et al. Diagnosis and treatment of persistent pain after trauma to the head and neck. J Oral Maxillofac Surg 1994;52: 1138–47 [discussion: 1147–8].

8. Polycarpou N, Ng YL, Canavan D, et al. Prevalence of persistent pain after endodontic treatment and factors affecting its occurrence in cases with complete radiographic healing. Int Endod J 2005;38:169–78.

9. Benoliel R, Eliav E, Tal M. No sympathetic nerve sprouting in rat trigeminal ganglion following painful and non-painful infraorbital nerve neuropathy. Neurosci Lett 2001;297:151–4.

10. Fried K, Bongenhielm U, Boissonade FM, et al. Nerve injury-induced pain in the trigeminal system. Neuroscientist 2001;7:155–65.

11. Beniczky S, Tajti J, Timea Varga E, et al. Evidence-based pharmacological treatment of neuropathic pain syndromes. J Neural Transm 2005;112:735–49.

12. Macrae WA. Chronic pain after surgery. Br J Anaesth 2001;87:88–98.

13. Ardekian L, Dodson TB. Complications associated with the placement of dental implants. Oral Maxillofac Surg Clin North Am 2003;15:243–9.

14. Schmidt R, Schmelz M, Forster C, et al. Novel classes of responsive and unresponsive C nociceptors in human skin. J Neurosci 1995;15:333–41.

15. Renton T, Thexton A, Hankins M, et al. Quantitative thermosensory testing of the lingual and inferior alveolar nerves in health and after iatrogenic injury. Br J Oral Maxillofac Surg 2003;41:36–42.

16. Albrektsson T. A multicenter report on osseointegrated oral implants. J Prosthet Dent 1988;60:75–84.

17. Albrektsson T, Dahl E, Enbom L, et al. Osseointegrated oral implants. A Swedish multicenter study of 8139 consecutively inserted Nobelpharma implants. J Periodontol 1988;59:287–96.

18. Gregg JM. Neuropathic complications of mandibular implant surgery: review and case presentations. Ann R Australas Coll Dent Surg 2000;15: 176–80.

19. Higuchi KW, Folmer T, Kultje C. Implant survival rates in partially edentulous patients: a 3-year prospective multicenter study. J Oral Maxillofac Surg 1995;53:264–8.

20. Lazzara R, Siddiqui AA, Binon P, et al. Retrospective multicenter analysis of 3i endosseous dental implants placed over a five-year period. Clin Oral Implants Res 1996;7:73–83.

21. Haas DA, Lennon D. A 21 year retrospective study of reports of paresthesia following local anesthetic administration. J Can Dent Assoc 1995;61:319–20, 323–16, 329–30.

22. Barron RP, Benoliel R, Zeltser R, et al. Effect of dexamethasone and dipyrone on lingual and inferior alveolar nerve hypersensitivity following third molar extractions: preliminary report. J Orofac Pain 2004;18:62–8.

23. Valmaseda-Castellon E, Berini-Aytes L, Gay-Escoda C. Inferior alveolar nerve damage after lower third molar surgical extraction: a prospective study of 1117 surgical extractions. Oral Surg Oral Med Oral Pathol Oral Radiol Endod 2001;92: 377–83.

24. Gomes AC, Vasconcelos BC, de Oliveira e Silva ED, et al. Lingual nerve damage after mandibular third molar surgery: a randomized clinical trial. J Oral Maxillofac Surg 2005;63:1443–6.

25. Queral-Godoy E, Figueiredo R, Valmaseda-Castellon E, et al. Frequency and evolution of lingual nerve lesions following lower third molar extraction. J Oral Maxillofac Surg 2006;64:402–7.

26. Robert RC, Bacchetti P, Pogrel MA. Frequency of trigeminal nerve injuries following third molar removal. J Oral Maxillofac Surg 2005;63:732–5 [discussion: 736].

27. Berge TI. Incidence of chronic neuropathic pain subsequent to surgical removal of impacted third molars. Acta Odontol Scand 2002;60:108–12.

28. Valmaseda-Castellon E, Berini-Aytes L, Gay-Escoda C. Lingual nerve damage after third

lower molar surgical extraction. Oral Surg Oral Med Oral Pathol Oral Radiol Endod 2000;90:567–73.

29. von Ohle C, ElAyouti A. Neurosensory impairment of the mental nerve as a sequel of periapical periodontitis: case report and review. Oral Surg Oral Med Oral Pathol Oral Radiol Endod 2010;110: e84–9.

30. Ozkan BT, Celik S, Durmus E. Paresthesia of the mental nerve stem from periapical infection of mandibular canine tooth: a case report. Oral Surg Oral Med Oral Pathol Oral Radiol Endod 2008; 105:e28–31.

31. Singh PK. Root canal complications: 'the hypochlorite accident'. SADJ 2010;65:416–9.

32. Motta MV, Chaves-Mendonca MA, Stirton CG, et al. Accidental injection with sodium hypochlorite: report of a case. Int Endod J 2009;42:175–82.

33. Witton R, Henthorn K, Ethunandan M, et al. Neurological complications following extrusion of sodium hypochlorite solution during root canal treatment. Int Endod J 2005;38:843–8.

34. Lopez-Lopez J, Estrugo-Devesa A, Jane-Salas E, et al. Inferior alveolar nerve injury resulting from overextension of an endodontic sealer: nonsurgical management using the GABA analogue pregabalin. Int Endod J 2012;45:98–104.

35. Gambarini G, Plotino G, Grande NM, et al. Differential diagnosis of endodontic-related inferior alveolar nerve paraesthesia with cone beam computed tomography: a case report. Int Endod J 2011;44: 176–81.

36. Marbach JJ, Hulbrock J, Hohn C, et al. Incidence of phantom tooth pain: an atypical facial neuralgia. Oral Surg Oral Med Oral Pathol 1982;53:190–3.

37. Lobb WK, Zakariasen KL, McGrath PJ. Endodontic treatment outcomes: do patients perceive problems? J Am Dent Assoc 1996;127:597–600.

38. Campbell RL, Parks KW, Dodds RN. Chronic facial pain associated with endodontic therapy. Oral Surg Oral Med Oral Pathol 1990;69:287–90.

39. Klasser GD, Kugelmann AM, Villines D, et al. The prevalence of persistent pain after nonsurgical root canal. Quintessence Int 2011;42:259–69.

40. Nixdorf DR, Moana-Filho EJ, Law AS, et al. Frequency of persistent tooth pain after root canal therapy: a systematic review and meta-analysis. J Endod 2010;36:224–30.

41. Nasri-Heir C, Khan J, Benoliel R, et al. Altered pain modulation in patients with persistent postendodontic pain. Pain 2015;156:2032–41.

42. Smith MH, Lung KE. Nerve injuries after dental injection: a review of the literature. J Can Dent Assoc 2006;72:559–64.

43. Sambrook PJ, Goss AN. Severe adverse reactions to dental local anaesthetics: prolonged mandibular and lingual nerve anaesthesia. Aust Dent J 2011; 56:154–9.

44. Moon S, Lee SJ, Kim E, et al. Hypoesthesia after IAN block anesthesia with lidocaine: management of mild to moderate nerve injury. Restor Dent Endod 2012;37:232–5.

45. Renton T, Adey-Viscuso D, Meechan JG, et al. Trigeminal nerve injuries in relation to the local anaesthesia in mandibular injections. Br Dent J 2010;209:E15.

46. Pogrel MA. Permanent nerve damage from inferior alveolar nerve blocks: an update to include articaine. J Calif Dent Assoc 2007;35: 271–3.

47. Haas DA. Articaine and paresthesia: epidemiological studies. J Am Coll Dent 2006;73:5–10.

48. Hillerup S, Jensen RH, Ersboll BK. Trigeminal nerve injury associated with injection of local anesthetics: needle lesion or neurotoxicity? J Am Dent Assoc 2011;142:531–9.

49. Benoliel R, Zadik Y, Eliav E, et al. Peripheral painful traumatic trigeminal neuropathy: clinical features in 91 cases and proposal of novel diagnostic criteria. J Orofac Pain 2012;26:49–58.

50. Renton T, Yilmaz Z, Gaballah K. Evaluation of trigeminal nerve injuries in relation to third molar surgery in a prospective patient cohort. Recommendations for prevention. Int J Oral Maxillofac Surg 2012;41:1509–18.

51. Pigg M, Svensson P, Drangsholt M, et al. Seven-year follow-up of patients diagnosed with atypical odontalgia: a prospective study. J Orofac Pain 2013;27:151–64.

52. Baad-Hansen L, Leijon G, Svensson P, et al. Comparison of clinical findings and psychosocial factors in patients with atypical odontalgia and temporomandibular disorders. J Orofac Pain 2008;22:7–14.

53. Renton T, Yilmaz Z. Profiling of patients presenting with posttraumatic neuropathy of the trigeminal nerve. J Orofac Pain 2011;25:333–44.

54. Svensson P, Baad-Hansen L, Pigg M, et al. Guidelines and recommendations for assessment of somatosensory function in oro-facial pain conditions–a taskforce report. J Oral Rehabil 2011;38: 366–94.

55. Baad-Hansen L, Pigg M, Ivanovic SE, et al. Chairside intraoral qualitative somatosensory testing: reliability and comparison between patients with atypical odontalgia and healthy controls. J Orofac Pain 2013;27:165–70.

56. Baad-Hansen L, Pigg M, Ivanovic SE, et al. Intraoral somatosensory abnormalities in patients with atypical odontalgia: a controlled multicenter quantitative sensory testing study. Pain 2013;154: 1287–94.

57. List T, Leijon G, Svensson P. Somatosensory abnormalities in atypical odontalgia: a case-control study. Pain 2008;139:333–41.

58. Siqueira SR, Siviero M, Alvarez FK, et al. Quantitative sensory testing in trigeminal traumatic neuropathic pain and persistent idiopathic facial pain. Arq Neuropsiquiatr 2013;71:174–9.

59. Penarrocha MA, Penarrocha D, Bagan JV, et al. Post-traumatic trigeminal neuropathy. A study of 63 cases. Med Oral Patol Oral Cir Bucal 2012;17: e297–300.

60. Smith JG, Elias LA, Yilmaz Z, et al. The psychosocial and affective burden of posttraumatic neuropathy following injuries to the trigeminal nerve. J Orofac Pain 2013;27:293–303.

61. Pogrel MA, Jergensen R, Burgon E, et al. Long-term outcome of trigeminal nerve injuries related to dental treatment. J Oral Maxillofac Surg 2011; 69:2284–8.

62. International Association for the Study of Pain (IASP). IASP taxonomy. 2nd edition. IASP; 2012. Available at: http://www.iasp-pain.org/Taxonomy. Accessed April 14, 2016.

63. Rasmussen PV, Sindrup SH, Jensen TS, et al. Symptoms and signs in patients with suspected neuropathic pain. Pain 2004;110:461–9.

64. Baad-Hansen L, List T, Kaube H, et al. Blink reflexes in patients with atypical odontalgia and matched healthy controls. Exp Brain Res 2006; 172:498–506.

65. Jaaskelainen SK. The utility of clinical neurophysiological and quantitative sensory testing for trigeminal neuropathy. J Orofac Pain 2004;18:355–9.

66. Salter MW, Beggs S. Sublime microglia: expanding roles for the guardians of the CNS. Cell 2014;158: 15–24.

67. Lee MC, Tracey I. Imaging pain: a potent means for investigating pain mechanisms in patients. Br J Anaesth 2013;111:64–72.

68. von Hehn CA, Baron R, Woolf CJ. Deconstructing the neuropathic pain phenotype to reveal neural mechanisms. Neuron 2012;73:638–52.

69. Nitzan-Luques A, Devor M, Tal M. Genotype-selective phenotypic switch in primary afferent neurons contributes to neuropathic pain. Pain 2011;152: 2413–26.

70. Devor M. Ectopic discharge in Abeta afferents as a source of neuropathic pain. Exp Brain Res 2009; 196:115–28.

71. Woolf CJ, Salter MW. Neuronal plasticity: increasing the gain in pain. Science 2000;288:1765–9.

72. Mogil JS. Pain genetics: past, present and future. Trends Genet 2012;28:258–66.

73. Salter MW. Deepening understanding of the neural substrates of chronic pain. Brain 2014;137:651–3.

74. Eliav E, Benoliel R, Tal M. Inflammation with no axonal damage of the rat saphenous nerve trunk induces ectopic discharge and mechanosensitivity in myelinated axons. Neurosci Lett 2001; 311:49–52.

75. Benoliel R, Eliav E, Tal M. Strain-dependent modification of neuropathic pain behaviour in the rat hindpaw by a priming painful trigeminal nerve injury. Pain 2002;97:203–12.

76. Chacur M, Milligan ED, Gazda LS, et al. A new model of sciatic inflammatory neuritis (SIN): induction of unilateral and bilateral mechanical allodynia following acute unilateral peri-sciatic immune activation in rats. Pain 2001;94:231–44.

77. Dworkin RH, McDermott MP, Raja SN. Preventing chronic postsurgical pain: how much of a difference makes a difference? Anesthesiology 2010; 112:516–8.

78. Haviv Y, Zadik Y, Sharav Y, et al. Painful traumatic trigeminal neuropathy: an open study on the pharmacotherapeutic response to stepped treatment. J Oral Facial Pain Headache 2014; 28:52–60.

79. Attal N, Cruccu G, Baron R, et al. EFNS guidelines on the pharmacological treatment of neuropathic pain: 2010 revision. Eur J Neurol 2010;17: 1113–e1188.

80. Dworkin RH, O'Connor AB, Audette J, et al. Recommendations for the pharmacological management of neuropathic pain: an overview and literature update. Mayo Clin Proc 2010;85:S3–14.

81. Finnerup NB, Sindrup SH, Jensen TS. The evidence for pharmacological treatment of neuropathic pain. Pain 2010;150:573–81.

82. Sindrup SH, Jensen TS. Antidepressants in the treatment of neuropathic pain. In: Hanson PT, Fields HL, Hill RG, et al, editors. Neuropathic pain: pathophysiology and treatment. Seattle (WA): IASP Press; 2001. p. 169–83.

83. Lunn MP, Hughes RA, Wiffen PJ. Duloxetine for treating painful neuropathy, chronic pain or fibromyalgia. Cochrane Database Syst Rev 2014;(1):CD007115.

84. Moore RA, Derry S, Aldington D, et al. Amitriptyline for neuropathic pain and fibromyalgia in adults. Cochrane Database Syst Rev 2012;(12):CD008242.

85. Gilron I, Bailey JM, Tu D, et al. Nortriptyline and gabapentin, alone and in combination for neuropathic pain: a double-blind, randomised controlled crossover trial. Lancet 2009;374:1252–61.

86. Simpson DA. Gabapentin and venlafaxine for the treatment of painful diabetic neuropathy. J Clin Neuromuscul Dis 2001;3:53–62.

87. Chaparro LE, Wiffen PJ, Moore RA, et al. Combination pharmacotherapy for the treatment of neuropathic pain in adults. Cochrane Database Syst Rev 2012;(7):CD008943.

88. Hanna M, O'Brien C, Wilson MC. Prolonged-release oxycodone enhances the effects of existing gabapentin therapy in painful diabetic neuropathy patients. Eur J Pain 2008;12:804–13.

89. Gilron I, Bailey JM, Tu D, et al. Morphine, gabapentin, or their combination for neuropathic pain. N Engl J Med 2005;352:1324–34.

90. Heir G, Karolchek S, Kalladka M, et al. Use of topical medication in orofacial neuropathic pain: a retrospective study. Oral Surg Oral Med Oral Pathol Oral Radiol Endod 2008;105:466–9.

91. Wetering EJ, Lemmens KM, Nieboer AP, et al. Cognitive and behavioral interventions for the management of chronic neuropathic pain in adults: a systematic review. Eur J Pain 2010;14:670–81.

92. Ziccardi VB. Microsurgical techniques for repair of the inferior alveolar and lingual nerves. Atlas Oral Maxillofac Surg Clin North Am 2011;19:79–90.

93. Ziccardi VB, Steinberg MJ. Timing of trigeminal nerve microsurgery: a review of the literature. J Oral Maxillofac Surg 2007;65:1341–5.

94. Farole A, Jamal BT. A bioabsorbable collagen nerve cuff (NeuraGen) for repair of lingual and inferior alveolar nerve injuries: a case series. J Oral Maxillofac Surg 2008;66:2058–62.

95. Pogrel MA. The results of microneurosurgery of the inferior alveolar and lingual nerve. J Oral Maxillofac Surg 2002;60:485–9.

96. Ziccardi VB, Rivera L, Gomes J. Comparison of lingual and inferior alveolar nerve microsurgery outcomes. Quintessence Int 2009;40:295–301.

97. Susarla SM, Kaban LB, Donoff RB, et al. Functional sensory recovery after trigeminal nerve repair. J Oral Maxillofac Surg 2007;65:60–5.

98. Susarla SM, Kaban LB, Donoff RB, et al. Does early repair of lingual nerve injuries improve functional sensory recovery? J Oral Maxillofac Surg 2007; 65:1070–6.

99. Caissie R, Goulet J, Fortin M, et al. Iatrogenic paresthesia in the third division of the trigeminal nerve: 12 years of clinical experience. J Can Dent Assoc 2005;71:185–90.

100. Rutner TW, Ziccardi VB, Janal MN. Long-term outcome assessment for lingual nerve microsurgery. J Oral Maxillofac Surg 2005;63:1145–9.

101. Strauss ER, Ziccardi VB, Janal MN. Outcome assessment of inferior alveolar nerve microsurgery: a retrospective review. J Oral Maxillofac Surg 2006; 64:1767–70.

102. Renton T, Yilmaz Z. Managing iatrogenic trigeminal nerve injury: a case series and review of the literature. Int J Oral Maxillofac Surg 2012;41:629–37.

103. Renton T, Dawood A, Shah A, et al. Post-implant neuropathy of the trigeminal nerve. A case series. Br Dent J 2012;212:E17.

104. Han SR, Yeo SP, Lee MK, et al. Early dexamethasone relieves trigeminal neuropathic pain. J Dent Res 2010;89:915–20.

105. Bullard DE, Nashold BS Jr. The caudalis DREZ for facial pain. Stereotact Funct Neurosurg 1997;68: 168–74.

106. Kanpolat Y, Savas A, Ugur HC, et al. The trigeminal tract and nucleus procedures in treatment of atypical facial pain. Surg Neurol 2005; 64(Suppl 2):S96–100 [discussion: S100–1].

Burning Mouth Syndrome

Gary D. Klasser, DMD[a],*, Miriam Grushka, MSc, DDS, PhD[b], Nan Su, BSc, MBBS[c]

KEYWORDS

• Burning mouth syndrome • Glossodynia • Oral burning • Neuropathic

KEY POINTS

- Despite the current knowledge gained from the scientific literature, burning mouth syndrome (BMS) remains an enigmatic, misunderstood, and under-recognized painful condition.
- Symptoms associated with BMS can be varied, which provides a challenge for practitioners and has a negative impact on oral health–related quality of life for patients.
- Management of BMS is a challenge for practitioners, because it is currently only targeted for symptom relief without a definitive cure.
- There is a desperate need for further investigations into management, with larger patient samples and longer duration of intervention and follow-up using multicenter trials.

INTRODUCTION

Burning mouth syndrome (BMS) is an enigmatic, idiopathic, chronic, often painful clinical entity for which there are yet to be well established standardized and validated definitions, diagnostic criteria, or classifications. First described by Fox[1] in 1935, BMS has several different definitions that depend on interpretations from several organizations that review this ambiguous condition. The American Academy of Orofacial Pain[2] defines BMS as a burning sensation in the oral mucosa despite the absence of clinical findings and abnormalities in laboratory testing or imaging. The International Association for the Study of Pain (IASP)[3] defines BMS as a burning pain in the tongue or other oral mucous membrane associated with normal signs and laboratory findings lasting at least 4 to 6 months.[4,5] The current (tenth) version of the International Classification of Diseases of the World Health Organization (the preeminent tool for coding diagnoses within the health care systems of many countries) uses the term glossodynia (K14.6), which includes additional terms such as glossopyrosis and painful tongue and describes the condition as painful sensations in the tongue, including a sensation of burning.[6]

The International Headache Society (IHS) in The International Classification of Headache Disorders III-beta (ICHD-III-beta)[7] classifies BMS in Part 3: painful cranial neuropathies, other facial pains and other headaches within the section concerning painful cranial neuropathies and other facial pains. BMS (ICHD-III-beta: 13.10), previously labeled as stomatodynia, or glossodynia when confined to the tongue, is currently defined as an intraoral burning or dysesthetic sensation, recurring daily for more than 2 hours per day over more than 3 months, without clinically evident causative lesions. It is further commented that pain is usually bilateral and its intensity fluctuates, with the most common site of presentation being the tip of the tongue. Subjective dryness of the mouth, dysesthesia, and altered taste often are accompanying symptoms. There is a high menopausal female prevalence, and some studies show comorbid psychosocial and psychiatric disorders, whereas recent laboratory and brain imaging investigations have indicated changes in the central and peripheral nervous systems.

Nomenclature related to BMS has created much confusion because this condition has been given many different names, often based on the quality

a Department of Diagnostic Sciences, Louisiana State University Health Sciences Center, School of Dentistry, 1100 Florida Avenue, Box 140, New Orleans, LA 70119, USA; b William Osler Health Centre, 974 Eglinton Avenue West, Toronto, Ontario M6C 2C5, Canada; c 974 Eginton Ave W, Toronto, Ontario M6C 2C5, Canada
* Corresponding author.
E-mail address: gklass@lsuhsc.edu

Oral Maxillofacial Surg Clin N Am 28 (2016) 381–396
http://dx.doi.org/10.1016/j.coms.2016.03.005
1042-3699/16/$ – see front matter © 2016 Elsevier Inc. All rights reserved.

and/or location of pain in the oral cavity. Some of the nomenclature applied is as follows: glossodynia, glossopyrosis, glossalgia, stomatodynia, stomatopyrosis, sore tongue, burning tongue, scalded mouth syndrome, oral dysesthesia, burning mouth condition, and BMS.[8,9] From the usage of these terms it is unclear whether or not the oral mucosa appeared normal and therefore whether these terms were describing BMS or just an oral burning sensation. Clearly, the use of these multiple and heterogeneous terms attests to the confusion and uncertainty that exists in the scientific literature and in clinical practice regarding this condition.

Furthermore, there is debate among researchers and clinicians as to whether burning mouth is a syndrome or a disorder.[8,10–13] By definition, a syndrome (a disease unto itself) is a collection of several simultaneous signs and symptoms of varying intensity, which, in the case of BMS, is a normal-appearing oral mucosa with a burning sensation, a feeling of oral dryness, and taste disturbances.[8,14–16] A disorder is defined as a condition manifesting symptoms of other diseases, such as the complaint of dry mouth being the cause of the burning sensation often reported by patients with BMS.[11] Overall, BMS is likely more than 1 disease process with a multifactorial cause, thereby making it a diagnosis of exclusion.

From these various definitions and multiple names applied to BMS it is easy to comprehend the frustration experienced by the patients and the difficulties encountered by practitioners in evaluating these individuals, because the patients are usually experiencing continuous burning pain in the mouth and the practitioners are struggling to identify any obvious clinical signs even with the accompaniment of additional diagnostic testing or imaging. This situation often produces a dilemma when developing and presenting a definitive diagnose. This article helps oral and maxillofacial surgeons in recognizing, understanding, and managing BMS.

EPIDEMIOLOGY

The prevalence of BMS is thought to range from 0.7% up to 15% of the population depending on the diagnostic criteria used.[17–19] The condition is most commonly reported in postmenopausal women, generally in the fifth to sixth decade of life. Men may also develop BMS, with a reported ratio of approximately 1:5 to 1:7 compared with women, depending on the study population.[17,20] Prevalence seems to increase with age in both men and women.[21]

DIAGNOSTIC CRITERIA

Over the years there have been several formal diagnostic criteria applied to BMS. Scala and colleagues[9] provided diagnostic criteria as the first step in an initial diagnosis of BMS by assessing the symptom pattern experienced by each patient. They reported the identification of full-blown forms of BMS to not be problematic, whereas the detection of either oligosymptomatic or monosymptomatic variants to be much more complex and the investigators thought their criteria would alleviate difficulties in the diagnostic process. Fortuna and colleagues[12] suggested renaming BMS as complex oral sensitivity disorder, which they described as an oropharyngeal discomfort caused by 1 or more symptoms for which no specific cause of any type can be identified. The IHS in the ICHD-III-beta and the IASP also present criteria to be used for the diagnosis of BMS.[3,7] **Table 1** provides the proposed diagnostic criteria used to identify BMS. Even though there are similarities among some components of these criteria there is no absolute consensus, nor has there been validation of any specific criteria.

CLASSIFICATION

Several classification systems have been proposed with the goal of improving the characterization for BMS. Lamey[8] and Lamey and Lewis[22] proposed a classification system that comprises 3 subtypes based on variations in pain intensity over 24 hours. Type 1 is characterized by patients having burning every day. However, the burning is absent on waking, but presents as the day goes on, being maximal in the evening. This type may be linked to systemic disorders such as nutritional deficiencies and endocrine disorders.[23] Approximately 35% of patients with BMS give such a history. Type 2 is characterized by burning that occurs every day, is present on awakening, and often makes falling asleep at night difficult. This subgroup of patients often reports mood changes, alterations in eating habits, and decreased desire to socialize, which seems to be caused by an altered sleep pattern.[4,24] Approximately 55% of patients with BMS describe this type of history. Type 3 is characterized by intermittent burning, present only on some days, with burning affecting unusual sites such as the floor of the mouth, buccal mucosa, and throat. Frequently, these patients display anxiety and allergic reactions, particularly to food additives.[25] About 10% of patients with BMS report this pattern of symptoms. In a demographic study by Killough and colleagues[26] comparing BMS populations in the United

Table 1
Proposed diagnostic criteria to identify BMS

Source, Year	Criteria
Fortuna et al,[12] 2013	1. Any type of oropharyngeal symptom that can be persistent or intermittent with possible phases of remission/exacerbation during the day 2. Absence of any clinically and instrumentally detectable oropharyngeal lesion 3. Absence of any type of local and/or systemic factors, such as oral diseases, drugs, trauma, hypersensitivity reactions, physical/chemical agents In addition (but not mandatory): state of being symptomatic is persistent (typically ≥3 mo)

ICHD-III-beta,[7] 2013	1. Oral pain fulfilling criteria B and C
	2. Recurring daily for >2 h per day for >3 mo
	3. Pain has both of the following characteristics:
	  a. Burning quality
	  b. Felt superficially in the oral mucosa
	4. Oral mucosa is of normal appearance and clinical examination, including sensory testing, is normal
	5. Not better accounted for by another ICHD-III diagnosis

IASP,[3] 1994, revised 2011	Burning tongue or other parts of oral mucosa, usually bilateral, dysgeusic taste and/or altered taste perception, dry mouth, and denture intolerance
Scala et al,[9] 2003	1. Daily deep burning sensation of oral mucosa (bilateral) 2. Pain is unremitting for at least 4–6 mo 3. Continuous throughout all or almost all the day 4. Seldom interferes with sleep 5. Characteristic symptoms are not getting worse/sometimes there may be an improvement over the ingestion of food and liquid Additional inclusion symptomatic criteria are: 6. Occurrence of other oral symptoms, such as dysgeusia and/or xerostomia 7. Presence of sensory/chemosensory anomalies 8. Presence of mood changes and/or specific disruptions in patient personality traits

Data from Refs.[3,7,9,12]

Kingdom and United States, there were similar prevalence rates using these subtypes within these 2 populations. Gremeau-Richard and colleagues[27] classified BMS as being peripherally or centrally mediated according to the results of a lingual nerve injection with local anesthesia. Another classification schema differentiated BMS into 3 distinct categories based on neuropathic pain statuses that may overlap in individual patients.[28] The first was a peripheral small fiber neuropathy within the intraoral mucosa (50%–65%), the second was categorized as a subclinical major trigeminal neuropathy (20%–25%), and the third was related to a central pain that may be caused by hypofunction of dopaminergic neurons in the basal ganglia resulting in deficient dopaminergic top-down inhibition (20%–40%). Note that these classification schemes are not universally accepted, nor are they essential for the management of patients with BMS.

A more pragmatic approach in classifying patients with BMS is to divide patients into either primary (essential/idiopathic) BMS (no other evident disease) or secondary BMS (oral burning from other clinical abnormalities).[9] Because secondary BMS is associated with a preexisting condition or cause, it should be remembered that once such a condition is treated the symptoms will either improve or disappear. Danhauer and colleagues[29] examined 69 patients with BMS (83% female; average age of 62 years; pain duration of 2.45 years; visual analog scale pain rating of 49 mm rated from 0 to 100 mm) with all patients completing pain (Multidimensional Pain Inventory [MPI]) and psychological (Symptom Checklist 90-Revised [SCL-90R]) questionnaires in addition to having a clinical examination. There were no differences between patients with primary and secondary BMS with respect to age, pain duration, pain intensity, or levels of psychological distress. However, there were substantial differences in burning symptom cessation with treatment because the patients with secondary BMS improved if the underlying clinical abnormality was treated, whereas the primary BMS group did not report such positive outcomes.

CLINICAL SIGNS AND SYMPTOMS

Most patients with BMS describe their symptoms in the oral mucosa using the following words: painful, burning, tender, tingling, hot, scalding, and numbness, but sometimes the sensation is merely described as discomfort, raw, and annoying. BMS is characterized by both positive (burning pain, dysgeusia, and dysesthesia) and negative (taste loss and paresthesia) sensory symptoms.[30] The pain is mainly located bilaterally, and symmetrically in the anterior two-thirds of the tongue (71%–78%) followed by the dorsum and lateral borders of the tongue (72%), the anterior aspect of the hard palate (25%), and the labial mucosa of the lips (24%), and often occurs in multiple sites.[5,14,31–33] There have been suggestions that burning of the lips should be considered as a single entity because this has been described featuring a thinned labial mucosa and inactive minor labial salivary glands.[34] Other less commonly reported sites include the buccal mucosa, floor of the mouth, hard and soft palate, and the throat (36%).[31] Unlike other painful conditions (trigeminal neuralgia [TN]), the burning pain does not follow peripheral nerve distributions. The sites of pain do not seem to affect the course of the disorder or the response to treatments.[35,36] Approximately 50% of patients with BMS experience a spontaneous onset of symptoms without any identifiable triggering factor.[15,37] However, about 17% to 33% of the patients attribute the onset of their symptoms to a previous illness, such as an upper respiratory tract infection, previous dental procedure, or medication use (including antibiotic therapy),[37–40] suggesting the possibility of neurologic alterations preceding the onset of burning in some patients.[41–43] Other individuals claim the onset of symptoms relate to traumatic life stressors.[15,32,37] Typically, the symptoms occur continuously for months or years without periods of cessation or remission,[37] with some reports suggesting an average duration of 2 to 3 years.[44,45] There have been reports[37] of complete/partial remission (with or without intervention) in approximately 50% of patients and a complete spontaneous remission in approximately 20% of patients within 6 to 7 years of onset. The remission of symptoms, either complete or partial, is often characterized by a change in pain pattern from a constant to an episodic form.[37,46] Contrary to these optimistic findings, Sardella and colleagues,[47] in an investigation to specifically evaluate the spontaneous remission rate in BMS,

reported that a complete spontaneous remission was observed in only 3% of the patients within 5 years after BMS onset.

The pattern of daily symptoms is reportedly constant with fluctuation in pain intensity and with approximately one-third of patients experiencing symptoms both day and night.[5,32,48] Most patients report minimal symptoms on awakening, after which the symptoms gradually increase during the day and become more severe toward the evening.[4,5] About one-third of the patients have difficulty with sleep onset and some awaken during the night because of the burning pain.[19,32] The intensity of the burning pain has been described as moderate to severe, and in some cases it is comparable with the intensity of toothache pain with regard to severity but not quality.[24] In most patients, the burning sensation intensifies in the presence of personal stressors, fatigue, and with the intake of hot/spicy/acidic foods, and in about half the patients the intake of food or liquids and distraction seem to reduce or alleviate the symptoms (dissimilar to pain caused by organic lesions or neuralgia).[5,30,49,50] It is unclear what the effects of tobacco, ethanol, or dietary factors are on the symptoms of BMS. Patients with BMS have a significantly higher incidence of dry mouth, thirst, and taste disturbances but they do not differ from healthy controls regarding changes in oral mucosa or dental problems.[5,15,51,52] Furthermore, patients had no greater prevalence of medical conditions such as diabetes, arthritis, and cardiovascular and gastrointestinal disorders compared with age-matched and sex-matched controls.[5]

Patients with BMS have more nonspecific health complaints and more severe menopausal symptoms compared with healthy controls.[5] Headaches, dizziness, neck and back pain, dermatologic disorders, irritable bowel syndrome, anxiety, depression, personality disorders, and other psychiatric disorders are reported more frequently in these patients.[32,38,40,51–55] However, many of these studies are unclear as to whether these symptoms are risk factors for development of BMS or a consequence of the syndrome, indicating a need for longitudinal cohort studies.

CAUSE

At present, the cause for primary BMS has remained largely unknown. The presumed cause is best explained as being multifactorial, involving the interaction between biological (neurophysiologic mechanisms) and psychological factors.[16] Even though multiple local, systemic, and psychological factors have been found related to BMS, several of these factors should be considered as conditions important to the differential diagnosis of oral burning rather than as causal factors implicated in BMS.

Local Factors

Several local factors (physical, chemical, or biological) have been considered as possible causal factors for BMS. Some of these are:

- Xerostomia, which is the subjective sensation of dry mouth and is found to be a frequent complaint (25% of patients with BMS)[23,44,56] in addition to drug-induced xerostomia[44,57]
- Hyposalivation, which denotes objectively reduced salivary flow measured by sialometry[15,23,31,58]
- Taste disturbances involving either an alteration in taste perception, a persistently altered taste, or a combination of these[5,18,59,60]
- Oral bacterial, viral, and/or fungal (candidiasis) infections[61–68]
- Oral mucosal abnormalities, such as benign migratory glossitis (geographic tongue), scalloped and fissured tongue,[14,44,69] and diseases such as lichen planus[57,70]
- Parafunctional oral habits, such as clenching, bruxing, or tongue posturing[47,71]
- Mechanical and chemical irritations, such as galvanism and denture-related problems[23,72]
- Allergic reactions[23,73]

Grushka[5] reported no significant differences on clinical examination between subjects with BMS and controls with any intraoral soft or hard tissue findings. The discrepancy between this study and the studies that found higher prevalences of oral change may be caused by differences in definitions of BMS and/or its diagnosis or may be a result of the condition creating these changes rather than being causative of the condition.

Systemic Factors

Many systemic factors have been considered for explaining the cause of BMS. Some of these are:

- Autoimmune, gastrointestinal, and endocrine disorders, such as connective tissue diseases, gastroesophageal reflux disease, diabetes, and thyroid disorders[15,30,46,73–80]
- Hormonal deficiencies and menopausal alterations[5,74,81]
- Drug-induced conditions, especially involving angiotensin-converting enzyme inhibitors such as captopril, enalapril, and lisinopril[82,83]
- Nutritional deficiencies involving vitamins and minerals, especially those associated with

anemia (iron and vitamin B_{12} deficiency), zinc, and vitamin B complexes[84–88]

However, despite some evidence from these studies supporting a possible association of these systemic factors as causal agents, there are many inconsistencies within the literature.[5,14,23,56,89–91] Studies have also reported a relationship between other facial pains,[72] pains in other parts of the body,[72] and headache pain[5] as being more frequent in patients with BMS. However, the meaning and relevance of these associations remain unclear.

Psychological Factors

Psychological phenomena such as alterations in states of anxiety and depression, somatization, and certain aberrant personality traits, are common findings in patients with BMS,[45,92–95] thereby supporting psychological factors as major causal factors for BMS. At least one-third of patients may have an underlying psychiatric diagnosis.[44] A phobic concern regarding cancer is also found in 20% of patients[23] and is often manifested as repeated self-examination by the patient.[8] Although BMS may be a somatic symptom of depression, the association does not always equate to a causal relationship. Carlson and colleagues[96] used the MPI and SCL-90R on 33 BMS cases and compared the data with those from population samples that included both patients without BMS but with chronic pain and a normal nonclinical sample. They concluded that there was no evidence for significant clinical increases on any of the SCL-90R subscales, including depression, anxiety, and somatization. Moreover, BMS patients reported significantly fewer disruptions in normal activities as a result of their oral burning pain than did a large sample of patients with chronic pain. It was noted that 21% of the BMS cases had substantially increased psychological distress. Despite the presence of psychological issues and the need for treatment of these underlying issues, BMS may also occur in the absence of a psychological diagnosis.[97] The uniqueness of the frequency of occurrence of these psychological conditions in the BMS population as being consistent with that of other chronic painful conditions has not been well documented. It is possible for these psychological conditions to be comorbidities, modifiers of the burning mouth condition, or a behavioral consequence of having BMS rather than causal factors. Regardless, these psychological issues must be addressed because of their impact on the quality of life as well on treatment outcomes.[98] Hence, appropriate management should therefore include referral to health professionals who may assist these patients with their mental health status.[99,100] Another factor to consider is that many of the medications used in the treatment of these psychological conditions may be responsible for the side effects, such as dry mouth and taste alterations, that may induce or exacerbate BMS symptoms.

ASSOCIATED FEATURES
Saliva

Many patients with BMS also have an associated feeling of dry mouth (xerostomia). Resting whole salivary flow is reduced, whereas stimulated whole salivary flow is usually normal.[58,101–103] In addition to changes in rate of unstimulated whole salivary flow, alterations in the composition of saliva have been reported and include increased total protein, interleukin (IL)-6, 17-β estradiol, cortisol, and α-amylase levels, decreased secretory immunoglobulin A (SIgA) level, and minor increases in salivary elements, including iron, magnesium, and zinc.[102–105]

Taste

Up to 70% of patients with BMS experience some form of taste distortion, usually as bitter or metallic, or altered perception.[21] Taste thresholds, measured by whole mouth taste, have been found to be increased, resulting in decreased sensitivities to salt, sweet, sour, and bitter, and leading to difficulty in identification, especially for salt and sour.[50,103,106] Electric taste threshold, measured by gustometry and often reported to be perceived as a sour taste, has also been found to be significantly increased in BMS.[106,107] In contrast with these studies, Bergdahl and Bergdahl,[108] in reviewing perceived taste disturbances from a large population-based study, found only a weak correlation between burning mouth and taste disturbances, with perceived taste disturbances being more prevalent in female than in male patients.

Psychosocial Comorbidities

Psychiatric disorders in BMS have been studied using various methods, including questionnaires. Patients with BMS often have a significantly higher frequency of major depressive disorder, generalized anxiety disorder, hypochondria, and cancerphobia, and often take more psychotropic medications.[99] Patients with BMS also had decreased openness, higher neurotism, and poor sleep quality.[104] Additional studies suggest that depression and anxiety can be both the result and the cause for sleep disturbance, and

interrupted sleep seems to be associated with increased pain, which in turn contributes to poor sleep quality.[109,110] The pain and poor sleep can lead to decreased quality of life, including increased functional limitation and physical disability, and decreased vitality and social function.[98] One case study suggests that the pain can become so severe and unbearable that suicidal tendencies can develop.[111] Therefore, it was suggested that sleep dysfunction may be a risk factor for BMS and a possible target for treatment.[112]

PATHOPHYSIOLOGIC THEORIES

The pathophysiology of BMS continues to be unclear, especially with the lack of any visible oral mucosal changes on examination. Current suggested pathophysiology is multifactorial and encompasses changes to taste, changes in hormone levels, nerve damage, central nervous system changes, autoimmune disorders, and psychological factors.

Taste and Sensory System Interactions

One current mechanism of burning mouth pain is thought to be the loss of inhibition on the trigeminal nerve as a result of damage to the chorda tympani.[113] The chorda tympani innervates the anterior two-third of the tongue and, together with the greater petrosal nerve and cranial nerve IX (the glossopharyngeal nerve), provides taste sensations.[114] Thermal and pain thresholds of the anterior tongue are mediated by the trigeminal nerve through the thinly myelinated Aδ and unmyelinated C fibers.[115,116] Changes in thermal, tactile, and pain threshold have been reported in BMS, as well as the taste disturbances described earlier, suggesting impairment of both the taste system and trigeminal nerve.[50,117,118]

Patients with BMS often report a decrease in their burning pain with eating, chewing gum, or sucking on candy, suggesting that food may provide an inhibitory effect on the burning pain or that the stimulation of taste buds may result in central inhibition of the trigeminal sensory system, thereby decreasing the pain. Schöbel and colleagues[116] offered evidence of a central loss of inhibition on the trigeminal nerve, thereby supporting this theory. In adult humans, sugar seems to inhibit the pain caused by capsaicin, mediated by the trigeminal nerve. In addition, when the subjects underwent unilateral blocking to the chorda tympani, the pain intensity induced by capsaicin was reduced ipsilateral to the procedure but increased contralaterally.[116]

Contrarily, Boucher and colleagues[119] argued against the loss-of-inhibition theory when they found, based on animal models, that bilateral chorda tympani dissection did not result in capsaicin avoidance but sensitivity to capsaicin seemed to decrease. One possible explanation for these results may be that chorda tympani damage may alter lingual nerve function, causing decreased capsaicin sensitivity or, alternatively, that loss of innervation by chorda tympani may cause hyperkeratinization of the dorsal tongue, thus reducing capsaicin sensitivity.[116] Another explanation may be a reduction of both the number and size of taste buds as a result of loss of chorda tympani innervation, thus resulting in decreased sensitivity.[120]

Supporting the role of involvement of a loss of central inhibition processes is a functional MRI study that reported thalamic hypofunction in the brain in patients with BMS.[121]

Hormonal Alterations

Because BMS predominantly affects women of postmenopausal age, changes in gonadal hormones seem to be a predisposing factor. In menopause, ovarian function declines and estrogen levels decrease, resulting in increased levels of follicle-stimulating hormone (FSH), leading to various menopausal symptoms. Oral mucosa and salivary glands contain estrogen receptors and the oral mucosa is histologically similar to the vaginal mucosa and responds to estrogen in a similar fashion. Postmenopausal patients with high FSH levels and low estradiol levels seem to have more complaints of burning.[122] Estrogen receptors have also been found in the trigeminal complex. In animal models, ovariectomy has been shown to lead to long-term hyperalgesia and an increase in numbers of nociceptive neurons in the trigeminal subnucleus caudalis,[119] suggesting that changes in gonadal hormone levels can alter neuron expression and may predispose perimenopausal/postmenopausal women to BMS. Levels of dehydroepiandrosterone, a precursor for androgen and estrogen, in morning saliva samples of patients with BMS have also been found to be low.[123]

It has been suggested that increased salivary 17-β estradiol and salivary cortisol levels, and decreased plasma adrenaline levels found in BMS may therefore represent neuroendocrine changes in association with the depression/anxiety in patients with BMS.[102,124,125]

The hypothalamus-pituitary-adrenal (HPA) axis is densely populated with estrogen receptors, and hypothalamus-pituitary-gonadal axis hormones can control the release of adrenal stress hormones at the level of the hypothalamus. Increased 17-β estradiol has been shown to attenuate functions within the HPA axis[126] and androgen deprivation treatment in men for prostate cancer has been shown to lead to increased emotional liability and depressed mood.[127]

Neuropathic Consideration

Peripheral small fiber neuropathy
The peripheral nerve fibers are classified by size into large, medium, and small fibers. Large fibers mediate motor strength, vibration, and touch sensation. Small fibers, including thinly myelinated A-δ and unmyelinated C fibers, innervate the skin through somatic fibers, and innervate the smooth muscles though autonomic fibers. When damage occurs to the small somatic nerve fibers, pain, burning, tingling, and numbness can result, with symptoms usually worst at night.[128] When damage occurs to the autonomic fibers, facial symptoms can include dry eyes and dry mouth.[128] Small fiber neuropathy can occur with many medical conditions, including metabolic disorders, endocrine disorders, vitamin B_{12} deficiency, viral infection, and autoimmune disorders such as Sjögren syndrome.[128]

Recent studies report that patients with BMS have altered sensitivity to cold and hot, whereas the mechanical tongue function remains intact, suggesting damage to small fibers of the tongue only with conserved motor function mediated by the large nerve fibers.[117,129,130] In normal tongue, there are numerous small nerve fibers in the subepithelial region with fewer fibers normally in the epithelial tissue of the tongue. In patients with BMS, both myelinated and unmyelinated fibers have been found to be significantly reduced in the tongue, especially in symptomatic areas.[131,132]

Nociceptive channels and neuropeptides
Transient receptor potential vanniloid channel type 1 (TRPV-1), a member of a family of nonselective cation channels, is involved in nociception.[132] TRPV-1 upregulation has been documented in rectal hypersensitivity, inflammation of the bowel, vulvodynia, and overactive bladder.[132,133] In BMS, its numbers are significantly increased in the papillae of the tongue but not on the epithelium.[132,134]

The voltage-gated sodium channel 1 and 8 (Na_v 1, 8), another ion channel associated with pain sensation, has also been found to be in slightly increased numbers in the subepithelial region of the tongue in BMS.[132] Both TRPV-1 and Na_v 1, 8 are under the regulation of nerve growth factor (NGF), which has been found to be at increased levels in BMS in both subepithelium and basal tongue epithelium. Because NGF is not produced by the nerve fibers, the increase in NGF level may be the result of increased uptake into a decreased population of remaining nerve fibers.[132]

NGF, synthesized in the areas of the trigeminal distribution, the dental pulp, and the cornea,[135] supports the growth and maintenance of nociceptive neurons during development and interacts with immune cells such as mast cells to release inflammatory mediators.[136] Substance P is a neuropeptide released by nerve fibers and is an indication of nerve fiber presence. Salivary examination of the presence of neuropeptides in BMS has found increased NGF levels but decreased substance P[136] levels, suggesting loss of normal nerve fiber with regeneration and maintenance of nociceptive fibers.[135]

Subclinical trigeminal neuralgia

There has been some suggestion that BMS is a subclinical type of TN.[18] Evidence of trigeminal nerve involvement in BMS includes increased heat and pain thresholds, the sensations of which are carried by the mandibular branch of the trigeminal nerve (V3), and altered sensitivity to the 4 taste modalities[50,115,118,137]; abnormal blink reflex, mediated by the ophthalmic nerve (V1) of the trigeminal nerve[97]; and findings of peripheral trigeminal neuropathy, mostly lingual or mandibular nerve lesion, in approximately 20% of patients with BMS. In addition, lingual branch damage can produce intraoral trigeminal neuropathy with clinical symptoms indistinguishable from BMS.[18]

Although symptoms of trigeminal nerve damage may be present in patients with BMS, TN and BMS have different clinical presentations. The pain quality in TN is often described as a sudden, severe, brief, lancinating episodic pain lasting from seconds to minutes within the distribution of the trigeminal nerve, and often unilateral,[138,139] whereas BMS is a chronic burning pain with the pain progressively increasing in intensity throughout the day, often affecting multiple oral sites and not restricted to a nerve distribution.[19] Pain has been reported to be more intense in TN than in BMS with no difference in intensity between acute and chronic TN, whereas patients with chronic BMS reported more intense pain than those with acute BMS.[139] Physically, compression of the trigeminal nerve root can be found in 90% to 95% of TN, whereas BMS is mostly idiopathic with no visible physical changes.[139] Given the difference in presentation and cause of TN and BMS, it is less likely that BMS is a subclinical type of TN. It is more likely that some patients with BMS have damage to the trigeminal system peripherally and/or centrally.

Central pain related to deficient dopaminergic inhibition

Autonomic nervous function studies, including deep breathing heart rate, heart rate variability, and sympathetic skin responses, have shown that some patients with BMS have changes in heart rate variability and exhalation/inhalation ratio, suggesting sympathetic dysfunction, and prolonged latency in skin response suggesting parasympathetic dysfunction.[97,140] These finding are similar to those found in Parkinson disease, a cerebral degenerative disease associated with dysfunction of the dopaminergic system, with up to 40% of patients with Parkinson disease reporting burning in the oral cavity.[140] This has led some clinicians to suggest the involvement of the central dopaminergic system in BMS. In some patients with BMS, PET studies have shown a reduction in dopamine levels in the nigrostriatal neurons as well as the basal ganglion, especially the putamen.[28] Several cases have been reported in which BMS has been successfully treated with levodopa,[141] supporting the possible involvement of the dopaminergic system in at least a subpopulation of BMS.

Autoimmune disorder (lichen planus)

Oral burning that arises from peripheral small fiber neuropathy can be caused by autoimmune disorders such as Sjögren syndrome, lupus erythema, inflammatory bowel disease, sarcoidosis, and fibromyalgia.[142] Burning can also be a complaint in oral lichen planus, an immunologically medicated mucocutaneous disease.[143] Burning can also occur as a result of a delayed contact sensitivity reaction, with 67% of patients with burning mouth showing a positive reaction.[144] Some clinicians therefore suggest a connection between activation of the immune system and development of neuropathy leading to burning pain. The exact mechanism of how this damage occurs remains to be established. It is likely that T-cell stimulation may lead to secretion of cytokines,[142] promoting increased inflammatory response, whereas B-cell stimulation may release autoimmune antibodies, which may react against nerve tissue antigens.[142] Immunologic work-up in BMS has shown changes in levels of salivary and plasma immune factors, including increased expression of IL-6 and IL-8 in areas of peripheral small fiber neuropathy; decreased levels of serum IL-2 and tumor necrosis factor alpha; increased levels of salivary IL-6, and decreased levels of salivary SIgA; and increased salivary tryptase levels (released from mast cells on stimulation by NGF).[103,104,136,142,145] A decrease in CD8(+) cells has also been found in BMS leading to an increase in CD4/CD8 ratio, although this may be more the result of aging and psychological stress causing a shift from cell-mediated response to humoral response.[124] Although the immune system may play a role in the onset of burning mouth pain through immune-mediated nerve damage, there is currently little evidence to support this.

DIAGNOSIS

BMS has for many years remained a diagnosis of exclusion. At present, as a result of the increase in knowledge with regard to burning mouth pain, diagnosis has been facilitated.

When mucosa changes are evident, they must be addressed and ruled out to ensure that the burning pain is not the result of a disorder such as lichen planus or fungal infection. Once the mucosal tissues are returned to their normal state, and if the burning persists, the presence of burning mouth pain associated with BMS is suggested.

Although in the past there have been no good criteria on which to base the diagnosis of burning mouth pain, diagnosis, based on the recent literature, is now facilitated. Testing for burning mouth pain can now include studies of salivary flow, taste function, blood tests to rule out systemic factors, contact sensitivity, as well as a clinical history that suggests pain that is usually reduced by stimulation and function.

Taste testing should show changes in whole mouth threshold; decreased bitter at the tongue tip and even altered oral burning elicited by ethanol application based on the results of stimulation with capsaicin.[113] Salivary flows have shown decreased unstimulated flow with normal stimulated flow.[58] Other more sophisticated testing can include thresholds for cold, hot, and touch, although there are fewer data on an individual level than for some of the other testing. Facilitation of the diagnosis is also important for research studies that include diagnostic criteria, making the studies easier to compare across groups.

MANAGEMENT

Distinct recommendations for the management of patients with BMS are scarce in the literature. From a clinical perspective, clinicians must initially determine whether the patient is experiencing signs and symptoms consistent with primary (essential/idiopathic) BMS or secondary BMS in which symptoms are caused by underlying local or systemic conditions.[146] Secondary BMS requires appropriate diagnosis and treatment of the underlying conditions. In primary BMS, the cause is unclear, so management options are based on the patient's symptoms, often yielding unsatisfactory results. A retrospective study evaluated 53 patients who had BMS for at least 18 months. A variety of treatment modalities were administered, for which moderate improvement was reported in 28.3% of the subjects, and spontaneous remission occurred in 3.7%. All other patients reported no change or worsening symptoms of BMS after a mean of 5 years after having been diagnosed with the condition.[47]

Before initiating a management strategy, it is important for clinicians to educate and reassure their patients regarding the characteristics of the condition and to elucidate the existing therapeutic difficulties with a meaningful discussion as to the possibilities of symptom relief. Depending on the outcome after therapeutic trials, patients need to be aware that management may involve a multidisciplinary team approach, often requiring multiple modifications of the management plan until an effective protocol is achieved. The importance of this approach cannot be overstated because often these patients are frustrated by a lack of understanding of this condition among health practitioners. Mignona and colleagues[147] reported that the mean delay from the onset of symptoms to a definitive diagnosis was 34 months (range, 1–348 months; median, 13 months). Furthermore, the mean number of medical and dental practitioners consulted by each patient with BMS (n = 59) over this period and who initially misdiagnosed BMS was 3.1 (range, 0–12; median, 3). In about 30% of the cases, no diagnosis of the oral symptoms was made or explanation given. In a similar study with an American population, it was reported that, on average, patients reported oral burning symptoms for 41 months (range, 2–360 months; median, 20 months), and 38 (n = 49 subjects with BMS) of the patients received/trialed 71 various interventions (mean = 1.9) before receiving a definitive diagnosis for their BMS symptoms.[148]

At present, clinicians have the choice of 3 approaches or combinations thereof as considerations in management.

Behavioral Strategies

Behavioral strategies to be considered consist of self-help measures, such as cessation of parafunctional habits (clenching, bruxism, tongue protrusion), and/or modification of oral care product usage, such as alcohol-free mouthwashes, and the use of products without flavoring agents or irritating components (cinnamic aldehyde, sodium lauryl sulfate, tooth whitening agents,

Table 2
Recommendations from BMS systematic reviews (since 2005)

Author, Year	Number of Studies Reviewed	Study Design	First-line Therapy Evidence	Alternative Therapy
Zakrzewska et al,[156] 2005	9 studies	RCT + controlled clinical trials	*Insufficient evidence: analgesics, hormones, or antidepressants* Behavioral: CBT Topical: clonazepam Systemic: alpha-lipoic acid	—
Patton et al,[146] 2007	10 studies	Meta-analyses, systematic reviews, RCT+ crossover studies	*Recommendations based on RCT* Behavioral: CBT Topical: clonazepam Systemic: SSRI (paroxetine, sertraline),antipsychotics (amisulpride)	*Suggestions based on expert opinion + common clinical practice but not yet evaluated* Topical: capsaicin, doxepine, lidocaine Systemic: TCA, SNRI, anticonvulsants, opioids, benzodiazepines (clonazepam, alprazolam)
de Moraes et al,[157] 2012	12 studies	RCT	Topical: capsaicin, clonazepam Systemic: alpha-lipoic acid	—
Ducasse et al,[158] 2013	16 studies	RCT	Behavioral: psychotherapy[a] Topical: clonazepam, tongue protector Systemic: clonazepam, SSRI (paroxetine, sertraline)	Systemic: antipsychotics (amisulpride), Catuama (mixture of guarana, catuaba, ginger, and muirapuama) Interventional: lingual nerve block
Kuten-Shorrer et al,[159] 2014	12 studies Note: evaluated the placebo effect in BMS	RCT	The mean placebo response as a fraction of drug response over 10 studies was 72%, suggesting a robust placebo response	2 studies reported no improvement between active intervention + placebo

Abbreviations: CBT, cognitive behavior therapy; RCT, randomized controlled trial; SNRI, selective norepinephrine reuptake inhibitor; SSRI, selective serotonin reuptake inhibitor; TCA, tricyclic antidepressant.
[a] Only if Hospital Anxiety and Depression score is high.
Data from Refs.[146,156–159]

anticalculus ingredients).[149,150] Other products for consideration in discontinuing their use include mints, gum, or other breath aids.[151] Stress management approaches, such as moderate exercise regimens, yoga, and tai chi, may be attempted. In addition, desensitizing appliances may be considered to reduce oral burning and may also be used as habit-breaking appliances.[152] Behavioral strategies using professional assistance, including cognitive behavioral approaches (focus on how beliefs and thoughts influence behavior) used alone or in combination with other therapies and/or group psychotherapy, have shown efficacy in decreasing pain intensity.[153–155]

Topical Therapies

Topical therapies using the following have all been trialed, with various rates of success:

- Anxiolytics (clonazepam)
- Anesthetics (lidocaine, bupivacaine)
- Antidepressants (doxepin)
- Atypical analgesics (capsaicin)
- Nonsteroidal antiinflammatory (benzydamine; not US Food and Drug Administration [FDA] approved for use in the United States)
- Antimicrobials (lysozyme, lactoperoxidase)
- Mucosal protectants (sucralfate, aloe vera, lycopene virgin oil)
- Artificial sweeteners (sucralose)
- Low-level laser therapy

Systemic Therapies

Systemic approaches using a vast number of medications from various medication categories include:

- Antidepressants (amitriptyline, imipramine, nortriptyline, desipramine, trazodone, paroxetine, sertraline, duloxetine, milnacipran)
- Anxiolytics (clonazepam, diazepam, chlordiazepoxide)
- Anticonvulsants (gabapentin, pregabalin, topiramate)
- Antioxidants (alpha-lipoic acid)
- Atypical analgesics/antipsychotics (capsaicin, olanzapine: amisulpride, levosulpiride; both medications are not FDA approved for use in the United States)
- Histamine receptor antagonists (lafutidine; not FDA approved for use in the United States)
- Monoamine oxidase inhibitors (moclobemide; not FDA approved for use in the United States)
- Salivary stimulants (pilocarpine, cevimeline)
- Dopamine agonists (pramipexole)
- Herbal supplements (*Hypericum perforatum* or St John's wort, Catuama)

- Vitamin supplementation (vitamin B, C)
- Transcranial magnetic stimulation
- Acupuncture

Since 2005, there have been 5 systematic reviews reported in the scientific literature that have exclusively reported on interventions used in the management of BMS.[146,156–159] However, there is only a minor consensus among these specific systematic reviews as to the therapy of choice and rankings thereof to guide clinicians in providing an evidence-based approach for the management of this condition. **Table 2** provides a summary of the recommendations provided by each of these systematic reviews.

SUMMARY

Even with the current knowledge gained from the scientific literature, BMS remains an enigmatic, misunderstood, and under-recognized painful condition. Symptoms associated with BMS can be varied, thereby providing a challenge for practitioners and having a negative impact on oral health–related quality of life for patients. Management also remains a challenge for practitioners because it is currently only targeted for symptom relief without a definitive cure. Despite having randomized clinical trials reviewing management approaches and providing evidence-based treatment algorithms, the results remain inconclusive. Clearly, there is an urgent need for further investigations with larger patient samples and longer duration of intervention and follow-up using multicenter trials. These approaches are necessary to determine the efficacy of different therapies because this is the only way viable therapeutic options can be established for patients with this chronic and painful syndrome.

REFERENCES

1. Fox H. Burning tongue glossodynia. N Y State J Med 1935;35:881–4.
2. American Academy of Orofacial Pain. Continuous neuropathic pain. In: de Leeuw R, Klasser GD, editors. Orofacial pain: guidelines for assessment, diagnosis and management. 5th edition. Chicago: Quintessence; 2013. p. 95–6.
3. Merskey H, Bogduk N. Descriptions of chronic pain syndromes and definitions of pain terms. Classification of chronic pain. 2nd edition. Seattle (WA): IASP Press; 1994. p. 74–5.
4. Grinspan D, Fernandez Blanco G, Allevato MA, et al. Burning mouth syndrome. Int J Dermatol 1995;34(7):483–7.

5. Grushka M. Clinical features of burning mouth syndrome. Oral Surg Oral Med Oral Pathol 1987;63(1):30–6.

6. Available at: http://www.icd10data.com/Search.aspx?search=glossodynia. Accessed December 1, 2015.

7. Headache Classification Committee of the International Headache Society (IHS). The International Classification of Headache Disorders, 3rd edition (beta version). Cephalalgia 2013;33(9):629–808.

8. Lamey PJ. Burning mouth syndrome. Dermatol Clin 1996;14(2):339–54.

9. Scala A, Checchi L, Montevecchi M, et al. Update on burning mouth syndrome: overview and patient management. Crit Rev Oral Biol Med 2003;14(4):275–91.

10. Zakrzewska JM, Hamlyn PJ. Facial pain. In: Crombie IK, editor. Epidemiology of pain. Seattle (WA): IASP press; 1999. p. 175–82.

11. Rhodus NL, Carlson CR, Miller CS. Burning mouth (syndrome) disorder. Quintessence Int 2003;34(8):587–93.

12. Fortuna G, Di Lorenzo M, Pollio A. Complex oral sensitivity disorder: a reappraisal of current classification of burning mouth syndrome. Oral Dis 2013;19(7):730–2.

13. Markman S, Eliav E. Are we ready for a new definition? Oral Dis 2013;19(7):728–9.

14. Gorsky M, Silverman S, Chinn H. Burning mouth syndrome: a review of 98 cases. J Oral Med 1987;42(1):7–9.

15. Grushka M, Sessle BJ. Burning mouth syndrome. Dent Clin North Am 1991;35(1):171–84.

16. Zakrzewska JM. The burning mouth syndrome remains an enigma. Pain 1995;62(3):253–7.

17. Coculescu EC, Tovaru S, Coculescu BI. Epidemiological and etiological aspects of burning mouth syndrome. J Med Life 2014;7(3):305–9.

18. Kolkka-Palomaa M, Jaaskelainen SK, Laine MA, et al. Pathophysiology of primary burning mouth syndrome with special focus on taste dysfunction: a review. Oral Dis 2015;21(8):937–48.

19. Grushka M, Epstein JB, Gorsky M. Burning mouth syndrome. Am Fam Physician 2002;65(4):615–20.

20. Kohorst JJ, Bruce AJ, Torgerson RR, et al. A population-based study of the incidence of burning mouth syndrome. Mayo Clin Proc 2014;89(11):1545–52.

21. Forssell H, Jaaskelainen S, List T, et al. An update on pathophysiological mechanisms related to idiopathic oro-facial pain conditions with implications for management. J Oral Rehabil 2015;42(4):300–22.

22. Lamey PJ, Lewis MA. Oral medicine in practice: orofacial pain. Br Dent J 1989;167(11):384–9.

23. Lamey PJ, Lamb AB. Prospective study of aetiological factors in burning mouth syndrome. Br Med J (Clin Res Ed) 1988;296(6631):1243–6.

24. Grushka M, Sessle BJ, Miller R. Pain and personality profiles in burning mouth syndrome. Pain 1987;28(2):155–67.

25. Lamey PJ, Lamb AB, Hughes A, et al. Type 3 burning mouth syndrome: psychological and allergic aspects. J Oral Pathol Med 1994;23(5):216–9.

26. Killough S, Rees T, Lamey PJ. Demographic study of sub-types of burning mouth syndrome in a UK and USA population. J Dent Res 1995;74:892.

27. Gremeau-Richard C, Dubray C, Aublet-Cuvelier B, et al. Effect of lingual nerve block on burning mouth syndrome (stomatodynia): a randomized crossover trial. Pain 2010;149(1):27–32.

28. Jaaskelainen SK. Pathophysiology of primary burning mouth syndrome. Clin Neurophysiol 2012;123(1):71–7.

29. Danhauer SC, Miller CS, Rhodus NL, et al. Impact of criteria-based diagnosis of burning mouth syndrome on treatment outcome. J Orofac Pain 2002;16(4):305–11.

30. Suarez P, Clark GT. Burning mouth syndrome: an update on diagnosis and treatment methods. J Calif Dent Assoc 2006;34(8):611–22.

31. Gorsky M, Silverman S, Chinn H. Clinical characteristics and management outcome in the burning mouth syndrome. An open study of 130 patients. Oral Surg Oral Med Oral Pathol 1991;72(2):192–5.

32. van der Ploeg HM, van der Wal N, Eijkman MA, et al. Psychological aspects of patients with burning mouth syndrome. Oral Surg Oral Med Oral Pathol 1987;63(6):664–8.

33. Svensson P, Bjerring P, Arendt-Nielsen L, et al. Sensory and pain thresholds to orofacial argon laser stimulation in patients with chronic burning mouth syndrome. Clin J Pain 1993;9(3):207–15.

34. Brown RS, Flaitz CM, Hays GL, et al. Five cases of burning lips syndrome. Compend Contin Educ Dent 1996;17(10):927–30.

35. Lamey PJ, Lamb AB. Lip component of burning mouth syndrome. Oral Surg Oral Med Oral Pathol 1994;78(5):590–3.

36. Grushka M. Burning mouth syndrome: evolving concepts. Oral Maxillofac Surg Clin North Am 2000;12(2):287–95.

37. Grushka M, Katz RL, Sessle BJ. Spontaneous remission in burning mouth syndrome. J Dent Res 1987;66:274.

38. Hammaren M, Hugoson A. Clinical psychiatric assessment of patients with burning mouth syndrome resisting oral treatment. Swed Dent J 1989;13(3):77–88.

39. Tammiala-Salonen T, Hiidenkari T, Parvinen T. Burning mouth in a Finnish adult population. Community Dent Oral Epidemiol 1993;21(2):67–71.

40. Donetti E, Bedoni M, Guzzi G, et al. Burning mouth syndrome possibly linked with an amalgam

tattoo: clinical and ultrastructural evidence. Eur J Dermatol 2008;18(6):723–4.

41. Formaker BK, Mott AE, Frank ME. The effects of topical anesthesia on oral burning in burning mouth syndrome. Ann N Y Acad Sci 1998;855: 776–80.

42. Haas DA, Lennon DA. A 21 year retrospective study of reports of paresthesia following local anesthetic administration. J Can Dent Assoc 1995; 61(1):319 20.

43. Sandstedt P, Sorensen S. Neurosensory disturbances of the trigeminal nerve: a long-term follow-up of traumatic injuries. J Oral Maxillofac Surg 1995;53(5):498–505.

44. Drage LA, Rogers RS. Clinical assessment and outcome in 70 patients with complaints of burning or sore mouth symptoms. Mayo Clin Proc 1999; 74(3):223–8.

45. Browning S, Hislop S, Scully C, et al. The association between burning mouth syndrome and psychosocial disorders. Oral Surg Oral Med Oral Pathol 1987;64(2):171–4.

46. Ship JA, Grushka M, Lipton JA, et al. Burning mouth syndrome: an update. J Am Dent Assoc 1995;126(7):842–53.

47. Sardella A, Lodi G, Demarosi F, et al. Burning mouth syndrome: a retrospective study investigating spontaneous remission and response to treatments. Oral Dis 2006;12(2):152–5.

48. Bergdahl M, Bergdahl J. Burning mouth syndrome: prevalence and associated factors. J Oral Pathol Med 1999;28(8):350–4.

49. Torgerson RR. Burning mouth syndrome. Dermatol Ther 2010;23(3):291–8.

50. Just T, Steiner S, Pau HW. Oral pain perception and taste in burning mouth syndrome. J Oral Pathol Med 2010;39(1):22–7.

51. Feinmann C, Harris M, Cawley R. Psychogenic facial pain: presentation and treatment. Br Med J (Clin Res Ed) 1984;288(6415):436–8.

52. Hampf G, Vikkula J, Ylipaavalniemi P, et al. Psychiatric disorders in orofacial dysaesthesia. Int J Oral Maxillofac Surg 1987;16(4):402–7.

53. Jerlang BB. Burning mouth syndrome (BMS) and the concept of alexithymia–a preliminary study. J Oral Pathol Med 1997;26(6):249–53.

54. Eli I, Baht R, Littner MM, et al. Detection of psychopathologic trends in glossodynia patients. Psychosom Med 1994;56(5):389–94.

55. Mignogna MD, Pollio A, Fortuna G, et al. Unexplained somatic comorbidities in patients with burning mouth syndrome: a controlled clinical study. J Orofac Pain 2011;25(2):131–40.

56. Main DM, Basker RM. Patients complaining of a burning mouth. Further experience in clinical assessment and management. Br Dent J 1983; 154(7):206–11.

57. Maresky LS, van der Bijl P, Gird I. Burning mouth syndrome. Evaluation of multiple variables among 85 patients. Oral Surg Oral Med Oral Pathol 1993;75(3):303–7.

58. Poon R, Su N, Ching V, et al. Reduction in unstimulated salivary flow rate in burning mouth syndrome. Br Dent J 2014;217(7):E14.

59. Grushka M, Sessle BJ, Howley TP. Psychophysical evidence of taste dysfunction in burning mouth syndrome. Chem Senses 1986;11(4):485–98.

60. Formaker BK, Frank ME. Taste function in patients with oral burning. Chem Senses 2000;25(5):575–81.

61. Katz J, Benoliel R, Leviner E. Burning mouth sensation associated with fusospirochetal infection in edentulous patients. Oral Surg Oral Med Oral Pathol 1986;62(2):152–4.

62. Samaranayake LP, Lamb AB, Lamey PJ, et al. Oral carriage of Candida species and coliforms in patients with burning mouth syndrome. J Oral Pathol Med 1989;18(4):233–5.

63. Osaki T, Yoneda K, Yamamoto T, et al. Candidiasis may induce glossodynia without objective manifestation. Am J Med Sci 2000;319(2):100–5.

64. Vitkov L, Weitgasser R, Hannig M, et al. Candida-induced stomatopyrosis and its relation to diabetes mellitus. J Oral Pathol Med 2003;32(1):46–50.

65. Adler I, Denninghoff VC, Alvarez MI, et al. Helicobacter pylori associated with glossitis and halitosis. Helicobacter 2005;10(4):312–7.

66. Terai H, Shimahara M. Glossodynia from Candida-associated lesions, burning mouth syndrome, or mixed causes. Pain Med 2010;11(6):856–60.

67. Nagel MA, Choe A, Traktinskiy I, et al. Burning mouth syndrome due to herpes simplex virus type 1. BMJ Case Rep 2015;2015.

68. Epstein JB, Grushka M, Sherlock C, et al. Burning mouth: an initial examination of a potential role of herpes virus infection. Oral Med Pathol 2006; 11(2):45–8.

69. Powell FC. Glossodynia and other disorders of the tongue. Dermatol Clin 1987;5(4):687–93.

70. Srinivasan M, Kodumudi KN, Zunt SL. Soluble CD14 and toll-like receptor-2 are potential salivary biomarkers for oral lichen planus and burning mouth syndrome. Clin Immunol 2008;126(1):31–7.

71. Paterson AJ, Lamb AB, Clifford TJ, et al. Burning mouth syndrome: the relationship between the HAD scale and parafunctional habits. J Oral Pathol Med 1995;24(7):289–92.

72. Svensson P, Kaaber S. General health factors and denture function in patients with burning mouth syndrome and matched control subjects. J Oral Rehabil 1995;22(12):887–95.

73. Brody HA, Prendergast JJ, Silverman S. The relationship between oral symptoms, insulin release, and glucose intolerance. Oral Surg Oral Med Oral Pathol 1971;31(6):777–82.

74. Basker RM, Sturdee DW, Davenport JC. Patients with burning mouths. A clinical investigation of causative factors, including the climacteric and diabetes. Br Dent J 1978;145(1):9–16.

75. Bergdahl J, Anneroth G, Perris H. Personality characteristics of patients with resistant burning mouth syndrome. Acta Odontol Scand 1995; 53(1):7–11.

76. Brailo V, Vueiaeeviae-Boras V, Alajbeg IZ, et al. Oral burning symptoms and burning mouth syndrome-significance of different variables in 150 patients. Med Oral Patol Oral Cir Bucal 2006; 11(3):E252–5.

77. Carrington J, Getter L, Brown RS. Diabetic neuropathy masquerading as glossodynia. J Am Dent Assoc 2001;132(11):1549–51.

78. Femiano F, Lanza A, Buonaiuto C, et al. Burning mouth syndrome and burning mouth in hypothyroidism: proposal for a diagnostic and therapeutic protocol. Oral Surg Oral Med Oral Pathol Oral Radiol Endod 2008;105(1):e22–7.

79. Femiano F, Gombos F, Esposito V, et al. Burning mouth syndrome (BMS): evaluation of thyroid and taste. Med Oral Patol Oral Cir Bucal 2006;11(1): E22–5.

80. Moore PA, Guggenheimer J, Orchard T. Burning mouth syndrome and peripheral neuropathy in patients with type 1 diabetes mellitus. J Diabetes Complications 2007;21(6):397–402.

81. Forabosco A, Criscuolo M, Coukos G, et al. Efficacy of hormone replacement therapy in postmenopausal women with oral discomfort. Oral Surg Oral Med Oral Pathol 1992;73(5):570–4.

82. Savino LB, Haushalter NM. Lisinopril-induced "scalded mouth syndrome". Ann Pharmacother 1992;26(11):1381–2.

83. Brown RS, Krakow AM, Douglas T, et al. "Scalded mouth syndrome" caused by angiotensin converting enzyme inhibitors: two case reports. Oral Surg Oral Med Oral Pathol Oral Radiol Endod 1997;83(6):665–7.

84. Lamey PJ, Hammond A, Allam BF, et al. Vitamin status of patients with burning mouth syndrome and the response to replacement therapy. Br Dent J 1986;160(3):81–4.

85. Hugoson A, Thorstensson B. Vitamin B status and response to replacement therapy in patients with burning mouth syndrome. Acta Odontol Scand 1991;49(6):367–75.

86. Cho GS, Han MW, Lee B, et al. Zinc deficiency may be a cause of burning mouth syndrome as zinc replacement therapy has therapeutic effects. J Oral Pathol Med 2010;39(9):722–7.

87. De Giuseppe R, Novembrino C, Guzzi G, et al. Burning mouth syndrome and vitamin B12 deficiency. J Eur Acad Dermatol Venereol 2011;25(7): 869–70.

88. Sun A, Wang YP, Lin HP, et al. Significant reduction of homocysteine level with multiple B vitamins in atrophic glossitis patients. Oral Dis 2013;19(5): 519–24.

89. Wardrop RW, Hailes J, Burger H, et al. Oral discomfort at menopause. Oral Surg Oral Med Oral Pathol 1989;67(5):535–40.

90. Sardella A, Lodi G, Demarosi F, et al. Causative or precipitating aspects of burning mouth syndrome: a case-control study. J Oral Pathol Med 2006; 35(8):466–71.

91. Vucicevic-Boras V, Topic B, Cekic-Arambasin A, et al. Lack of association between burning mouth syndrome and hematinic deficiencies. Eur J Med Res 2001;6(9):409–12.

92. Rojo L, Silvestre FJ, Bagan JV, et al. Psychiatric morbidity in burning mouth syndrome. Psychiatric interview versus depression and anxiety scales. Oral Surg Oral Med Oral Pathol 1993;75(3):308–11.

93. Nicholson M, Wilkinson G, Field E, et al. A pilot study: stability of psychiatric diagnoses over 6 months in burning mouth syndrome. J Psychosom Res 2000;49(1):1–2.

94. Maina G, Albert U, Gandolfo S, et al. Personality disorders in patients with burning mouth syndrome. J Personal Disord 2005;19(1):84–93.

95. Amenabar JM, Pawlowski J, Hilgert JB, et al. Anxiety and salivary cortisol levels in patients with burning mouth syndrome: case-control study. Oral Surg Oral Med Oral Pathol Oral Radiol Endod 2008;105(4):460–5.

96. Carlson CR, Miller CS, Reid KI. Psychosocial profiles of patients with burning mouth syndrome. J Orofac Pain 2000;14(1):59–64.

97. Mendak-Ziolko M, Konopka T, Bogucki ZA. Evaluation of select neurophysiological, clinical and psychological tests for burning mouth syndrome. Oral Surg Oral Med Oral Pathol Oral Radiol 2012; 114(3):325–32.

98. Souza FT, Santos TP, Bernardes VF, et al. The impact of burning mouth syndrome on health-related quality of life. Health Qual Life Outcomes 2011;9:57.

99. de Souza FT, Teixeira AL, Amaral TM, et al. Psychiatric disorders in burning mouth syndrome. J Psychosom Res 2012;72(2):142–6.

100. Lopez-Jornet P, Camacho-Alonso F, Lucero-Berdugo M. Quality of life in patients with burning mouth syndrome. J Oral Pathol Med 2008;37(7): 389–94.

101. Spadari F, Venesia P, Azzi L, et al. Low basal salivary flow and burning mouth syndrome: new evidence in this enigmatic pathology. J Oral Pathol Med 2015;44(3):229–33.

102. Kim HI, Kim YY, Chang JY, et al. Salivary cortisol, 17beta-estradiol, progesterone, dehydroepiandrosterone, and alpha-amylase in patients with

burning mouth syndrome. Oral Dis 2012;18(6): 613–20.

103. Imura H, Shimada M, Yamazaki Y, et al. Characteristic changes of saliva and taste in burning mouth syndrome patients. J Oral Pathol Med 2015;45(3): 231–6.

104. de Souza FT, Kummer A, Silva ML, et al. The association of openness personality trait with stress-related salivary biomarkers in burning mouth syndrome. Neuroimmunomodulation 2015;22(4): 250–5.

105. Lopez-Jornet P, Juan H, Alvaro PF. Mineral and trace element analysis of saliva from patients with BMS: a cross-sectional prospective controlled clinical study. J Oral Pathol Med 2014;43(2):111–6.

106. Nasri-Heir C, Gomes J, Heir GM, et al. The role of sensory input of the chorda tympani nerve and the number of fungiform papillae in burning mouth syndrome. Oral Surg Oral Med Oral Pathol Oral Radiol Endod 2011;112(1):65–72.

107. Eliav E, Kamran B, Schaham R, et al. Evidence of chorda tympani dysfunction in patients with burning mouth syndrome. J Am Dent Assoc 2007; 138(5):628–33.

108. Bergdahl M, Bergdahl J. Perceived taste disturbance in adults: prevalence and association with oral and psychological factors and medication. Clin Oral Investig 2002;6(3):145–9.

109. Lopez-Jornet P, Lucero-Berdugo M, Castillo-Felipe C, et al. Assessment of self-reported sleep disturbance and psychological status in patients with burning mouth syndrome. J Eur Acad Dermatol Venereol 2015;29(7):1285–90.

110. Adamo D, Schiavone V, Aria M, et al. Sleep disturbance in patients with burning mouth syndrome: a case-control study. J Orofac Pain 2013; 27(4):304–13.

111. Kontoangelos K, Koukia E, Papanikolaou V, et al. Suicidal behavior in a patient with burning mouth syndrome. Case Rep Psychiatry 2014;2014: 405106.

112. Chainani-Wu N, Madden E, Silverman S. A case-control study of burning mouth syndrome and sleep dysfunction. Oral Surg Oral Med Oral Pathol Oral Radiol Endod 2011;112(2):203–8.

113. Bartoshuk LM, Snyder DJ, Grushka M, et al. Taste damage: previously unsuspected consequences. Chem Senses 2005;30(Suppl 1):i218–9.

114. Su N, Ching V, Grushka M. Taste disorders: a review. J Can Dent Assoc 2013;79:d86.

115. Kaplan I, Levin T, Papoiu AD, et al. Thermal sensory and pain thresholds in the tongue and chin change with age, but are not altered in burning mouth syndrome. Skin Res Technol 2011;17(2): 196–200.

116. Schobel N, Kyereme J, Minovi A, et al. Sweet taste and chorda tympani transection alter capsaicin-induced lingual pain perception in adult human subjects. Physiol Behav 2012;107(3): 368–73.

117. Grushka M, Sessle BJ, Howley TP. Psychophysical assessment of tactile, pain and thermal sensory functions in burning mouth syndrome. Pain 1987; 28(2):169–84.

118. Siviero M, Teixeira MJ, Siqueira JT, et al. Central mechanisms in burning mouth syndrome involving the olfactory nerve: a preliminary study. Clinics (Sao Paulo) 2011;66(3):509–12.

119. Boucher Y, Simons CT, Carstens MI, et al. Effects of gustatory nerve transection and/or ovariectomy on oral capsaicin avoidance in rats. Pain 2014;155(4): 814–20.

120. Li YK, Yang JM, Huang YB, et al. Shrinkage of ipsilateral taste buds and hyperplasia of contralateral taste buds following chorda tympani nerve transection. Neural Regen Res 2015;10(6):989–95.

121. Albuquerque RJ, de Leeuw R, Carlson CR, et al. Cerebral activation during thermal stimulation of patients who have burning mouth disorder: an fMRI study. Pain 2006;122(3):223–34.

122. Suri V. Menopause and oral health. J Midlife Health 2014;5(3):115–20.

123. Dias Fernandes CS, Salum FG, Bandeira D, et al. Salivary dehydroepiandrosterone (DHEA) levels in patients with the complaint of burning mouth: a case-control study. Oral Surg Oral Med Oral Pathol Oral Radiol Endod 2009;108(4):537–43.

124. Koike K, Shinozaki T, Hara K, et al. Immune and endocrine function in patients with burning mouth syndrome. Clin J Pain 2014;30(2):168–73.

125. Belmaker RH, Agam G. Major depressive disorder. N Engl J Med 2008;358(1):55–68.

126. Jacobs EG, Holsen LM, Lancaster K, et al. 17beta-estradiol differentially regulates stress circuitry activity in healthy and depressed women. Neuropsychopharmacology 2015;40(3):566–76.

127. Donovan KA, Walker LM, Wassersug RJ, et al. Psychological effects of androgen-deprivation therapy on men with prostate cancer and their partners. Cancer 2015;121(24):4286–99.

128. Tavee J, Zhou L. Small fiber neuropathy: a burning problem. Cleve Clin J Med 2009;76(5):297–305.

129. Mo X, Zhang J, Fan Y, et al. Thermal and mechanical quantitative sensory testing in Chinese patients with burning mouth syndrome - a probable neuropathic pain condition? J Headache Pain 2015; 16(1):84.

130. de Siqueira SR, Teixeira MJ, de Siqueira JT. Somatosensory investigation of patients with orofacial pain compared with controls. J Neuropsychiatry Clin Neurosci 2014;26(4):376–81.

131. de Tommaso M, Lavolpe V, Di Venere D, et al. A case of unilateral burning mouth syndrome of neuropathic origin. Headache 2011;51(3):441–4.

132. Yilmaz Z, Renton T, Yiangou Y, et al. Burning mouth syndrome as a trigeminal small fibre neuropathy: increased heat and capsaicin receptor TRPV1 in nerve fibres correlates with pain score. J Clin Neurosci 2007;14(9):864–71.

133. Tatsumi E, Katsura H, Kobayashi K, et al. Changes in transient receptor potential channels in the rat geniculate ganglion after chorda tympani nerve injury. Neuroreport 2015;26(14):856–61.

134. Borsani E, Majorana A, Cocchi MA, et al. Epithelial expression of vanilloid and cannabinoid receptors: a potential role in burning mouth syndrome pathogenesis. Histol Histopathol 2014;29(4):523–33.

135. Smith KG, Yates JM, Robinson PP. The effect of nerve growth factor on functional recovery after injury to the chorda tympani and lingual nerves. Brain Res 2004;1020(1–2):62–72.

136. Borelli V, Marchioli A, Di Taranto R, et al. Neuropeptides in saliva of subjects with burning mouth syndrome: a pilot study. Oral Dis 2010;16(4):365–74.

137. Sinay VJ, Bonamico LH, Dubrovsky A. Subclinical sensory abnormalities in trigeminal neuralgia. Cephalalgia 2003;23(7):541–4.

138. Bangash TH. Trigeminal neuralgia: frequency of occurrence in different nerve branches. Anesth Pain Med 2011;1(2):70–2.

139. Komiyama O, Obara R, Uchida T, et al. Pain intensity and psychosocial characteristics of patients with burning mouth syndrome and trigeminal neuralgia. J Oral Sci 2012;54(4):321–7.

140. Koszewicz M, Mendak M, Konopka T, et al. The characteristics of autonomic nervous system disorders in burning mouth syndrome and Parkinson disease. J Orofac Pain 2012;26(4):315–20.

141. Prakash S, Ahuja S, Rathod C. Dopa responsive burning mouth syndrome: restless mouth syndrome or oral variant of restless legs syndrome? J Neurol Sci 2012;320(1–2):156–60.

142. Pavlakis PP, Alexopoulos H, Kosmidis ML, et al. Peripheral neuropathies in Sjogren's syndrome: a critical update on clinical features and pathogenetic mechanisms. J Autoimmun 2012;39(1–2):27–33.

143. Au J, Patel D, Campbell JH. Oral lichen planus. Oral Maxillofac Surg Clin North Am 2013;25(1):93–100, vii.

144. Lynde CB, Grushka M, Walsh SR. Burning mouth syndrome: patch test results from a large case series. J Cutan Med Surg 2014;18(3):174–9.

145. Pekiner FN, Gumru B, Ozbayrak S. Efficacy of moclobemide in burning mouth syndrome: a non-randomized, open-label study. J Orofac Pain 2008;22(2):146–52.

146. Patton LL, Siegel MA, Benoliel R, et al. Management of burning mouth syndrome: systematic review and management recommendations. Oral Surg Oral Med Oral Pathol Oral Radiol Endod 2007;103(Suppl):S39.e1–13.

147. Mignogna MD, Fedele S, Lo Russo L, et al. The diagnosis of burning mouth syndrome represents a challenge for clinicians. J Orofac Pain 2005;19(2):168–73.

148. Klasser GD, Epstein JB, Villines D, et al. Burning mouth syndrome: a challenge for dental practitioners and patients. Gen Dent 2011;59(3):210–20 [quiz: 221–2].

149. Endo H, Rees TD. Cinnamon products as a possible etiologic factor in orofacial granulomatosis. Med Oral Patol Oral Cir Bucal 2007;12(6):E440–4.

150. Minor JS, Epstein JB. Burning mouth syndrome and secondary oral burning. Otolaryngol Clin North Am 2011;44(1):205–19, vii.

151. Lopez-Jornet P, Camacho-Alonso F, Andujar-Mateos P. A prospective, randomized study on the efficacy of tongue protector in patients with burning mouth syndrome. Oral Dis 2011;17(3):277–82.

152. Axell T. Treatment of smarting symptoms in the oral mucosa by appliance of lingual acrylic splints. Swed Dent J 2008;32(4):165–9.

153. Bergdahl J, Anneroth G, Perris H. Cognitive therapy in the treatment of patients with resistant burning mouth syndrome: a controlled study. J Oral Pathol Med 1995;24(5):213–5.

154. Femiano F, Gombos F, Scully C. Burning mouth syndrome: open trial of psychotherapy alone, medication with alpha-lipoic acid (thioctic acid), and combination therapy. Med Oral 2004;9(1):8–13.

155. Miziara ID, Filho BC, Oliveira R, et al. Group psychotherapy: an additional approach to burning mouth syndrome. J Psychosom Res 2009;67(5):443–8.

156. Zakrzewska JM, Forssell H, Glenny AM. Interventions for the treatment of burning mouth syndrome. Cochrane Database Syst Rev 2005;(1):CD002779.

157. de Moraes M, do Amaral Bezerra BA, da Rocha Neto PC, et al. Randomized trials for the treatment of burning mouth syndrome: an evidence-based review of the literature. J Oral Pathol Med 2012;41(4):281–7.

158. Ducasse D, Courtet P, Olie E. Burning mouth syndrome: current clinical, physiopathologic, and therapeutic data. Reg Anesth Pain Med 2013;38(5):380–90.

159. Kuten-Shorrer M, Kelley JM, Sonis ST, et al. Placebo effect in burning mouth syndrome: a systematic review. Oral Dis 2014;20(3):e1–6.

Orofacial Movement Disorders

Glenn T. Clark, DDS, MS[a], Saravanan Ram, DDS, MS[b],*

KEYWORDS

- Orofacial dystonia • Orofacial dyskinesia • Tardive dyskinesia • Bruxism
- Drug-induced extrapyramidal reactions

KEY POINTS

- Orofacial dystonia is a specific movement disorder characterized by an intermittent involuntary momentarily sustained contraction of the jaw or orofacial muscles.
- Orofacial dyskinesia is a continuous repetitive movement disorder of the jaw or tongue, lips, or tongue and can be tardive or spontaneous.
- Botulinum toxin injections are the most effective means of managing orofacial movement disorders and are often used in conjunction with medications.
- Drug-induced extrapyramidal reactions refer to dystonia, akathisia, or parkinsonian type movements caused by antipsychotic medications.

OROFACIAL MOVEMENT DISORDERS

Multiple disorders that affect the motor system need to be considered when the trigeminal, facial, or genioglossal muscles become dysfunctional. The focus of this article is on 4 orofacial movement disorders (OMDs) including: (1) orofacial dystonia, (2) orofacial dyskinesia, (3) drug-induced extrapyramidal reaction, and (4) sleep bruxism (**Table 1**).[1–4]

OROFACIAL DYSTONIA

Orofacial dystonia affects the orofacial region and involves the jaw openers (both lateral pterygoids and anterior digastric), tongue muscles, facial muscles (especially orbicularis oris and buccinator), and platysma. It is a specific movement disorder that is considered to be present when an intermittent involuntary momentarily sustained contraction of the jaw or orofacial muscles occurs. When this occurs in association with blepharospasm (focal dystonia of the orbicularis oculi muscles), it is called Meige syndrome.[5]

Prevalence of Orofacial Dystonia

Most dystonias are idiopathic and the focal form of dystonia occurs 10 times more often than the generalized systemic form. The prevalence of all forms of idiopathic dystonia ranges between 3 and 30 per 100,000.[6] Focal dystonias can be primary or secondary and the secondary form of dystonias occurs as a result of a trauma (peripheral or central), brainstem lesion, systemic disease (eg, multiple sclerosis, Parkinson disease), vascular disease (eg, basal ganglia infarct), or drug use.[7] Most dystonias are primary or idiopathic, and demonstrate no specific central nervous system (CNS) disease.

Pathophysiology of Orofacial Dystonia

Of course, various pathophysiologic mechanisms have been proposed to explain dystonia, including

Disclosure statement: The authors have nothing to disclose.
[a] Orofacial Pain Graduate Residency Program, Herman Ostrow School of Dentistry of USC, Los Angeles, CA 90089-0641, USA; [b] Oral Medicine Graduate Residency Program, 925 West 34th Street, Herman Ostrow School of Dentistry of USC, Los Angeles, CA, 90089-0641, USA
* Corresponding author.
E-mail address: saravanr@usc.edu

Table 1
Five oral motor disorders

Oral Motor Disorders	Definition	Clinical Features	Management
Orofacial Dystonia	• Involuntary • Repetitive • Briefly sustained muscle contraction • Results in an abnormal posturing of structure	• Involuntary jaw opening • Lateral or open jaw motion • Protrusion of the tongue • Present during the day • Disappears during sleep • Dystonic spasms increase in intensity during stress, emotional upset, or fatigue	• Pharmacologic treatment • Transient help with botulinum toxin injections • Select use of neurosurgical treatment
Orofacial Dyskinesia	• Repetitive and stereo-typic oral movements • Onset with neuroleptic medications • Persists or worsens after withdrawal of neuroleptics	• Facial grimacing • Tongue protrusion • Puckering, smacking, and licking of lips • Side-to-side jaw motion	No effective treatment
Drug-induced Dystonic-type Extrapyramidal Reactions	• Medications-induced • Illegal drugs–induced • Unspecified extrapyramidal syndrome reaction	• Dystonic • Akathisia • Parkinsonism	Withdraw offending drug
Sleep Bruxism	• Stereotyped movement • Grinding or clenching of the teeth during sleep	• Dental attrition • Tooth pain • Temporomandibular joint dysfunction • Headaches	• Pharmacologic treatment data not convincing • Most cases managed with an occlusal appliance • Only most severe cases treated with botulinum toxin injections

basal ganglia dysfunction, hyperexcitability of interneurons involved in motor signaling, reduced inhibition of spinal cord and brainstem signals coming from supraspinal input, and dysfunction of neurochemical systems involving dopamine, serotonin, and noradrenaline.[8] All dystonias are involuntary but tend to be more intermittent than dyskinesias (see later discussion) and are composed of short but sustained muscle contractions that produce twisting and repetitive movements or abnormal postures.[9,10]

Almost pathognomonic for dystonia in the orofacial region is that many patients can partially control or suppress the movement with the use of tactile stimulation, such as touching the chin in the case of orofacial dystonia or holding an object in their mouth. This suppressive effect has been called geste antagonistique.[11] These tactile maneuvers may mislead physicians to the erroneous diagnosis of malingering or hysteria. Other examples of sensory tricks include placing a hand on the side of the face, the chin, or the back of the head; or touching these areas with 1 or more fingers, which at times will reduce neck contractions associated with cervical dystonia. Sometimes patients will have discovered that placing an object in the mouth, such as a toothpick or a piece of gum, may reduce dystonia of the jaw, mouth, and lower face. Finally, almost all of the focal and segmental dystonias only occur during waking periods and disappear entirely during sleep.[12]

Management of Dystonia

For most OMDs, there is no well-defined treatment protocol except (1) rule out CNS disease and local pathologic conditions; (2) try 1 or more of the medications that may be helpful in these cases; (3) if the disorder is severe enough and focal enough to consider, and the medications are not adequate, consider botulinum toxin injections; and (4) for those that cannot be helped with the previous steps, it is reasonable to consider neurosurgical therapy or implanted medication pumps that can deliver intrathecal medications.

Botulinum toxin type A for dystonia

In 1989, Blitzer and colleagues[13] first described the injection of botulinum toxin for orofacial dystonia. Their article described injecting many of the orofacial muscles in 20 orofacial dystonias and claimed that masseter and temporalis injections helped with suppressing the overall orofacial dystonia. In 1991, Blitzer and colleagues[14] described the first use of botulinum toxin in patients with lingual dystonia but cautioned clinicians that dysphagia was a problem in some of their cases.

There are many variations of orofacial dystonia, but involuntary jaw-opening dystonia is common. One complication of jaw-opening dystonia is that the temporomandibular joint (TMJ) can become physically locked in the wide-open position so that even after the dystonic contraction stops, the jaw will not easily close back to the normal position. In 1997, Moore and Wood described the management of recurrent, involuntary TMJ dislocation using botulinum toxin type A (BoTN-A).[15] The injected target was each of the lateral pterygoid muscle and the injections were performed using electromyogram (EMG) guidance. The investigators describe that the effect lasted for 10 months. The lateral pterygoid is the muscle most responsible for opening and it is a difficult injection that has a high potential for misplacement of the solution into other adjacent muscles.

BoTN-A is often considered first-line therapy for focal dystonia. A recent systematic review of the literature evaluated the effect of BoTN-A versus anticholinergic medications for cervical dystonia.[16] Specifically this study identified only 1 clinical trial suitable for inclusion in the review and, based on this article, the investigators concluded that the existing evidence suggests that BoTN-A injections provide more objective and subjective benefit than trihexyphenidyl to patients with cervical dystonia.

Medications for orofacial dystonia

A list of commonly used medications for the management of OMDs is listed in **Table 2**.

Anticholinergic therapy The anticholinergic drugs, such as trihexyphenidyl hydrochloride, biperiden, benztropine (Cogentin), or ethopropazine (Parsitan), which block the neurotransmitter acetylcholine, are the first line of motor-suppressive medications used for dystonia, although they are only partially effective when compared with botulinum toxin injections.[16,17] It is critical to start at a low dose and increase the dose very slowly to try to minimize the adverse effects. Use of these drugs is often limited by central side effects such as confusion, drowsiness, hallucination, personality change, and memory difficulties; and peripheral side effects such as dry mouth, blurred vision, urinary retention, and constipation.

Dopamine therapy Specific subsets of dystonias that have a childhood onset have been shown to respond remarkably well to low-dosage L-Dopa such as carbidopa or levodopa. These dystonias are referred to as dopa-responsive dystonia.[18,19] Some patients with primary dystonia respond to drugs that increase the neurotransmitter dopamine. These drugs are dopaminergic agents and include levodopa (Sinemet) and bromocriptine (Parlodel). Side effects may include parkinsonism, hypotension, and depression. Ironically, however, many patients respond to agents that block or deplete dopamine. Many of these drugs are antipsychotic agents such as clozapine (Clozaril) and tetrabenazine (Nitoman).

Benzodiazepine therapy Drugs such as diazepam (Valium), clonazepam (Klonopin), and lorazepam (Ativan) affect the nervous system's ability to process the neurotransmitter γ-aminobutyric acid (GABA)-A. A primary side effect is sedation but may also include depression, personality change, and drug addiction. Rapid discontinuation can result in a withdrawal syndrome. Some dystonia patients tolerate very high doses without apparent adverse effects.

γ-Aminobutyric acid agonist therapy Baclofen (Lioresal) stimulates the body's ability to process a neurotransmitter called GABA-B. Intrathecal forms of baclofen, in which a steady dose of medication is fed into the nervous system by a surgically implanted device, are also available. Side effects may include confusion, dizziness or lightheadedness, drowsiness, nausea, and muscle weakness.

Miscellaneous drugs for movement disorder therapy There are several miscellaneous drugs that have been reported to suppress motor disorders. One medication used to suppress motor activity is buspirone, which is a nonbenzodiazepine anxiolytic drug.[20,21] Another drug in which the mechanism is unclear is amantadine, which is used to suppress extrapyramidal reactions.[22] Other drugs that suppress motor activity are diphenhydramine[23] and clonidine.[24]

Surgery for orofacial dystonia

Owing to the increased morbidity of surgery, it is usually reserved as a last resort for those patients

Table 2
Medications used for management of orofacial movement disorders

Drug	Group	Indications	Receptor Action
Trihexyphenidyl hydrochloride (Artane)	Cholinergic antagonists	Idiopathic Parkinson Extrapyramidal reactions Primary dystonias	Antagonizes acetylcholine receptors
Benztropine (Cogentin)	Cholinergic antagonists	Parkinsonism Extrapyramidal reactions Acute onset secondary dystonias	Antagonizes acetylcholine and histamine receptors
Biperiden (Akineton)	Cholinergic antagonists	Parkinsonism Extrapyramidal disorders	Antagonizes acetylcholine receptors
Baclofen (Lioresal)	GABA agonist or antispasmodic	Spasticity	Mechanism unclear but most likely a GABA effect
Clonazepam (Klonopin)	GABA agonist or tricyclic antidepressant	Seizures, absence Anxiety, panic disorder Periodic leg movements, neuralgia	Binds to benzodiazepine receptors and enhances GABA effect
Tiagabine (Gabitril)	Anticonvulsant	Partial seizures	GABA reuptake inhibitor
Buspirone (Buspar)	Anxiolytic or hypnotic	Anxiety	Nonbenzodiazepine but mechanism unclear
Amantadine (Symmetrel)	Antiviral or antiparkinsonian	Influenza A Extrapyramidal reactions Parkinsonism	Mechanism unclear
Carbidopa or levodopa (Sinemet)	Antiparkinsonian	Parkinson-associated tremor	Inhibits peripheral dopamine decarboxylation Dopamine precursor
Diphenhydramine (Benadryl)	Antihistamine	Dystonic reactions	Antagonizes central and peripheral H1 receptors (nonselective)
Clonidine (Catapres)	Alpha-2 adrenergic agonist	Shown helpful for tardive dyskinesia	Stimulates alpha-2 adrenergic receptor
BoTN-A (Botox)	Neuromuscular blocker	Focal dystonia	Blocks release of acetylcholine from motor end plate

who fail to respond to medications or for those who develop resistance to BoTN-A injections. Surgery for dystonia can be peripheral or central. Peripheral surgery is usually indicated for those cases of blepharospasm and cervical dystonia that fail to respond to BoTN-A. Selective peripheral denervation and myectomy are the 2 peripheral surgical procedures. The former is widely used in the management of cervical dystonias with well-established safety and efficacy.[25] Surgical removal of the affected muscle is referred to as myectomy and is usually done for patients with blepharospasm who fail to respond to conservative management.[26]

Central surgery involves the globus pallidus region of the brain. The 3 central surgeries include deep brain stimulation (DBS), pallidotomy, and microvascular decompression surgery. DBS uses an implanted electrode to deliver continuous high-frequency electrical stimulation to the thalamus, globus pallidus, or any part of the brain involved with the control of movement.[27] Pallidotomy is an invasive procedure that involves creating a surgical lesion in the globus pallidus and may be done unilaterally or bilaterally.[28,29] Hemifacial spasm secondary to compression of the facial nerve by a nearby blood vessel can be relieved by microvascular decompression surgery.[30] A summary of orofacial dystonia is presented in **Box 1**.

OROFACIAL DYSKINESIA

The word dyskinesia means abnormal movement and is used to describe a continuous repetitive movement disorder of the jaw or tongue, lips, or tongue, which can be drug-induced (tardive) or occur without clear cause (spontaneous). Unfortunately, there is no more specific diagnostic test for dyskinesia other than clinical observation and history. Risk factors for the development of tardive dyskinesia are older age, female gender, and the presence of affective disorders.[31]

Prevalence of Orofacial Dyskinesia

For spontaneous dyskinesias, the prevalence rate is 1.5% to 38% of elderly individuals, depending on age and definition. Elderly women are twice as likely to develop the disorder.[32] Specifically, it affects 1.5% to 4% in healthy elderly,[33,34] 18% to 31.7% of elderly living in retirement homes,[35–37] and 3.7% of elderly in daycare centers.[38] When this disorder is associated with drug use, the medications most commonly implicated are the neuroleptic medications now in widespread use as a component of behavioral therapy. The prevalence rate of drug-induced dyskinesia (tardive form) is approximately 15% to 30% in patients who receive long-term treatment with neuroleptic medications.[39]

Pathophysiology of Orofacial Dyskinesia

These neuroleptic medications chronically block dopamine receptors in the basal ganglia. The result would be a chemically induced denervation supersensitivity of the dopamine receptors, leading to excessive movement. However, other neurotransmitter abnormalities in GABAergic and cholinergic pathways have been suggested as underlying changes.

Management of Orofacial Dyskinesia

Treatment of orofacial dyskinesia is largely with medications that, unfortunately, are not highly successful. Less than 10% of patients experienced sustained benefit from anticholinergic agents and, although neuroleptic medication may have better efficacy, the side effects and the risk of tardive manifestations prevented their general use. Benzodiazepines, particularly clonazepam, seemed particularly promising, with sustained benefit in 67% of subjects from one study.[40]

The general rule is to (1) withdraw the offending medication and (2) hope that the dyskinesia or dystonic reaction will go away.[41] If the suspected medication cannot be stopped or is severe, the following methods are used: diphenhydramine 50 mg or benztropine 2 mg, intravenous (IV) or intramuscular (IM).[42–44] The preferred route of administration is IV. If this is not feasible, IM drug administration can be used. Finally, both amantadine 200 to 400 mg/d by mouth[45] and diazepam 5 mg IV[46] have been shown to be effective for recurrent neuroleptic-induced dystonic reactions. A summary of orofacial dyskinesia is presented in **Box 2**.

DRUG-INDUCED EXTRAPYRAMIDAL REACTIONS

There are patients who develop a medication-induced oral motor hyperactivity that does not fit into the dyskinesia category.[47] Most often, it is a form of dystonia that is induced by antipsychotic medications.

Prevalence of Extrapyramidal Syndrome

Medications, typically dopamine receptor-blocking agents for the treatment of psychosis, are the main culprits causing drug-induced extrapyramidal syndrome (EPS). Despite the advent of newer atypical antipsychotic drugs that promised a low side-effect profile than conventional antipsychotics, drug-induced EPS continues to be a significant problem. Less than 5% of patients exposed to antipsychotics develop dystonic reactions that manifest years after exposure to the medication.[48] The craniocervical region is the site most affected by these reactions.[49]

Pathophysiology of Extrapyramidal Syndrome

The medications and illegal drugs produce a motor response that is better classified as an unspecified EPS reaction. EPS responses typically have 3 presentations; dystonia, akathisia, and parkinsonism.

Dystonic reactions consist of involuntary, tonic contractions of skeletal muscles.[50–52] Akathisia reactions occur as a subjective experience of motor restlessness.[53,54] Patients may complain of an inability to sit or stand still, or a compulsion to pace or cross and uncross their legs. Parkinsonian reactions manifest themselves as tremor, rigidity, and akinesia, which shows as a slowness in initiating motor tasks and fatigue when performing activities requiring repetitive movements (bradykinesia). When a medication or drug induces a dystonic EPS reaction, it typically involves the muscles of the head, face, and jaw, producing spasm, grimacing, tics, or trismus.

Most of the literature has focused on the more severe acute dystonic EPS reactions that occur with the use of antipsychotic medications. In addition to the antipsychotics, several antiemetics with dopamine receptor–blocking properties have also been associated with drug-induced EPS. These include prochlorperazine, promethazine, and metoclopramide. Of course, other less severe reactions do occur that vary in intensity and even wax and wane over time. The most commonly reported offending agents that are not neuroleptics are the selective serotonin reuptake inhibitors (SSRIs), stimulant medications, and illegal drugs.

SSRIs such as fluoxetine, fluvoxamine, paroxetine, sertraline, citalopram, escitalopram are used for depression and a variety of other mental illness. Unfortunately, these drugs are reported to produce the side effect of increased clenching and bruxism.[55–58] The term SSRI-induced bruxism has been used to describe this condition but may not be accurate in that the actual motor behavior does not present as brief strong sleep state–related contractions as seen in bruxism. The motor abnormalities are more of an increased sustained nonspecific activation of the jaw and tongue musculature.[59]

Illegal drugs, such as methamphetamine, cocaine, and 3,4-methylenedioxymethamphetamine (Ecstasy), and legal prescription stimulants, such as methylphenidate, phentermine, pemoline, dextroamphetamine, amphetamines, and diethylpropion, have all been reported to induce bruxism and dystonic extrapyramidal reactions.[60–64]

Management of Drug-Induced Extrapyramidal Reactions

The primary approach is either removing medications (if a suspected drug-related motor disorder is present) or adding additional medications that suppress the motor system. If a patient has a proven tardive dyskinesia that does not stop with withdrawal of the offending medications, or if these medications cannot be stopped, this is managed as a spontaneous movement disorder with motor suppressive medications. These medications work well for acute onset spasms of the jaw but often only a small effect is seen and side effects can be substantial in patients with hyperkinetic oral movement disorders.

Fortunately, acute dystonic reactions secondary to neuroleptic drugs are infrequent and disappear on discontinuation of the medication but this may take days to months, depending on the drug, its dose, and the patient. The same goes for less severe dystonic EPS reactions associated with SSRIs and stimulant drugs. If the suspected medication cannot be stopped or it is severe, the following methods are used: diphenhydramine 50 mg or benztropine 2 mg IV or IM. The preferred route of administration is IV. If this is not feasible, IM drug administration can be used. Both amantadine 200 to 400 mg/d by mouth and diazepam 5 mg IV have been shown to be effective for recurrent neuroleptic-induced dystonic reactions.

Some patients with SSRI-induced dystonic EPS have relief when the dose of SSRI or the other stimulant drug is reduced. For example, when fluoxetine changes from 20 mg/d to 10 mg/d. Other patients respond to the addition of buspirone in doses of 5 to 15 mg/d.[65] Other patients developed bruxism within the first few weeks of SSRI therapy; however, they were successfully treated with buspirone in doses of 10 mg 2 to 3 times daily. Buspirone seems to be an effective treatment based on a few case reports. This drug may have an additional benefit of relieving anxiety if it is present. It is usually well tolerated and carries a low risk of significant side effects. A summary of drug-induced EPS is presented in **Box 3**.

BRUXISM

Bruxism is usually described as a stereotyped movement disorder characterized by grinding or clenching of the teeth during sleep. It involves strong contractions of the jaw muscles during sleep, and these contractions can be rhythmic or continuous isometric contractions lasting from several seconds to as often as 10 minutes each night.[66]

Prevalence of Bruxism

The prevalence of chronic bruxism is unknown because no large probability-based random sample study has been performed using polysomnography (PSG), which is needed to measure bruxism. The prevalence in the general adult population has been reported between 3% and 90% and among children, prevalence ranges from 7% to 88%.[67–75] Of course, many bruxers do not have substantial attrition and many also do not make tooth grinding sounds during sleep, so sleep partner or parental reports are not always accurate.

Pathophysiology of Bruxism

The pathophysiology of bruxism is unknown. Various factors have been associated with bruxism. The most cogent theories describe bruxism as a neuromotor dysregulation disorder. This theory proposes that bruxism occurs due to the failure to inhibit jaw motor activity during a sleep state arousal. There are numerous clear-cut neuromotor diseases that exhibit bruxism as a feature of the disease (eg, cerebral palsy). The disorder of periodic limb movements is thought to be quite similar to bruxism except that it occurs in the leg muscles rather than in the jaw.[76] Bruxism has been reported during each stage of sleep; however, most episodes appear during stage II sleep.[77,78] Bruxism also occurs frequently when the patient moves from a deeper to a lighter stage of sleep and can be induced by attempts at waking the sleeping subject.[79]

Consequently, some bruxism episodes seem to be part of an arousal phenomenon that includes an increase in heart rate and respiration, galvanic skin resistance changes, and the appearance of the K-complex on the electroencephalogram. Although most bruxism episodes seem to occur during stage II sleep and during arousal, others have reported that bruxism may occur during rapid eye movement (REM) sleep.[80–82] The presence of rhythmic masticatory muscle activity (RMMA) during sleep does not seem to cause sleep disruption. Sleep macrostructure (eg, total sleep time, sleep latency, number of awakenings or sleep stage shifts, and sleep stage duration) is similar between groups.

Differences in sleep microstructure between bruxism patients and normals have been investigated in only a few studies. In 2002, Lavigne and colleagues[83] quantified the number of microarousals, K-complexes, K-alphas, electroencephalographic (EEG) spindles, and the density of slow wave activity (SWA) in both bruxers and control groups to better understand the pathophysiology of bruxism. Bruxism subjects showed 6 times more RMMA episodes per hour of sleep than

---

Box 3
Recommendations for diagnosis and management of drug-induced extrapyramidal syndrome

- EPS or reactions (usually the dystonic type) cause tightening, spasm, grimacing, tics, or outright trismus in the orofacial region due to prescribed and illegal medications.

- The difference between an EPS and a tardive dyskinesia is that the latter diagnosis is only made if the motor disorder is still present 3 months after the suspected medication has been withdrawn.

- Common offending prescription medications for EPS include antipsychotic medications, several anti-emetics with dopamine receptor blocking properties, serotonin and norepinephrine reuptake inhibitor, and SSRI medications.

- Stimulant medications also cause EPS activity in the orofacial region (methamphetamine, cocaine, 3,4-methylenedioxymethamphetamine, methylphenidate, phentermine, pemoline, dextroamphetamine, amphetamines and diethylpropion).

- The primary approach is either removing medications and/or protect the teeth with an occlusal appliance if the cessation of the medication is not appropriate.

- In some cases, adding a second motor-suppressive medication may be necessary to treat drug-induced EPS if the medication cannot be stopped or lowered in dose.

controls, with a higher frequency in the second and third non-REM to REM cycles. Bruxism subjects presented 42.7% fewer K-complexes per hour of stage II sleep but only normals showed a decline from the first to fourth non-REM episode. Only 24% of bruxism RMMA episodes were associated with K-complexes in 60 seconds. The number of K-alphas was 61% lower in bruxism subjects and no change across non-REM episodes was noted. Although no difference in EEG spindles or SWA was observed between groups, EEG spindles increased and SWA decreased linearly over consecutive non-REM to REM cycles. The investigators concluded that good sleep in bruxism patients is characterized by a low incidence of K-complexes or K-alphas and by the absence of any difference in other sleep microstructure variables or sleep wave activity. In 2006, a study showed a shift in sympathovagal balance towards increased sympathetic activity started 8 minutes preceding bruxism onset. In moderate to severe bruxism subjects, a clear increase in sympathetic activity precedes bruxism onset.[84] Moreover, the onset of RMMA and bruxism episodes during sleep were shown to be under the influences of brief and transient activity of the brainstem arousal-reticular ascending system, contributing to the increase of activity in autonomic-cardiac and motor modulatory networks.[85]

Management of Bruxism

The primary management method for strong bruxism and clenching is still with the use of a full arch occlusal appliance during sleep, plus clear instructions to the patient to make sure they try to avoid any and all clenching habits.[86] In some cases, it is also advisable to have the patient use the occlusal appliance a few hours each day during which they consciously never close their teeth on the appliance. The literature is clear that at best the appliance does not stop the bruxism behavior but limits its dental damage.

Buspirone might be a suppressive agent of SSRI-induced bruxism. In 1999, a case report involving 4 patients was published that described the successful treatment of SSRI-induced bruxism with buspirone.[20] Currently, there is no study that has tested the effect of buspirone on standard bruxism; it is only known that it may have an inhibitory effect on SSRI-induced bruxism.

Clonazepam, a benzodiazepine, was mentioned as an effective bruxism suppression agent but its therapeutic value is limited due to the known dependency issues induced by this class of drug and the short-term nature of its proven effects.[87]

A controlled randomized blinded study examined the effect 1 mg of clonazepam before sleep on bruxism and concluded that clonazepam significantly decreased the levels of bruxism as a direct result of the clonazepam.[88]

Another, more rigorous, study examined bruxism levels before and during the use of propranolol (a beta adrenergic blocker) and clonidine (an alpha-2 adrenergic agonist) using a randomized controlled study design on 25 subjects with PSG-proven bruxism.[89] The subjects showed no effect of propranolol on bruxism; however, with clonidine, the sleep bruxism index score was reduced 61%.

Two systematic reviews examined the relative efficacy of various treatments for sleep bruxism.[90,91] These studies concluded that sleep bruxism can be managed by mandibular advancement devices, clonidine, and standard occlusal splints. Moreover, when these investigators included information such as adverse effects of various treatments they concluded that the standard occlusal splint was the treatment of choice for bruxism.

An innovative new method to suppress bruxism was developed and reported in 2001. This method involved using a vibratory stimulation-based inhibition system for nocturnal bruxism.[92] For the single subject tested to date, the bruxism-contingent vibratory-feedback system for occlusal appliances effectively inhibited bruxism without inducing substantial sleep disturbance. Whether the reduction in bruxism would continue if the device no longer provided feedback and whether the force levels applied are optimal to induce suppression remain to be determined. All occlusal appliances alter the behavior for a few weeks when first used; however, this treatment only offers a brief respite from some headaches and bruxism-induced TMJ derangement and/or arthritis problems.

In 2008, another study appeared that described the effect of conditioning electrical stimuli on temporalis electromyographic activity during sleep.[93] Specifically, the study reported on 14 volunteers who were aware of jaw-clenching activity as indicated by complaints from sleep partners, soreness in the jaw-muscle on awakening, and tooth wear facets. The system used temporalis muscle activity to trigger an electrical square-wave pulse train, which was adjusted to noticeable but generally not painful intensity. The stimulus was applied through the EMG electrodes and subjects had baseline EMG recordings for 5 to 7 consecutive nights, followed by 3-week EMG recordings with the feedback turned on, 2 weeks without the feedback, and finally 3 weeks with the biofeedback on. The data clearly showed that during feedback the number of EMG episodes per hour sleep was significantly reduced; during the 2 sessions with biofeedback it was not suppressed.

SUMMARY

OMDs are a complex and challenging group of disorders affecting the jaw and facial muscles. Currently, medications and BoTN-A are the most commonly used means of management. For those patients who fail to respond to medical management, central or peripheral neurosurgery may be the last resort.

REFERENCES

1. Clark GT. Medical management of oral motor disorders: dystonia, dyskinesia and drug-induced dystonic extrapyramidal reactions. J Calif Dent Assoc 2006;34(8):657–67.
2. Kato T, Thie NM, Montplaisir JY, et al. Bruxism and orofacial movements during sleep. Dent Clin North Am 2001;45(4):657–84.
3. Clark GT, Koyano K, Browne PA. Oral motor disorders in humans. J Calif Dent Assoc 1993; 21(1):19–30.
4. Winocur E, Gavish A, Volfin G, et al. Oral motor parafunctions among heavy drug addicts and their effects on signs and symptoms of temporomandibular disorders. J Orofac Pain 2001;15(1):56–63.
5. Tolosa E, Marti MJ. Blepharospasm-oromandibular dystonia syndrome (Meige's syndrome): clinical aspects. Adv Neurol 1988;49:73–84.
6. Cardoso F, Jankovic J. Dystonia and dyskinesia. Psychiatr Clin North Am 1997;20(4):821–38.
7. Korczyn AD, Inzelberg R. Dystonia. Curr Opin Neurol Neurosurg 1993;6(3):350–7.
8. Richter A, Loscher W. Pathology of idiopathic dystonia: findings from genetic animal models. Prog Neurobiol 1998;54(6):633–77.
9. Defazio G, Abbruzzese G, Livrea P, et al. Epidemiology of primary dystonia. Lancet Neurol 2004; 3(11):673–8.
10. Le KD, Nilsen B, Dietrichs E. Prevalence of primary focal and segmental dystonia in Oslo. Neurology 2003;61(9):1294–6.
11. Gomez-Wong E, Marti MJ, Cossu G, et al. The 'geste antagonistique' induces transient modulation of the blink reflex in human patients with blepharospasm. Neurosci Lett 1998;251(2): 125–8.
12. Clark GT, Ram S. Four oral motor disorders: bruxism, dystonia, dyskinesia and drug-induced dystonic extrapyramidal reactions. Dent Clin North Am 2007;51(1):225–43.
13. Blitzer A, Brin MF, Greene PE, et al. Botulinum toxin injection for the treatment of oromandibular dystonia. Ann Otol Rhinol Laryngol 1989;98(2):93–7.
14. Blitzer A, Brin MF, Fahn S. Botulinum toxin injections for lingual dystonia. Laryngoscope 1991;101(7 Pt 1):799.
15. Moore AP, Wood GD. Medical treatment of recurrent temporomandibular joint dislocation using botulinum toxin A. Br Dent J 1997;183(11–12):415–7.
16. Costa J, Espírito-Santo CC, Borges AA, et al. Botulinum toxin type A versus anticholinergics for cervical dystonia. Cochrane Database Syst Rev 2005;(1):CD004312.
17. Bhidayasiri R. Dystonia: genetics and treatment update. Neurologist 2006;12(2):74–85.
18. Bressman SB. Dystonia update. Clin Neuropharmacol 2000;23(5):239–51.
19. Nygaard TG, Marsden CD, Fahn S. Dopa-responsive dystonia: long-term treatment response and prognosis. Neurology 1991;41:174–81.
20. Bostwick JM, Jaffee MS. Buspirone as an antidote to SSRI-induced bruxism in 4 cases. J Clin Psychiatry 1999;60(12):857–60.
21. Bonifati V, Fabrizio E, Cipriani R, et al. Buspirone in levodopa-induced dyskinesias. Clin Neuropharmacol 1994;17(1):73–82.
22. Konig P, Chwatal K, Havelec L, et al. Amantadine versus biperiden: a double-blind study of treatment efficacy in neuroleptic extrapyramidal movement disorders. Neuropsychobiology 1996; 33(2):80–4.
23. van't Groenewout JL, Stone MR, Vo VN, et al. Evidence for the involvement of histamine in the antidystonic effects of diphenhydramine. Exp Neurol 1995;134(2):253–60.
24. Wagner ML, Walters AS, Coleman RG, et al. Randomized, double-blind, placebo-controlled study of clonidine in restless legs syndrome. Sleep 1996; 19(1):52–8.
25. Braun V, Richter HP. Selective peripheral denervation for spasmodic torticollis: 13-year experience with 155 patients. J Neurosurg 2002;97(2 Suppl): 207–12.
26. Bates AK, Halliday BL, Bailey CS, et al. Surgical management of essential blepharospasm. Br J Ophthalmol 1991;75(8):487–90.
27. Bertrand C, Molina-Negro P, Martinez SN. Combined stereotactic and peripheral surgical approach for spasmodic torticollis. Appl Neurophysiol 1978;41(1–4):122–33.
28. Eltahawy HA, Saint-Cyr J, Giladi N, et al. Primary dystonia is more responsive than secondary dystonia to pallidal interventions: outcome after pallidotomy or pallidal deep brain stimulation. Neurosurgery 2004;54(3):613–9 [discussion: 619–21].
29. Bronte-Stewart H. Surgical therapy for dystonia. Curr Neurol Neurosci Rep 2003;3(4):296–305.
30. Yuan Y, Wang Y, Zhang SX, et al. Microvascular decompression in patients with hemifacial spasm: report of 1200 cases. Chin Med J (Engl) 2005; 118(10):833–6.

31. Tanner CM, Goldman SM. Epidemiology of movement disorders. Curr Opin Neurol 1994;7(4):340–5.

32. Jankovic J. Cranial-cervical dyskinesias: an overview. Adv Neurol 1988;49:1–13.

33. Kane JM, Weinhold P, Kinon B, et al. Prevalence of abnormal involuntary movements ("spontaneous dyskinesias") in the normal elderly. Psychopharmacology (Berl) 1982;77(2):105–8.

34. D'Alessandro R, Benassi G, Cristina E, et al. The prevalence of lingual-facial-buccal dyskinesias in the elderly. Neurology 1986;36(10):1350–1.

35. Delwaide PJ, Desseilles M. Spontaneous buccolinguofacial dyskinesia in the elderly. Acta Neurol Scand 1977;56(3):256–62.

36. Bourgeois M, Boueilh P, Tignol J. Spontaneous dyskinesia in the elderly and tardive dyskinesia of neuroleptics. A survey among 270 patients (author's transl). Encephale 1980;6(1):37–9 [in French].

37. Blowers AJ, Borison RL, Blowers CM, et al. Abnormal involuntary movements in the elderly. Br J Psychiatry 1981;139:363–4.

38. Blanchet PJ, Abdillahi O, Beauvais C, et al. Prevalence of spontaneous oral dyskinesia in the elderly: a reappraisal. Mov Disord 2004;19(8):892–6.

39. Brasic JR. Clinical assessment of tics. Psychol Rep 2001;89(1):48–50.

40. Hershey LA, Daroff RB. Medical management of benign essential blepharospasm. Adv Ophthalmic Plast Reconstr Surg 1985;4:183–94.

41. Scott BL. Evaluation and treatment of dystonia. South Med J 2000;93(8):746–51.

42. Raja M. Managing antipsychotic-induced acute and tardive dystonia. Drug Saf 1998;19(1):57–72.

43. Gelenberg AJ. Treating extrapyramidal reactions: some current issues. J Clin Psychiatry 1987; 48(Suppl):24–7.

44. Donlon PT, Stenson RL. Neuroleptic induced extrapyramidal symptoms. Dis Nerv Syst 1976;37(11): 629–35.

45. Borison RL. Amantadine in the management of extrapyramidal side effects. Clin Neuropharmacol 1983;6(Suppl 1):S57–63.

46. Gagrat D, Hamilton J, Belmaker RH. Intravenous diazepam in the treatment of neuroleptic-induced acute dystonia and akathisia. Am J Psychiatry 1978;135(10):1232–3.

47. Fernandez HH, Friedman JH. Classification and treatment of tardive syndromes. Neurologist 2003; 9(1):16–27.

48. Burke RE, Fahn S, Jankovic J, et al. Tardive dystonia: late-onset and persistent dystonia caused by antipsychotic drugs. Neurology 1982;32(12): 1335–46.

49. Kiriakakis V, Bhatia KP, Quinn NP, et al. The natural history of tardive dystonia. A long-term follow-up study of 107 cases. Brain 1998; 121(Pt 11):2053–66.

50. Chouinard G. New nomenclature for drug-induced movement disorders including tardive dyskinesia. J Clin Psychiatry 2004;65(Suppl 9):9–15.

51. Trosch RM. Neuroleptic-induced movement disorders: deconstructing extrapyramidal symptoms. J Am Geriatr Soc 2004;52(12 Suppl):S266–71.

52. Tarsy D, Baldessarini RJ, Tarazi FI. Effects of newer antipsychotics on extrapyramidal function. CNS Drugs 2002;16(1):23–45.

53. Tarsy D. Neuroleptic-induced extrapyramidal reactions: classification, description, and diagnosis. Clin Neuropharmacol 1983;6(Suppl 1):S9–26.

54. Van Putten T, May PR, Marder SR. Akathisia with haloperidol and thiothixene. Psychopharmacol Bull 1984;20(1):114–7.

55. Ellison JM, Stanziani P. SSRI-associated nocturnal bruxism in four patients. J Clin Psychiatry 1993; 54(11):432–4.

56. Romanelli F, Adler DA, Bungay KM. Possible paroxetine-induced bruxism. Ann Pharmacother 1996;30(11):1246–8.

57. Gerber PE, Lynd LD. Selective serotonin-reuptake inhibitor-induced movement disorders. Ann Pharmacother 1998;32(6):692–8.

58. Lobbezoo F, van Denderen RJ, Verheij JG, et al. Reports of SSRI-associated bruxism in the family physician's office. J Orofac Pain 2001;15(4):340–6.

59. Berry RB, Yamaura EM, Gill K, et al. Acute effects of Paroxetine on genioglossus activity in obstructive sleep apnea. Sleep 1999;22(8):1087–92.

60. Peroutka SJ, Newman H, Harris H. Subjective effects of 3,4-methylenedioxymethamphetamine in recreational users. Neuropsychopharmacology 1988;1(4):273–7.

61. Vollenweider FX, Gamma A, Liechti M, et al. Psychological and cardiovascular effects and short-term sequelae of MDMA ("Ecstasy") in MDMA-naive healthy volunteers. Neuropsychopharmacology 1998;19(4):241–51.

62. Fazzi M, Vescovi P, Savi A, et al. The effects of drugs on the oral cavity. Minerva Stomatol 1999;48(10): 485–92.

63. See SJ, Tan EK. Severe amphetamine-induced bruxism: treatment with botulinum toxin. Acta Neurol Scand 2003;107(2):161–3.

64. Winocur E, Gavish A, Voikovitch M, et al. Drugs and bruxism: a critical review. J Orofac Pain 2003;17(2): 99–111.

65. Pavlovic ZM. Buspirone to improve compliance in Venlafaxine-induced movement disorder. Int J Neuropsychopharmacol 2004;20:1–2.

66. Thorpy MJ. Sleep bruxism. The international classification of sleep disorders, revised. Am Acad Sleep Med 2001;182–5.

67. Negoro T, Briggs J, Plesh O, et al. Bruxing patterns in children compared to intercuspal clenching and chewing as assessed with dental models,

electromyography, and incisor jaw tracing: preliminary study. ASDC J Dent Child 1998;65(6):449–58.

68. Glaros AG. Incidence of diurnal and nocturnal bruxism. J Prosthet Dent 1981;45(5):545–9.

69. Cash RC. Bruxism in children: review of the literature. J Pedod 1988;12(2):107–27.

70. Seligman DA, Pullinger AG, Solberg WK. The prevalence of dental attrition and its association with factors of age, gender, occlusion, and TMJ symptomatology. J Dent Res 1988;67(10):1323 33.

71. Milosevic A, Young PJ, Lennon MA. The prevalence of tooth wear in 14-year-old school children in Liverpool. Community Dent Health 1994;11(2):83–6.

72. Tsolka P, Walter JD, Wilson RF, et al. Occlusal variables, bruxism and temporomandibular disorders: a clinical and kinesiographic assessment. J Oral Rehabil 1995;22(12):849–56.

73. Attanasio R. Nocturnal bruxism and its clinical management. Dent Clin North Am 1991;35(1):245–52.

74. Lobbezoo F, Lavigne GJ. Do bruxism and temporomandibular disorders have a cause-and-effect relationship? J Orofac Pain 1997;11(1):15–23.

75. Shetty SR, Munshi AK. Oral habits in children–a prevalence study. J Indian Soc Pedod Prev Dent 1998;16(2):61–6.

76. Wetter TC, Pollmacher T. Restless legs and periodic leg movements in sleep syndromes. J Neurol 1997;244(4 Suppl 1)):S37–45.

77. Reding GR, Zepelin H, Robinson JE, et al. Nocturnal teeth-grinding: all-night psychophysiologic studies. J Dent Res 1968;47(5):786–97.

78. Ware JC, Rugh JD. Destructive bruxism: sleep stage relationship. Sleep 1988;11(2):172–81.

79. Macaluso GM, Guerra P, Di Giovanni G, et al. Sleep bruxism is a disorder related to periodic arousals during sleep. J Dent Res 1998;77(4):565–73.

80. Powell RN. Tooth contact during sleep: association with other events. J Dent Res 1965;44(5):959–67.

81. Robinson BC. Masticatory muscle disturbances and their effect on the temporomandibular joint. Dent Stud 1969;48(2):125–6.

82. Kydd WL, Daly C. Duration of nocturnal tooth contacts during bruxing. J Prosthet Dent 1985;53(5):717–21.

83. Lavigne GJ, Rompre PH, Guitard F, et al. Lower number of k-complexes and k-alphas in sleep bruxism: a controlled quantitative study. Clin Neurophysiol 2002;113(5):686–93.

84. Huynh N, Kato T, Rompre PH, et al. Sleep bruxism is associated to micro-arousals and an increase in cardiac sympathetic activity. J Sleep Res 2006;15(3):339–46.

85. Lavigne GJ, Huynh N, Kato T, et al. Genesis of sleep bruxism: motor and autonomic-cardiac interactions. Arch Oral Biol 2007;52(4):381–4.

86. van der Zaag J, Lobbezoo F, Wicks DJ, et al. Controlled assessment of the efficacy of occlusal stabilization splints on sleep bruxism. J Orofac Pain 2005;19(2):151–8.

87. Saletu A, Parapatics S, Saletu B, et al. On the pharmacotherapy of sleep bruxism: placebo-controlled polysomnographic and psychometric studies with clonazepam. Neuropsychobiology 2005;51(4):214–25.

88. Saletu A, Parapatics S, Anderer P, et al. Controlled clinical, polysomnographic and psychometric studies on differences between sleep bruxers and controls and acute effects of clonazepam as compared with placebo. Eur Arch Psychiatry Clin Neurosci 2010;260(2):163–74.

89. Huynh N, Lavigne GJ, Lanfranchi PA, et al. The effect of 2 sympatholytic medications–propranolol and clonidine–on sleep bruxism: experimental randomized controlled studies. Sleep 2006;29(3):307–16.

90. Huynh N, Manzini C, Rompre PH, et al. Weighing the potential effectiveness of various treatments for sleep bruxism. J Can Dent Assoc 2007;73(8):727–30.

91. Huynh NT, Rompre PH, Montplaisir JY, et al. Comparison of various treatments for sleep bruxism using determinants of number needed to treat and effect size. Int J Prosthodont 2006;19(5):435–41.

92. Watanabe T, Baba K, Yamagata K, et al. A vibratory stimulation-based inhibition system for nocturnal bruxism: a clinical report. J Prosthet Dent 2001;85(3):233–5.

93. Jadidi F, Castrillon E, Svensson P. Effect of conditioning electrical stimuli on temporalis electromyographic activity during sleep. J Oral Rehabil 2008;35(3):171–83.

Medication Treatment Efficacy and Chronic Orofacial Pain

Glenn T. Clark, DDS, MS[a],*, Mariela Padilla, DDS, MEd[a],
Raymond Dionne, DDS, PhD[b]

KEYWORDS

- Trigeminal neuropathic pain • Chronic daily headaches • Myofascial pain
- Temporomandibular osteoarthritis • Medication efficacy

KEY POINTS

- This article discusses 4 types of chronic pain in the orofacial region, namely neuropathic pain (NPP), chronic daily headaches, myofascial pain, and osteoarthritis (OA).
- For trigeminal NPP, there are 3 medications (gabapentinoids, tricyclic antidepressants [TCAs], and serotonin-norepinephrine reuptake inhibitors [SNRIs]) plus topical anesthetics that have therapeutic efficacy.
- For chronic daily headaches (often migraine in origin), 3 prophylactic medications have reasonable therapeutic efficacy (β-blockers, TCAs, and various antiepileptic drugs [AEDs]).
- There are 3 Food and Drug Administration (FDA)-approved drugs for fibromyalgia (pregabalin, duloxetine, and milnacipran) but their efficacy is not robust.
- For osteoarthritis, nonsteroidal anti-inflammatory drugs (NSAIDs) have good therapeutic efficacy and when gastritis contraindicates them, corticosteriod injections are helpful.

CHRONIC OROFACIAL PAIN DISEASES AND PHARMACOLOGIC TREATMENT

There are a variety of chronic painful orofacial diseases that dentists must confront in practice. Specifically, these problems include trigeminal neuropathy, chronic daily headache, masticatory myofascial pain, and arthritic disease of the temporomandibular joint (TMJ). This article provides readers with an overview of medications that have reasonable treatment evidence and can be used to help manage these chronic pain problems. As a way of comparing these medications in this article, the associated numbers needed to treat (NNTs) a single patient and achieve a 50% reduction in symptoms are reported. Although most diseases are acute and resolve with time, there are a wide number of chronic conditions that manifest with pain in the orofacial region that are not managed by surgical intervention but do benefit from pharmacologic therapy. Some of the diseases this article addresses are presented in **Table 1**. The diseases listed in this table are not a complete inventory of all chronic conditions in the orofacial region and cancer pain, burning mouth syndrome, trigeminal neuralgia or masticatory muscle spasm, bruxism, and dystonia, for example, are not covered. Moreover, the focus of this article on pharmacologic therapies does not imply that medications are the only form or even the best form of treatment, just one that needs to be considered in an attempt to help a patient. Specifically excluded from this

Copyright (c) 2015 California Dental Association. Adapted with permission from the California Dental Association.
[a] Ostrow School of Dentistry, University of Southern California, 925 West 34th Street, Los Angeles, CA 90089, USA; [b] Department of Pharmacology, Brody School of Medicine, 6S19 Brody Medical Science Building, 600 Moye Boulevard, East Carolina University, Schools of Medicine and Dental Medicine, Greenville, NC 27834-4354, USA
* Corresponding author.
E-mail address: gtc@usc.edu

Oral Maxillofacial Surg Clin N Am 28 (2016) 409–421
http://dx.doi.org/10.1016/j.coms.2016.03.011

Table 1
Chronic orofacial pain diseases

Disease	Description
NPP/persistent dentoalveolar pain	NPP is a chronic pain resulting from injury to the nervous system. The injury can be to the central nervous system (brain and spinal cord) or the peripheral nervous system (nerves outside the brain and spinal cord). Persistent dentoalveolar pain is when there is persistent (chronic) continuous pain symptom located in the dentoalveolar region that cannot be explained within the context of other diseases or disorders.
Chronic daily headache/chronic migraine	Chronic daily headache is a descriptive term that includes disorders with headaches on more days than not and affects 4% of the general population. Chronic migraine is one of the most common forms of the chronic daily headache and occurs due to transformation of the episodic migraine to a chronic migraine.
Fibromyalgia/myofascial pain	Fibromyalgia is a chronic disorder characterized by widespread musculoskeletal pain, fatigue, and tenderness in localized areas. Myofascial pain refers to pain caused by muscular irritation. The large upper back muscles are prone to developing myofascial pain that radiates from sensitive points, called trigger points, throughout muscle tissue. Muscular irritation and upper back pain are due to muscle weakness and repetitive motions.
OA/RA/JIA	OA is a degeneration of joint cartilage and the underlying bone, most common from middle age onward. It causes pain and stiffness, especially in the hip, knee, and thumb joints. RA is a chronic progressive disease causing inflammation in the joints and resulting in painful deformity and immobility, especially in the fingers, wrists, feet, and ankles. JIA, also known as juvenile RA, is the most common form of arthritis in children and adolescents.

article, not because they do not deserve discussion but because of limited time and space, are platelet-rich plasma injections (reported to have therapeutic value in OA and tendinopathies), hyaluronic acid injections (used as an esthetic filler increasing soft tissue volume and as viscosupplementation of damaged joints), adipose-derived stromal cell therapy (adjuvant therapy for tissue regeneration), botulinum toxin (therapy for neurologic conditions, pain, and muscle spasms)/spasm, and marijuana (chronic pain and palliative care). Finally, although not advocating opioids for chronic orofacial pain (chronic headache, arthritis, and fibromyalgia) and orofacial NPP conditions, what is known about opioids for these problems is discussed.

MEDICATIONS FOR TRIGEMINAL NEUROPATHIC PAIN

The first problem addressed is chronic trigeminal NPP, which encompasses a multitude of trigeminal nerve problems due to trauma and/or inflammation. One of these is the disorder of atypical toothache, which is also called persistent dental

alveolar pain. The conventional dental approach for painful teeth that usually are given a diagnosis of irreversible pulpitis has been dental restoration, occlusal reduction, endodontics, and occasionally extraction. Unfortunately, these treatment methods have not resolved some patients' dental pain complaints, probably because the peripheral nerves and central sensory nerves have undergone neuropathic sensitization and are now firing spontaneously and ectopically.

Topical Medicines for Trigeminal Neuropathic Pain

It has been 16 years since the first article that discussed topical orofacial pain medications, was published in the *Journal of the American Dental Association*.[1] Since then, several research studies, case reports, and review articles have been published.[2–6] A recent review of the literature on topical treatments for chronic pain suggested that this modality has some distinct advantages, such as lower side effects, fewer drug-drug interactions, and improved patient tolerance.[7] This nonsystematic review made a suggestion on how to select and use topical agents for a patient's

NPP, but this form of therapy is often not used for chronic NPP because topical pain-suppressive medications have been shown less effective than other pharmacologic methods in rigorous research studies.[8] A 2015 review examined efficacy by performing a careful calculation of the NNT to achieve a 50% pain relief level for a multitude of NPP medications. By calculating the NNT, it is possible to compare medications that were not directly compared inside a randomized clinical trial. Specifically, this study reported an NNT of 10.6 for capsaicin high-concentration patches, which is quite poor. Unfortunately, this study did not determine the NNT for lidocaine patches and based on this, the investigators gave only a weak recommendation for use and proposed these topical agents could be a second-line therapy along with tramadol (a weak opioid) for peripheral NPP. The two most common drug classes administered topically in orofacial pain clinics include NSAIDs for arthritic disease (such as ketoprofen gel and diclofenac gel) and topical anesthetics (benzocaine and lidocaine) for NPP and various other topical agents, such as capsaicin or a mixture of anesthetic and an anticonvulsant agent. These agents are usually mixed into a skin-penetrating vehicle (Lipoderm or pluronic lecithin organogel) or if used intraorally, into a methylcellulose paste (Orobase) that allows transmucosal absorption and improved retention of the medication to the tissues. In a 2014 systematic review of the literature, the efficacy of topical medications as a treatment of NPP was examined.[9] The investigators included randomized, double-blind studies where topical lidocaine (5%) with placebo or another active treatment was used on chronic NPP patients (postherpetic neuralgia, trigeminal neuralgia, and postsurgical or posttraumatic neuralgia). The investigators included 12 studies where lidocaine was compared with a placebo or an active control. The results of this analysis found all studies had a high risk of bias and there was no clear evidence of an effect of topical lidocaine for NPP, although individual studies reviewed indicated that it was effective for relief of pain. In contrast, a 2003 study reported on the efficacy of lidocaine patches 5% in the treatment of focal peripheral NPP syndromes using a randomized, double-blind, placebo-controlled study design.[10] This study revealed that as an add-on therapy, the lidocaine patch 5% was effective in reducing ongoing pain and allodynia. The investigators calculated the NNT for lidocaine in this study was 4.4. Unfortunately, none of these studies or reviews specifically looked at the use of topical anesthetics for focal orofacial NPP or persistent dentoalveolar pain. This is an important distinction because using topical medications on more readily absorbent mucosal tissues might make a large difference in efficacy of the topicals used intraorally versus using them on skin. A 2008 case study showed that topical medications versus systemic medications can have a substantial effect and thus might be considered a first-line therapy for some chronic neuropathic oral pain patients.[11] Although the study provides only low level of evidence because it is a retrospective chart review of 39 patients treated for orofacial NPP, it showed that the pain was significantly reduced, even in those who had received only topical medications. The next logical question is, Who would benefit from a topical medication only approach? Many patients prefer a topical if it works well for its safety and convenience, but this question also raises the issue of the nocebo-responsive patient. Placebo analgesia makes individuals experience relief of their pain simply by virtue of the anticipation of a benefit. Placebos mimic the action of active treatments and promote the endogenous release of opioids. In contrast, the nocebo response is when a verbal suggestion of negative outcomes results in the amplification of pain. Anxiety is thought to influence positively the strength of nocebo response in those predisposed to it.[12] Often patients cannot take systemic medications due to side effects and in nocebo-responsive patients these side effects occur at very low doses. A systematic review recently examined to what degree adverse medications reactions to can be blamed on the nocebo response and not the medication itself.[13] Specifically this study examined randomized controlled trials (RCTs) with a parallel design of any drug therapy compared with pharmacologic placebo in patients with fibromyalgia and diabetic peripheral neuropathy. The investigators concluded that nocebo effects substantially accounted for adverse events in the reviewed drug trials. Identifying nocebo-responsive patients is easy because they readily tell, if asked, that they get all the adverse effects of medications and firmly wish to avoid systemic medications. It is a curiosity that the same patients often take nutraceuticals and use topical medications.

Gabapentinoids and Serotonin-Norepinephrine Reuptake Inhibitors Used to Treat Trigeminal Neuropathic Pain

The systematic review and meta-analysis by Finnerup and colleagues[8] in 2015 on pharmacologic treatments of NPP examined various oral medications in addition to the topical medications described previously. Specifically, this review calculated the NNT to achieve 50% pain relief level in 1 patient for several types of medications. The study found that for SNRIs (duloxetine and venlafaxine), the NNT was 6.4. For the gabapentinoids (pregabalin and gabapentin), the NNT was 7.2 to 7.7. For TCAs, the NNT was 3.6, which is clearly lower, but the investigators of this review did not consider TCAs a first-line therapy. Another study that examined pregabalin and gabapentin in matched patients with peripheral NPP was reported in 2010.[14] In particular, this study performed a cost-consequences analysis in a nested case-control design in patients with refractory chronic peripheral NPP. The study examined data from two 12-week long, observational, prospective studies in primary medical care involving 44 patients treated with gabapentin (cases) and 88 patients treated with pregabalin (controls) who were matched for age and gender. They concluded that the pregabalin seemed associated with greater reduction in mean weekly intensity of pain, but there were no significant differences in cost compared with gabapentin. As a result of these data, the investigators suggested that there was strong evidence for these 2 medications classes and they should be considered first-line treatments in NPP.

Tricyclic Antidepressants for Trigeminal Neuropathic Pain

In contrast to the review recommendations by Finnerup and colleagues,[8] who judged TCAs as more or less equivalent to gabapentinoids and SNRI class medications, a different systematic review looked at nortriptyline, a TCA class medication, as a treatment of NPP. This review found nortriptyline clearly better than placebo but the investigators could not recommend it as a highly efficacious medication.[15] This study included only randomized, double-blind studies of at least 2 weeks' duration comparing nortriptyline with placebo or another active treatment of chronic NPP. The investigators included 6 studies treating 310 participants (mean or median age 49–64 years) with various NPP conditions. Based on their analysis, the investigators found little evidence to support the use of nortriptyline to treat the NPP conditions; they suggested it was not a first-line treatment. These investigators suggested that other medicines, such as duloxetine and pregabalin, had stronger evidence than nortriptyline. Unfortunately none of these articles on oral medications NPP specifically evaluated trigeminal NPP, such as persistent dentoalveolar pain, and these medications are essentially used off-label when treating this or other trigeminal manifestations of NPP.

Opioids for Trigeminal Neuropathic Pain

There is little quality scientific literature that examines the use of opioids for neuropathic orofacial pain disorders, but there is adequate literature on NPP in other regions of the body. For example, a 2014 systematic review examined the efficacy of oxycodone for NPP in adults.[16] The review identified 3 qualified studies with 254 participants who had either painful diabetic neuropathy or postherpetic neuralgia. Controlled-release (CR) oxycodone was dispensed in all 3 studies, with doses titrated up to a maximum of between 60 mg and 120 mg daily compared with a placebo medication. The investigators concluded that all studies had 1 or more sources of potential major bias and although greater pain intensity reduction and better patient satisfaction was seen with oxycodone the evidence was considered third-tier evidence. At least 1 adverse event was experienced by 86% of participants taking oxycodone CR compared with 63% taking placebo. The investigators reported that the NNT to treat for an additional harmful effect (number needed to harm) was 4.3. They concluded that no convincing, unbiased evidence suggests that oxycodone (as oxycodone CR) is of value in treating people with painful diabetic neuropathy or postherpetic neuralgia. Another study examined the use of morphine in combination with nortriptyline for NPP.[17] This study was a randomized, double-blind, crossover trial that included patients with NPP. Patients were randomized to 1 of 3 groups to receive either oral nortriptyline, morphine, or their combination. During each of three 6-week periods, doses were titrated towards maximal tolerated dose; 52 patients were enrolled and 39 completed at least 2 of the 3 treatment periods. The results showed that the combination of both medications was better than each 1 individually. Combination treatment, however, also resulted in moderate to severe constipation and dry mouth. The investigators concluded that there was a superior efficacy of a nortriptyline-morphine combination over either monotherapy with constipation, dry mouth, and somnolence as the most frequent adverse effects. Finally the systematic review and meta-analysis by Finnerup and colleagues[8] on NPP medications did comment on opioids. Specifically they reviewed the evidence on efficacy and side effects of opioids when used for NPP and concluded that, although the NNTs were moderately low for both strong opioids and tramadol (a weaker opioid), they offered only a weak recommendation for use of both tramadol (second-line therapy) and strong opioids (third-line therapy). In 2014, the FDA issued a ruling that tramadol would not be an FDA schedule IV drug and be elevated to schedule III, and they described it as a centrally acting opioid analgesic.[18]

Table 2 summarizes evidence-based NPP treatments.

MEDICATIONS FOR CHRONIC DAILY HEADACHES
Is Naproxen a Good Medication for Treating Episodic Migraine?

For many patients with episodic migraine, the triptan-class medications (sumatriptan, zolmitriptan, rizatriptan, naratriptan, eletriptan, almotriptan, and frovatriptan) are a great solution to aborting their disabling migraine headaches (**Table 3**). Unfortunately, this class of medications has an FDA prescription limitation of 8 tablets a month maximum, which most insurance companies follow. If a patient's headaches are infrequent (less than 8 times per month), patients have an adequate supply of medication. In those cases of headaches more than 8 times per month, another approach is needed. In 2014, a study compared doses of sumitriptan plus naproxen in combination versus naproxen alone for the treatment of episodic migraine.[19] The study described a 2-center, double-blind, randomized, parallel-group study. Subjects were equally randomized to receive either 85 mg of sumatriptan plus 500 mg naproxen sodium (Group 1) or 500 mg of naproxen only daily for 1 month followed by 2 months of the same medications used for episodic acute treatment. The results of the study showed no significant group difference with regard to the number of migraine headache days. More subjects in the naproxen-only group, however, prematurely withdrew from the study more often because of lack of efficacy. The investigators concluded that there were subsets of patients who can use naproxen sodium alone and have a significant reduction in migraine headache days.

Table 2
Evidence-based neuropathic pain treatments

Treatments	Numbers Needed to Treat
1. Gabapentinoids	7.2–7.7
2. TCAs	3.6
3. SNRIs	6.4
4. Topical anesthetics	4.4
5. Opioids (strong and weak)	4.3

Table 3
Evidence-based chronic daily headache treatments

Treatments	Numbers Needed to Treat
1. Long-acting NSAID (Naproxen)	Not available
2. β-Blocker (Propranolol)	1.5
3. TCA (Amitriptyline)	3.2
4. AED (Valproate)	3.0–4.0
5. AED (Topiramate)	4.0
6. NMDA blocker (Memantine)	Not available
7. Opioids	Not available

Until recently, conventional wisdom suggested that any patient with possible medication overuse headache needed to stop all analgesics, including NSAIDs. This idea was examined in a 2012 study that looked at the evidence basis of using NSAIDs and other complementary treatments for episodic migraine prevention in adults.[20] Specifically, this report conducted a systematic review of published studies from June 1999 to May 2009 that focused on nontraditional therapies, NSAIDs, and other complementary therapies. Based on the studies reviewed, the investigators suggested that *Petasites* (butterbur) was effective for migraine prevention and that several NSAIDs were also helpful, including ibuprofen, ketoprofen, naproxen, and naproxen sodium.

How Effective Are Preventive Medications for Chronic Migraine?

When abortive medications (triptans and analgesics) are not adequate, most clinicians consider adding a preventive medication to suppress the headache. There are several types of preventive medications used for chronic migraine, including β-blockers, TCAs, and anticonvulsants, which are also known as AEDs. Of these, the one that is not FDA approved for migraine prophylaxis is amitriptyline. In a 2001 meta-analysis study, all types of antidepressants and their efficacy on chronic migraine were examined.[21] This study found 19 individual studies that included TCA class drugs and 12 of them used amitriptyline. The investigators concluded that patients treated with antidepressants were twice as likely to improve as those treated with placebo and that the overall NNT was 3.2 for TCAs. In 2014, a study examined the efficacy and mechanism of anticonvulsant drugs in migraine.[22] Efficacy has been demonstrated in randomized placebo-controlled trials for topiramate and valproic acid, including divalproex sodium. In the case of topiramate, efficacy has been demonstrated for chronic migraine and even medication overuse headache, questioning the established concept of medication withdrawal. Unfortunately, anticonvulsants often produce more side effects and sometimes adverse events that require treatment cessation. In 2013, a systematic review was published that examined valproate (valproic acid or sodium valproate or a combination of the 2) for the prophylaxis of episodic migraine.[23] This review assessed the efficacy and tolerability of these medications on prevention of migraine attacks in adult patients with episodic migraine. The investigators included only prospective, controlled trials of valproate taken regularly to prevent the occurrence of migraine attacks, to improve migraine-related quality of life, or both. Ten articles were included in the analysis and, of these, 2 trials showed that sodium valproate reduced headache frequency by approximately 4 headaches per 28 days compared with placebo. Four other trials showed that divalproex sodium more than doubled the proportion of responders relative to placebo, and 1 study of sodium valproate (34 participants) versus placebo supported these findings. There was no significant difference in the proportion of responder's divalproex sodium versus propranolol (1 trial). Pooled analysis of data from 2 clinical trials demonstrated a slight but significant advantage for topiramate (50 mg) over valproate (400 mg). The investigators concluded that valproate is effective in reducing headache frequency and is reasonably well tolerated in adult patients with episodic migraine and had an NNT between 3.0 and 4.0. With regard to propranolol, a 2003 systematic review examined 20 studies that evaluated medications for migraine prevention in adolescents and children under age 18.[24] Unfortunately, only 1 study examined propranolol and allowed the NNT to be calculated. This review claimed that propranolol was quite effective for headache prevention and reported an NNT of 1.5 to produce a two-thirds reduction in headache frequency. A different systematic review published in 2013 examined the efficacy of topiramate for the prophylaxis of episodic migraine in adults.[25] Twenty articles describing 17 unique trials met the inclusion criteria for this review. Analysis of data from 9 trials showed that topiramate reduced headache frequency by approximately 1.2 attacks per 28 days compared with placebo. Meta-analysis of those studies where different doses were used shows that 200 mg are no more effective than 100 mg in reducing headache frequency and had an NNT of 4.0. When topiramate was compared with either a TCA class drug (amitriptyline) or a β-blocker (propranolol), no significant difference was found in efficacy. There was a slight significant advantage of topiramate over valproate noted in 2 studies on reducing headache frequency. Behavioral therapy (relaxation) improved migraine-specific quality of life significantly more than topiramate. Adverse events were not uncommon when using topiramate but they were usually mild and of a nonserious nature. The investigators concluded that topiramate in a 100 mg/d dosage is effective in reducing headache frequency and reasonably well tolerated in adult patients with episodic migraine.

Use of an N-methyl-D-aspartate Receptor Blocking Agent for Chronic Migraines

There are many chronic migraine sufferers who are resistant to both the usual and customary abortive and preventive class medications. In 2014, a study examined if memantine was a logical and appropriate medication for the treatment of primary migraine and other primary headaches.[26] Memantine is a known N-methyl-D-aspartate (NMDA) blocking agent and although it has primarily been used to reduce the progressive loss of memory in Alzheimer disease, it has some off-label evidence that it can suppress migraine pain via its NMDA-suppressive effects. The investigators of this study included less rigorous studies (retrospective case reports) and 2 prospective clinical trials. From these data, they concluded that memantine (10–20 mg daily) may be a useful treatment option for the prevention of primary headache disorders used either as monotherapy or adjunctive therapy for refractory chronic migraine patients.

Do Chronic Migraine Patients Take Their Medications as Prescribed?

When suggesting that a patient take a medication daily, the biggest barrier to efficacy is often medication adherence. In 2014, a study described the how well chronic migraine patients adhered to their prescribed medication protocol.[27] The study looked at prescriptions from a US claim database (Truven Health MarketScan databases) and focused on patients (>18 years old) who were diagnosed with chronic migraine and had been prescribed one of the commonly used migraine preventive agents (antidepressants, β-blockers, or anticonvulsants). Medication usage was calculated and a cutoff of greater than or equal to 80% was used to classify adherence. The investigators found 8688 met the inclusion/exclusion criteria and adherence ranged between 26% and 29% at 6 months and 17% and 20% at 12 months.

They found that adherence was similar except for amitriptyline, nortriptyline, gabapentin, and divalproex, which had significantly lower odds of adherence compared with topiramate.

Opioids for Chronic Migraine and Chronic Daily Headache

Almost universally, headache specialists do not recommend opioid therapy for management of severe headache, except as a rescue medication when the headache is deemed an emergency. In 2015, there was a report on the use of various medications for management of headaches emergencies.[28] The investigators of this report, which was based on 9362 emergency room visits for headache, showed that 18% of the time a prescription for either an opioid or barbiturate was given. For most patients, headaches are not emergencies and in 2010, a task force of the European Federation of Neurological Societies stated that acetaminophen and NSAIDs are the recommended treatment of episodic tension-type headaches and that triptans, muscle relaxants, and opioids should not be used.[29]

MEDICATIONS FOR CHRONIC MYOFASCIAL PAIN/FIBROMYALGIA
Efficacy of Medications to Treat Fibromyalgia

There are several off-label medications used to help patients who have widespread myofascial pain and/or fibromyalgia (**Table 4**). The FDA approved pregabalin for the treatment of fibromyalgia in 2007 and within 2 years, 2 SNRIs, duloxetine hydrochloride and milnacipran hydrochloride, were also approved. Not approved but still commonly used in fibromyalgia are the TCA class drugs (amitriptyline and nortriptyline). In 2015, a review examined the use of various medications used for fibromyalgia.[30] The investigators of this study examined US commercial insurance claim data (2007–2009) and performed comparative effectiveness of amitriptyline, duloxetine, gabapentin, and pregabalin on health care use in patients with fibromyalgia. With these data, the study identified fibromyalgia patients who were prescribed amitriptyline, duloxetine, and gabapentin. These data were compared with fibromyalgia patients who were prescribed pregabalin. The number of outpatient visits, prescriptions, and hospitalizations decreased slightly after initiating 1 of the study drugs, but the number of emergency department visits increased after treatment initiation. Duloxetine was associated with a small but significant decrease in outpatient visits, number of other prescribed drugs, hospitalizations, and emergency department visits compared with pregabalin users. Few differences in health care use rates were noted among amitriptyline and gabapentin users compared with pregabalin. This study suggested that fibromyalgia patients still had high health care utilization before and after initiation of amitriptyline, duloxetine, gabapentin, or pregabalin but that duloxetine users had less health care utilization than pregabalin users. A 2012 study examined the role of TCAs and SNRIs in the treatment of fibromyalgia.[31] Only studies with an RCT design that tested the efficacy of various antidepressants were included; 35 studies, which included 3528 patients, were included in the meta-analysis. The investigators reported that 42.0% of these patients treated with SNRIs versus 32.0% patients with placebo reported a 30% pain reduction. The calculated the NNT of this medication class as 10.0. For tricyclic medications, the investigators reported that 48.3% of patients treated with TCAs versus 27.8% patients with placebo reported a 30% pain reduction. The calculated the NNT of this medication class as 4.9. This study concluded that amitriptyline and the SNRIs duloxetine and milnacipran are first-line options for the treatment of fibromyalgia syndrome patients. They also concluded, however, that a moderate number of patients drop out of therapy because of intolerable adverse effects or experience only a small relief of symptoms, which does not outweigh the adverse effects. Finally, a 2010 responder analysis study design examined the efficacy of pregabalin used for fibromyalgia.[32] This analysis obtained individual patient data from 4 randomized double-blind trials (2757 patients) of pregabalin in fibromyalgia lasting 8 to 14 weeks. From these data, an improvement response was calculated as well as the NNT for pregabalin (300 mg daily, 450 mg daily, and 600 mg daily) compared with placebo. The derived data showed that the maximum response occurred at 4 weeks to 6 weeks for and was

Table 4
Evidence-based fibromyalgia/myofascial pain treatments

Treatments	Numbers Needed to Treat
1. Gabapentinoids (Pregabalin)	13
2. TCA (Amitriptyline)	4.9
3. SNRI (Duloxetine)	10.0
4. Cognitive behavior therapy	Not available
5. Opioid therapy	Not available

unchanged after this. The NNTs for a greater than or equal to 50% improvement in pain intensity after 12 weeks were 22 for pregabalin (300 mg daily), 16 for pregabalin (450 mg daily), and 13 for pregabalin (600 mg daily). The investigators concluded that pregabalin helped with pain reduction compared with placebo in fibromyalgia and to a lesser degree with sleep disturbance. Unfortunately the NNTs were high.

Effective Dose and Cost-Benefit of Pregabalin for Fibromyalgia

With all medications that suppress nerve activity, there are issues with side effects and even adverse events, which must be balanced against the therapeutic benefit of the medication. This is true for the tricyclic medications, gabapentinoids, and the SNRI medications commonly used for fibromyalgia. If the patient takes too little of a medication because of side effects, it is not effective and its cost is not justified. Since pregabalin's approval for fibromyalgia in 2007, there have been multiple studies have examined its efficacy. In 2013, a systematic review of the literature examined what an effective daily dose would be as well as the cost effectiveness of pregabalin in the treatment of fibromyalgia.[33] This study identified 4 reports that allowed cost of therapy to be calculated and all 4 were RCTs with placebo controls. The study concluded that pregabalin (150 mg/d) did not have significant efficacy in comparison to placebo but generic pregabalin in the treatment doses of 450 mg/d or 600 mg/d is highly cost effective.

Behavioral Methods Versus Medication in the Treatment of Fibromyalgia

Because some fibromyalgia patients do not tolerate medications with moderate side effects, in 2014 the role of cognitive behavioral therapy (CBT) versus medications (pregabalin, duloxetine, and milnacipran) was examined in a review.[34] This study looked at the relative economic effect (cost-benefit) of patients in a randomized study comparing CBT (n = 57), medications (n = 56), and usual medical care (n = 55). The costs of health care use were estimated from patient self-reports and the investigators reported that total costs per patient in the CBT group were significantly lower than those in patients receiving either medications or usual medical care. The investigators also concluded that the CBT group was best in all of the comparisons performed assessing quality of life and pain levels. This finding was also supported by a 2014 systematic review style study that examined the treatment efficacy of nonpharmacologic versus pharmacologic treatment of fibromyalgia.[35] Outcomes examined in the review included pain, sleep disturbance, fatigue, affective symptoms (depression/anxiety), functional deficit, and cognitive impairment. The investigators included 21 pharmacologic studies and found that only amitriptyline demonstrated a significant effect on as many as 3 core fibromyalgia symptoms, but it exhibited many adverse effects, including tachyphylaxis. There were 64 studies that examined nonpharmacologic approaches to fibromyalgia and they were generally of poorer quality. Nevertheless, significant positive effects were shown on several symptom domains. These therapies included repetitive transcranial magnetic stimulation, balneotherapy exercise, cognitive behavior therapy and massage. The investigators speculated that few of the medications commonly used for fibromyalgia demonstrate significant relief across multiple fibromyalgia symptom domains, and additional research combining medications with nonpharmacologic treatment methods is needed.

Opioids for Fibromyalgia?

Like headaches, most rheumatologists do not recommend strong opioid therapy for the management of fibromyalgia, although there is some evidence that a weak opioid like tramadol has a role to play. In 2015, a survey was conducted on the use of opioids in fibromyalgia patients after hysterectomy surgery.[36] In this study they identified and studied 208 adult patients undergoing hysterectomy. The presurgery and postsurgery data collected included a fibromyalgia survey, pain severity survey, and miscellaneous psychological function questionnaires as well as preoperative opioid use. The investigators found that patients with a higher preoperative fibromyalgia survey scores were significantly more likely to exhibit increased postoperative opioid consumption. The speculation is that with higher fibromyalgia, the release of endogenous opioids may have altered patient tolerance to exogenous opioids. In 2015, a study examined value of long-term opioids for management of fibromyalgia.[37] Specifically, this study was a 12-month observational study, which included 1700 adult patients with fibromyalgia. Several questionnaires were collected on these patients to obtain information on their medication usage. The patients were then divided into (1) those taking an opioid (concurrent use of tramadol was permitted), (2) those taking tramadol (but no opioids), and (3) those not taking opioids or tramadol. The patients pain level was assessed periodically using the Brief Pain Inventory, Fibromyalgia Impact

Questionnaire, Patient Health Questionnaire, Insomnia Severity Index, Sheehan Disability Scale, and Generalized Anxiety Disorder Scale–7. The results of the study showed that the both nonopioid cohort and the tramadol-only cohort demonstrated significantly greater reductions in multiple pain and disability measures. The investigators concluded that those in the opioid cohort showed less improvement in pain-related interference with daily living, functioning, depression, and insomnia. Accordingly with their study, there is little support for the long-term use of opioid medications in patients with fibromyalgia. Finally in 2014, the British Pain Society published a guidelines article on the treatment of fibromyalgia.[38] This article describes in detail the potential pitfalls in the use of long-term opioids and rationale is provided why these medications are not recommended for fibromyalgia.

MEDICATIONS FOR TEMPOROMANDIBULAR ARTHRITIS

Nonsteroidal Anti-inflammatory Drugs for Temporomandibular Osteoarthritis

In 2012, a systematic review of RCTs examined which interventions worked best for the management of TMJ OA.[39] The review focused on studies of adults over the age of 18 and compared any form of nonsurgical or surgical therapy for TMJ OA. The review included 3 articles that qualified and, unfortunately, pooling of data for a meta-analysis was not possible. The findings derived from these 3 studies showed that diclofenac sodium given orally compared with occlusal splints were equivalent in efficacy. Moreover, using a glucosamine supplement seemed just as effective as ibuprofen for the management of TMJ OA. This review suggests that clinicians currently have 3 methods of helping their TMJ arthritis patients, including NSAIDs, occlusal splints, and glucosamine supplementation. Unfortunately, with only 3 studies that qualified for inclusion, it was not possible to compare and contrast the various NSAIDs available to select from when treating arthritis. In 2007, a comparative review on the relative efficacy of NSAIDs was published, which analyzed data from the Oxford Pain Group.[40] This group constructed a table for comparing analgesics commonly used for acute pain by calculating the NNT, which is the number of patients who need to receive the active drug to achieve at least 50% relief of pain compared with placebo over a 4-hour to 6-hour treatment period. The Oxford pain table shows that all NSAIDs have an NNT of 1.6 to 3.0 and in this table it is evident that NSAIDs are more

efficacious than acetaminophen for OA. In agreement with this observation is a meta-analysis on the relative efficacy of NSAIDs versus acetaminophen in reducing OA pain.[41] For a gastritis-susceptible patient, acetaminophen remains a good choice for relieving arthritis pain.

Temporomandibular Joint Corticosteroid Injections

It is becoming increasingly clear that TMJ injections with local anesthetic and corticosteroid can be an effective first-line modality for patients with limited mouth opening and for painful arthritis. In 2011, a case series based on 17 consecutive patients was published on the effectiveness of TMJ injections in patients with disc displacement without reduction (DDWOR).[42] The investigators claimed that active mouth opening before injection ranged between 15 mm and 40 mm (average 29 mm) and it increased by 10 mm after injection. The investigators concluded that TMJ injection with corticosteroid (20 mg of triamcinolone) and 1 mL of 2% lidocaine was recommended as an alternative first-line management modality for DDWOR. In 2012, another study examined the role of intra-articular (IA) corticosteroids for TMJ arthritis.[43] The subjects in the study were 63 children (68% female) who were diagnosed with juvenile idiopathic arthritis (JIA) who received 5 mg to 10 mg triamcinolone hexacetonide as an IA injection. Primary outcomes assessed in all subjects were the safety of the procedure and efficacy as determined by the change in maximal incisal opening. The investigators reported only 1 patient who developed the steroid complication of hypopigmentation and none developed degeneration or ankyloses, and their maximum interincisal opening was increased from 40.8 mm ± 0.93 mm to 43.5 mm ± 0.90 mm. In support of these findings is a systematic review of the literature, which examined IA injections of corticosteroid for the treatment of knee OA.[44] This review included 28 RCTs (single blind or double blind) and, among other findings, compared IA corticosteroid against placebo and against other IA corticosteroids. The overall consistent finding of these studies was that IA corticosteroid was more effective than IA placebo for pain reduction. The investigators showed that at 1 week postinjection this medication had an NNT of 3 to 4. This effect was short-lived, however, because at 4 weeks to 24 weeks postinjection, the investigators found that the effect on pain and function was not of statistical or clinical importance. Comparisons of IA corticosteroids showed triamcinolone hexacetonide was superior to betamethasone for number of patients reporting pain reduction up to 4 weeks postinjection. Comparisons between IA corticosteroid and joint lavage showed no differences in any of the efficacy or safety outcome measures.

Anticytokine Therapy for Rheumatoid Arthritis

In 2013, a study described the issue of immune modulators and OA.[45] The process of degrading the cartilage surface involves wear and tear with resulting inflammation as well as the activation of the immune system. Research shows that T cells, B cells, and macrophages all invade the degenerative joint and release cytokines, prostaglandin E2, metalloproteinases, and chemokines as well as activate the complement system.[46] In rheumatoid arthritis (RA), which is an acknowledged autoimmune disease, anticytokine therapies have a clear role but whether these medications should be used in OA is not clear.[47] The cytokines that promote inflammation are specifically targeted by medications that neutralize tumor necrosis factor (TNF)-α. In 2015, a study examined the role of anti-TNF therapy for RA.[48] The first biologic class drug for RA was a monoclonal antibody, infliximab, to human TNF. Since then, multiple other biologic class drugs have been developed although their use on patients with temporomandibular arthritis is largely restricted to patients with proved RA or idiopathic juvenile arthritis. In 2013, a study examined how effective the biologic class of immune modulators was in JIA patients.[49] This case series study examined both the less specific disease-modifying arthritic drugs and the more specific biologic class of immune modulators. The study included 154 patients attending a rheumatology clinic, and the eligible patients ranged in age from 16 to 24 years old with average disease duration of 8 years. The study reported that 29% of the patients were still on biologic therapies and had been for several years. Mild disease activity in the TMJ was detected in only 14% of these patients, suggesting this was an effective therapy that should be considered for use in the JIA population. A 2007 study examined the NNT to a 50% response rate, according to criteria put forth by the American College of Rheumatology, for adalimumab, etanercept, and infliximab when used on patients with RA.[50] There were 3 RCTs, 1 for each of the drugs included in the review. The calculated NNTs varied slightly depending on the method used but after adjustment the NNTs were adalimumab 4.0, etanercept 4.0, and infliximab in a double dosage 4.0. The

investigators concluded that these 3 anti-TNF therapies had equal efficacy for the treatment of RA.

Opioids for Arthritis

In 2015, a systematic review examined the role that opioids might play in the management of OA pain.[51] This review included 20 RCTs, which examined a variety of strong (oxycodone, buprenorphine, hydromorphone, morphine, fentanyl, and oxymorphone) and weak (tramadol, tapentadol, and codeine) opioids. The investigators found that overall, opioids were superior to placebo in reducing pain intensity in most studies but were not superior to placebo in achieving a 50% pain reduction in 2 studies. Patients dropped out more frequently with opioids than with placebo but there was no significant difference between opioids and placebo in the frequency of serious adverse events or deaths. The investigators concluded that opioids were superior to placebo in terms of efficacy and inferior in terms of tolerability. The suggested that short-term opioid therapy may be considered in selected chronic OA pain patients but that it is not a first-line treatment option for chronic OA pain. In 2011, an earlier systematic review examined the value of opioid therapy for RA pain.[52] This review included 11 studies (672 participants), which examined the efficacy of single doses of various opioid and nonopioid analgesics. The investigators reported that there were no differences between analgesic drug (opioid vs nonopioid) efficacies in these studies. One strong opioid investigated was CR morphine sulphate, in a single study with 20 participants. Six studies compared an opioid to placebo and they were found superior to placebo but also engendered more adverse events (most commonly nausea, vomiting, dizziness, and constipation). One study reviewed compared an opioid (codeine with paracetamol) to an NSAID (diclofenac) and found no difference in efficacy or safety between interventions. The investigators

| Table 5 |
| Evidence-based osteoarthritis or rheumatoid arthritis/juvenile idiopathic arthritis treatment |

Treatments	Numbers Needed to Treat
1. NSAIDs	1.6–3.0
2. Corticosteriod injections	3.0–4.0
3. Biologics[a]	4.0
4. Opioids	Not available

[a] For RA.

thus concluded that there is limited evidence that weak oral opioids may be effective analgesics for some patients with RA, but adverse effects are common and may offset the benefits of this class of medications.

Table 5 summarizes evidence-based OA and RA/JIA treatments.

SUMMARY REGARDING MEDICATIONS FOR CHRONIC OROFACIAL PAIN
Neuropathic Pain

When all these studies are taken into consideration, it seems that clinicians have at least 3 types of systemic medications (gabapentinoids, TCAs, and SNRIs) to use as well as topical anesthetics to use in patients with chronic trigeminal NPP. Unfortunately, the NNTs for all 3 of the systemic medications cannot be judged robust treatment because they range from 3.6 to 7.7. An NNT 2.0 or below is considered robust or very good. Nevertheless, it is important to have a 3-medication option because sometimes the side effects of the medications limit their usefulness. For some patients, opioids can be used infrequently for breakthrough pain, and those who do not want to take systemic pain-suppressive medications for their pain may get adequate relief with topical anesthetics applied directly to the NPP site. For those who start with topical and do not get full or adequate relief, they can use 1 or more of the systemic medications in addition to topical anesthetics. What are now needed are NNT calculations for combinations of medications, such as gabapentinoids and TCAs or gabapentinoids and topical anesthetic medications. Moreover, these studies need to be performed on patients who have a localized chronic continuous trigeminal nerve NPP disorder.

Chronic Daily Headache

For patients who have moderate to very frequent daily headaches, preventive medications are necessary and helpful. The preventive medications with reasonable evidence to support their use for chronic migraine, and clinicians have at least 3 types of systemic oral medications (β-blockers, TCAs, and AEDs) to use as well as an NMDA blocking agent to try to help patients manage their chronic continuous daily headaches and frequent migraines. The NNTs for these medications would be moderately low (3.0–4.0) but still not judged as robust treatments. In addition, for patients who do not want to take prescription medications, the evidence reviewed suggests that *Petasites* (butterbur) is a first-line therapy

along with naproxen sodium (500 mg). Opioids are and continue to be used (almost 20% of the time) in the emergency room when headache patients have a severe headache pain event and seek emergency help, but, in general, most expert think that opioids are not a logical treatment choice for either episodic or continuous headaches.

Fibromyalgia and Widespread Myofascial Pain

The data on the 3 medications approved by the FDA for fibromyalgia (pregabalin, duloxetine, and milnacipran) suggest that they are better than placebo but are not robust in their efficacy and that they are best judged as poor treatments (NNT >10). Fibromyalgia and widespread myofascial pain treatment will continue to involve combining medications with nonpharmacologic treatment methods, with the latter the preferred method of treatment. Lower-strength opioid therapy (eg, tramadol) is used with reasonable efficacy to help the most severely fibromyalgia syndrome–disabled patients.

Osteoarthritis, Rheumatoid Arthritis, and Juvenile Idiopathic Arthritis

The available data on NSAIDs show they are reasonably efficacious for OA. The NNTs for NSAIDs, corticosteriod injections, and the biologics range from 1.6 to 4.0 and, therefore, are judged as very good to fair. For gastritis-susceptible patients, acetaminophen remains a good choice for relieving arthritis pain. IA TMJ injection with corticosteroid (20 mg of triamcinolone) and 1 mL of 2% lidocaine is an alternative first-line management modality for both DDWOR and for most types of acute TMJ arthritis. Finally, for symptomatic RA and JIA patients, biologic therapies (anti–TNF-α) have been shown to diminish RA and JIA-related disease activity in the TMJ. Whether biologics should ever be used in adolescents or adults with severe OA disease of the TMJ is unclear. Finally, lower-strength opioid therapy (eg, tramadol) is used with reasonable efficacy to help the most severely OA-disabled patients.

REFERENCES

1. Padilla M, Clark GT, Merrill RL. Topical medications for orofacial neuropathic pain: a review. J Am Dent Assoc 2000;131(2):184–95.
2. Nasri-Heir C, Khan J, Heir GM. Topical medications as treatment of neuropathic orofacial pain. Dent Clin North Am 2013;57(3):541–53.

3. Haribabu PK, Eliav E, Heir GM. Topical medications for the effective management of neuropathic orofacial pain. J Am Dent Assoc 2013;144(6):612–4.

4. Bramwell BL. Topical medications for orofacial neuropathic pain. Int J Pharm Compd 2010;14(3): 200–3.

5. Ram S, Kumar SK, Clark GT. Using oral medications, infusions and injections for differential diagnosis of orofacial pain. J Calif Dent Assoc 2006;34(8):645–54.

6. Clark GT. Persistent orodental pain, atypical odontalgia, and phantom tooth pain: when are they neuropathic disorders? J Calif Dent Assoc 2006;34(8): 599–609.

7. Peppin JF, Albrecht PJ, Argoff C, et al. Skin matters: a review of topical treatments for chronic pain. Part two: treatments and applications. Pain Ther 2015; 4(1):33–50.

8. Finnerup NB, Attal N, Haroutounian S, et al. Pharmacotherapy for neuropathic pain in adults: a systematic review and meta-analysis. Lancet Neurol 2015; 14(2):162–73.

9. Derry S, Wiffen PJ, Moore RA, et al. Topical lidocaine for neuropathic pain in adults. Cochrane Database Syst Rev 2014;(7):CD010958.

10. Meier T, Wasner G, Faust M, et al. Efficacy of lidocaine patch 5% in the treatment of focal peripheral neuropathic pain syndromes: a randomized, double-blind, placebo-controlled study. Pain 2003; 106(1–2):151–8.

11. Heir G, Karolchek S, Kalladka M, et al. Use of topical medication in orofacial neuropathic pain: a retrospective study. Oral Surg Oral Med Oral Pathol Oral Radiol Endod 2008;105(4):466–9.

12. Ciaramella A, Paroli M, Poli P. An emerging dimension in psychosomatic research: the nocebo phenomenon in the management of chronic pain. ISRN Neurosci 2013;2013:574526.

13. Häuser W, Bartram C, Bartram-Wunn E, et al. Adverse events attributable to nocebo in randomized controlled drug trials in fibromyalgia syndrome and painful diabetic peripheral neuropathy: systematic review. Clin J Pain 2012;28(5):437–51.

14. Pérez C, Navarro A, Saldaña MT, et al. Pregabalin and gabapentin in matched patients with peripheral neuropathic pain in routine medical practice in a primary care setting: findings from a cost-consequences analysis in a nested case-control study. Clin Ther 2010;32(7):1357–70.

15. Derry S, Wiffen PJ, Aldington D, et al. Nortriptyline for neuropathic pain in adults. Cochrane Database Syst Rev 2015;(1):CD011209.

16. Gaskell H, Moore RA, Derry S, et al. Oxycodone for neuropathic pain and fibromyalgia in adults. Cochrane Database Syst Rev 2014;(6):CD010692.

17. Gilron I, Tu D, Holden RR, et al. Combination of morphine with nortriptyline for neuropathic pain. Pain 2015;156(8):1440–8.

18. Federal Register/Vol. 79, No. 127/Wednesday, July 2, 2014/Rules and Regulations pages 37623–9..

19. Cady R, Nett R, Dexter K, et al. Treatment of chronic migraine: a 3-month comparator study of naproxen sodium vs SumaRT/Nap. Headache 2014;54(1):80–93.

20. Holland S, Silberstein SD, Freitag F, et al. Evidence-based guideline update: NSAIDs and other complementary treatments for episodic migraine prevention in adults: report of the Quality Standards Subcommittee of the American Academy of Neurology and the American Headache Society. Neurology 2012; 78(17):1346–53.

21. Tomkins GE, Jackson JL, O'Malley PG, et al. Treatment of chronic headache with antidepressants: a meta-analysis. Am J Med 2001;111:54–63.

22. Hoffmann J, Akerman S, Goadsby PJ. Efficacy and mechanism of anticonvulsant drugs in migraine. Expert Rev Clin Pharmacol 2014;7(2):191–201.

23. Linde M, Mulleners WM, Chronicle EP, et al. Valproate (valproic acid or sodium valproate or a combination of the two) for the prophylaxis of episodic migraine in adults. Cochrane Database Syst Rev 2013;(6):CD010611.

24. Victor S, Ryan SW. Drugs for preventing migraine headaches in children. Cochrane Database Syst Rev 2003;(4):CD002761.

25. Linde M, Mulleners WM, Chronicle EP, et al. Topiramate for the prophylaxis of episodic migraine in adults. Cochrane Database Syst Rev 2013;(6):CD010610.

26. Huang L, Bocek M, Jordan JK, et al. Memantine for the prevention of primary headache disorders. Ann Pharmacother 2014;48(11):1507–11.

27. Hepp Z, Dodick DW, Varon SF, et al. Adherence to oral migraine-preventive medications among patients with chronic migraine. Cephalalgia 2015; 35(6):478–88.

28. Mafi JN, Edwards ST, Pedersen NP, et al. Trends in the ambulatory management of headache: analysis of NAMCS and NHAMCS Data 1999-2010. J Gen Intern Med 2015;30(5):548–55.

29. Bendtsen L, Evers S, Linde M, et al. EFNS guideline on the treatment of tension-type headache - report of an EFNS task force. Eur J Neurol 2010;17(11): 1318–25.

30. Kim SC, Landon JE, Lee YC. Patterns of health care utilization related to initiation of amitriptyline, duloxetine, gabapentin or pregabalin in fibromyalgia. Arthritis Res Ther 2015;17(1):18.

31. Häuser W, Wolfe F, Tölle T, et al. The role of antidepressants in the management of fibromyalgia syndrome: a systematic review and meta-analysis. CNS Drugs 2012;26(4):297–307.

32. Straube S, Derry S, Moore RA, et al. Pregabalin in fibromyalgia–responder analysis from individual patient data. BMC Musculoskelet Disord 2010;11:150.

33. Keshavarz K, Hashemi-Meshkini A, Gharibnaseri Z, et al. A systematic cost-effectiveness analysis of pregabalin in the management of fibromyalgia: an Iranian experience. Arch Med Sci 2013;9(6):961–7.

34. Luciano JV, D'Amico F, Cerdà-Lafont M, et al. Cost-utility of cognitive behavioral therapy versus U.S. Food and Drug Administration recommended drugs and usual care in the treatment of patients with fibromyalgia: an economic evaluation alongside a 6-month randomized controlled trial. Arthritis Res Ther 2014;16(5):451.

35. Perrot S, Russell IJ. More ubiquitous effects from non-pharmacologic than from pharmacologic treatments for fibromyalgia syndrome: a meta-analysis examining six core symptoms. Eur J Pain 2014; 18(8):1067–80.

36. Janda AM, As-Sanie S, Rajala B, et al. Fibromyalgia Survey criteria is associated with increased postoperative opioid consumption in women undergoing hysterectomy. Anesthesiology 2015;122(5): 1103–11.

37. Peng X, Robinson RL, Mease P, et al. Long-term evaluation of opioid treatment in fibromyalgia. Clin J Pain 2015;31(1):7–13.

38. Lee J, Ellis B, Price C, et al. Chronic widespread pain, including fibromyalgia: a pathway for care developed by the British Pain Society. Br J Anaesth 2014;112(1):16–24.

39. de Souza RF, Lovato da Silva CH, Nasser M, et al. Interventions for the management of temporomandibular joint osteoarthritis. Cochrane Database Syst Rev 2012;(4):CD007261.

40. Ong CK, Lirk P, Tan CH, et al. An evidence-based update on nonsteroidal anti-inflammatory drugs. Clin Med Res 2007;5(1):19–34.

41. Lee C, Straus WL, Balshaw R, et al. A comparison of the efficacy and safety of nonsteroidal antiinflammatory agents versus acetaminophen in the treatment of osteoarthritis: a meta-analysis. Arthritis Rheum 2004;51:746–54.

42. Samiee A, Sabzerou D, Edalatpajouh F, et al. Temporomandibular joint injection with corticosteroid and local anesthetic for limited mouth opening. J Oral Sci 2011;53(3):321–5.

43. Stoll ML, Good J, Sharpe T, et al. Intra-articular corticosteroid injections to the temporomandibular joints are safe and appear to be effective therapy in children with juvenile idiopathic arthritis. J Oral Maxillofac Surg 2012;70(8):1802–7.

44. Bellamy N, Campbell J, Robinson V, et al. Intraarticular corticosteroid for treatment of osteoarthritis of the knee. Cochrane Database Syst Rev 2006;(2):CD005328.

45. Haseeb A, Haqqi TM. Immunopathogenesis of osteoarthritis. Clin Immunol 2013;146(3):185–96.

46. Venkatesha SH, Dudics S, Acharya B, et al. Cytokine-modulating strategies and newer cytokine targets for arthritis therapy. Int J Mol Sci 2014; 16(1):887–906.

47. Reynolds G, Cooles FA, Isaacs JD, et al. Emerging immunotherapies for rheumatoid arthritis. Hum Vaccin Immunother 2014;10(4):822–37.

48. Monaco C, Nanchahal J, Taylor P, et al. Anti-TNF therapy: past, present and future. Int Immunol 2015;27(1):55–62.

49. Vidqvist KL, Malin M, Varjolahti-Lehtinen T, et al. Disease activity of idiopathic juvenile arthritis continues through adolescence despite the use of biologic therapies. Rheumatology (Oxford) 2013; 52(11):1999–2003.

50. Kristensen LE, Christensen R, Bliddal H, et al. The number needed to treat for adalimumab, etanercept, and infliximab based on ACR50 response in three randomized controlled trials on established rheumatoid arthritis: a systematic literature review. Scand J Rheumatol 2007;36(6):411–7.

51. Schaefert R, Welsch P, Klose P, et al. Opioids in chronic osteoarthritis pain: a systematic review and meta-analysis of efficacy, tolerability and safety in randomized placebo-controlled studies of at least 4 weeks duration. Schmerz 2015;29(1):47–59 [in German].

52. Whittle SL, Richards BL, Husni E, et al. Opioid therapy for treating rheumatoid arthritis pain. Cochrane Database Syst Rev 2011;(11):CD003113.

Injection Therapy for Headache and Facial Pain

Jonathan K. Kleen, MD, PhD[a], Morris Levin, MD[b],*

KEYWORDS

- Headache • Migraine • Injection • Local anesthetic • Onabotulinum toxin

KEY POINTS

- Injection therapy for peripheral nerve blockade is an increasingly viable treatment option for selected groups of patients with headache and facial pain that are refractory to medical therapy.
- Treatable headache types with injection therapy include chronic migraine, tension-type headache, chronic daily headache, cluster headache, occipital neuralgia, cervicogenic headache, trigeminal neuralgia, hemicrania continua, and even post–lumbar puncture headache.
- Injection therapies are conveniently administered in office appointments, with initial relief usually apparent before the patient leaves the clinic.
- Injection sites considered for anesthetic blockade include greater occipital nerve, lesser occipital nerve, auriculotemporal nerve, supraorbital supratrochlear nerves, infraorbital nerves, sphenopalatine ganglion, cervical facet and spinal nerve roots, and trigger point injections.
- Multisite onabotulinum toxin injections are increasingly used and effective for chronic migraine, and potentially other headache types pending further investigation.

INTRODUCTION

Despite the variety of acute and prophylactic pain-relieving medications that are often efficacious for headache and facial pain disorders, certain patients experience intolerable side effects to these agents. In others, the remaining pharmaceutical approaches may be too hazardous as a result of comorbid factors including psychiatric conditions, vascular disease (cardiovascular, cerebrovascular, or peripheral vascular disease), hepatic disease, or renal disease. Often these conditions involve the use of long-term medications that could interact negatively with pain-relieving agents. Other complicating contexts include transient contraindications, such as pregnancy, to regimens that are already established and effective for a given patient. In many of these patients,

medical therapies simply prove insurmountable. In addition, there is a subgroup of patients who are simply refractory to traditional modes of therapy.[1]

Peripheral nerve procedures, such as nerve blocks, can be dramatically effective for many of these patients and should always be included in the management repertoire. Peripheral nerve blockade for pain suppression is based on the ability of low concentrations of local anesthetics (LAs) to selectively block sensory fibers in mixed nerves. Ideally, motor function is spared or at least minimally affected. The duration of the block depends on the dose and the pharmacokinetic properties of the particular LA, but in practice one commonly observes a longer duration of benefits than expected. Blockade of

---

Conflicts of Interest: None (J.K. Kleen); Consultant for Allergan, Zogenix, MAP; participated in training physicians in injection techniques for Allergan (M. Levin).
[a] UCSF Department of Neurology, University of California San Francisco Medical Center, 505 Parnassus Avenue, Box 0114, San Francisco, CA 94143, USA; [b] UCSF Headache Center, UCSF Department of Neurology, University of California San Francisco Medical Center, 2330 Post Street, San Francisco, CA 94115, USA
* Corresponding author.
E-mail address: morris.levin@ucsf.edu

Oral Maxillofacial Surg Clin N Am 28 (2016) 423–434
http://dx.doi.org/10.1016/j.coms.2016.04.002

several nerves in the head and neck can also produce beneficial effects in pain syndromes involving regions outside of the territory served by these nerves. This result is often explained by the concept of convergence in the nociceptive system of the head and neck (discussed later), although not all observations are accounted for by this mechanism.

There is unfortunately a shortage of controlled studies on the effectiveness of LA procedures for headache and facial pain, and these procedures often carry a significant placebo effect.[2] Nevertheless, a large number of patients with facial pain and headaches (described by the International Classification of Headache Disorders[3]) obtain significant benefit from nerve block procedures, which are describe here.

CLINICAL CONDITIONS TREATED WITH INJECTION THERAPY

Injection therapy is a versatile tool in clinical practice, efficacious for diverse etiologies of facial pain and headaches. For instance, multiple painful cranial neuropathy conditions, such as trigeminal neuralgia and occipital neuralgia, are alleviated by such techniques as infraorbital nerve blockade, or blocking one or more of the occipital nerves. This tactic could extend to treatment of musculoskeletal syndromes whose painful foci may lie among the distributions of similar nerves. Alternatively, direct trigger point injections of the affected areas are effective, such as in temporomandibular joint dysfunction or myofascial pain syndrome.

We foresee an increasing number of patients using injection therapy in clinical practice in the coming years, particularly for headache disorders. This is in part from the slow build of clinical trials providing sound evidence for anesthetic blocks and even onabotulinum toxin A (Botox) injections in refractory headache conditions. These include chronic migraine, tension-type headache, chronic daily headache, and cervicogenic headache. Other debilitating conditions, such as cluster headache, hemicrania continua, and even post–lumbar puncture headache, can also be alleviated with certain injection therapies. In addition, some patients may suffer from mixed etiologies (eg, chronic migraine exacerbated by occipital neuralgia). The etiologic versatility of nerve block treatments could be particularly useful in treating these otherwise convoluted cases.

The bulk of this article is dedicated to describing the evidence for treating these conditions under the corresponding injection therapies techniques.

OVERVIEW OF PHARMACOLOGY

LAs chemically are weak bases, produced as salts to promote stability and solubility, and have hydrophilic and lipophilic components. They inhibit neural activity (neuropathic pain signaling) by interfering with sodium and potassium currents, preventing depolarization.[4] The ester LAs (including procaine and cocaine) were discovered and used first, although they are slightly more allergenic and shorter acting than amide LAs. The amide LAs are relatively hypoallergenic and well tolerated, hence their current prevalence in clinical practice. These include prilocaine, lidocaine, mepivacaine, and bupivacaine (listed in increasing order of anesthetic effect duration). The first three have similar potency (approximately one-quarter that of bupivacaine) and mid-range duration of action. Lidocaine in 1% solution is the most common choice, with an onset of action at around 4 to 8 minutes after injection and duration of about 1 to 2 hours. Bupivacaine in 0.25% or 0.50% solution offers more prolonged action, with an onset in about 8 to 12 minutes and duration between 4 and 8 hours. Many clinicians choose to combine lidocaine with bupivacaine in a mixture.

Epinephrine-containing LA formulations come with their own potential side effect profile and they are neither necessary nor recommended for nerve blocks. Alternately, some practitioners add a corticosteroid medication to the injected solution, often triamcinolone (Kenalog) or methylprednisolone (Depo-medrol). Some studies suggest efficacy of local steroid injections for cervicogenic headache and potentially migraine or cluster headaches,[5,6] although some results are mixed or are occasionally questioned in methodology. A more recent double-blind randomized controlled trial[7] found no significant difference from steroids on transformed migraine severity in the short- or long-term. Local corticosteroid injections also bring a host of additional potential side effects, such as slow injection site healing, alopecia, or cutaneous atrophy (lipoatrophy) at the injection site (particularly with triamcinolone, which can be mitigated by using methylprednisolone or betamethasone).[8,9] Although rare, even systemic effects embodying Cushing syndrome have been reported after serial injections.[10]

MECHANISMS OF NERVE BLOCK EFFECTS IN PRIMARY HEADACHE AND FACIAL PAIN DISORDERS

LAs seem to attenuate pain-transmitting neural signals, which are often carried by nociceptive C fibers.[11] The mechanism of therapeutic nerve blocks in headaches stemming from cervical, occipital, or trigeminal nerve injury or dysfunction (eg, posttraumatic damage or vascular compression) is likely via anesthesia of the irritated, pain-producing nerves.

In contrast, the exact mechanisms by which injection therapies alleviate primary headache disorders are unclear. Both migraine and cluster headache are thought to be centrally mediated, primary neuropathic disorders. The mechanism for their acute pain relief may be through reducing afferent input, leading to a decrease in activity at the level of the trigeminal nucleus caudalis, cervical dorsal horn, and their converging circuits.[12–15] Attenuating neural transmission at the first synapse of the nociceptive pathways that oversee head and neck pain could conceivably reduce the perception of pain in broader areas that are served by more proximal circuits of that nerve.

Nerve block therapies are also thought to help to break clinical "pain cycles," which could correlate with physiologic factors that underlie chronic pain. Sensitization of central or peripheral nervous system pain signaling could be an explanation for persistent neuropathic pain. The reduction of nociceptive signaling via nerve block injection therapy could help reduce this persistent aberrant activity, and even increase the threshold for pain signaling of other converging sensitized nociceptors in those circuits. This theoretic mechanism could allow for more long-term pain alleviation, and provide a better window of opportunity to start a prophylactic headache medication.

CONTRAINDICATIONS TO PERIPHERAL NERVE BLOCKADE

There are several contraindications or relative contraindications to peripheral nerve block procedures. Major examples from the literature[16,17] are cited in **Box 1**. However, providers should always be vigilant and assess for other potential risks for each individual patient.

PROCEDURAL TECHNIQUE FOR NERVE BLOCKS
Preparation and Patient Positioning

During the consent process the procedure should be explained to the patient, who should be allowed to ask questions. A few follow-up questions from the provider regarding the material discussed (ie, "teachback") can verify understanding and ensure that expectations are appropriate.

The syringe size should be 3 to 5 mL, for common injection volumes of 1 to 2 mL (occasionally

---

Box 1
Contraindications and conditions requiring precautions for nerve blockade therapies

Contraindications

- Infection (eg, nearby cellulitis or abscess)
- Nearby open skull defect (to avoid intracranial diffusion)
- Allergy to anesthetic
- Poorly cooperative patient (eg, unpredictable behavior risking accidental needle trauma)

Conditions requiring precautions

- Anticoagulant use (eg, if international normalized ratio is >3.0)
- Pregnancy (lidocaine is preferable over bupivacaine; Food and Drug Administration Category B and C, respectively)
- Obesity with unclear anatomic landmarks
- Propensity to vasovagal events

---

more for larger distributions). The preferred needle gauge is usually between 25 and 30. Standard procedural gloves should be used to help minimize infection risk; sterile gloves are not usually necessary, provided sufficient cleaning of the area (see later).

The patient should be seated on a chair of sufficient height so that the provider can perform the injection in a comfortable accessible position. The head should be positioned to expose the planned nerve (eg, neck flexed forward for an occipital nerve block).

Surgical Approach

Procedure

Step One: Following assessment of the anatomy and palpation of nearby vessels to avoid (see individual block descriptions), thorough cleaning of the area should be performed using povidone-iodine or alcohol preparation pads. Injections are usually approximately 1 to 2 mL of lidocaine, bupivacaine, or a mixture of the two but can be deferred to provider preference.

Step Two: The needle should be inserted at a shallow angle directed at the intended subcutaneous injection site. To avoid nerve damage, it is also helpful to advance the tip slowly and aim for a perineural distribution. Patients usually report lancinating pain if nerves are directly impinged on, at which point the needle should be redirected.

Step Three: Gently pull back the plunger of the syringe to evaluate for aspiration of any blood to signal that the needle may be in a lumen of a blood vessel. Redirect the needle elsewhere near the nerve target if so, repeating this evaluation each time. Pulling back too hard may rupture local capillaries and produce a false-positive, whereas pulling back too softly may give false reassurance.

Step Four: The injection should be administered at a moderate rate (eg, 1 mL over 10–20 seconds), to allow steady distribution and prevent hydraulic mechanical damage from the volume. The injection can also be given in a fanned spread or repeated in multiple sites, although this could increase risk for local damage and is often unnecessary given that LAs tend to diffuse well throughout the dermis.

Immediate postoperative care
The injection area may be rubbed or massaged for 10 to 20 seconds afterward; this does not likely improve efficacy but can improve patient comfort. To reduce inflammation, local measures (particularly cold application) are usually sufficient.

Patient care postprocedure
Patients should ideally wait in the office until the effects of the anesthetic are apparent and stable. This also allows for brief initial monitoring for adverse events (and to offer reassurance for benign associated symptoms). Sensation testing should reveal an area of anesthesia corresponding to the usual distribution of the nerves injected. If suboptimal, additional local injection can be pursued (if deemed necessary).

Possible Complications and Management

Mechanical nerve trauma
Paresthesias or prolonged numbness in the targeted nerve's distribution could occur, suggesting mechanical trauma to the nerve. About 97% of these cases resolve within a few weeks, and nearly all within a year. The incidence of block-related nerve injury is about 0.4 per 1000 procedures.[18]

Systemic side effects
Systemic distribution of LAs is how some clinical adverse effects can arise, although toxicity is rare (about 1 in 1000 procedures).[18] The most severe systemic side effects include seizures or alterations in consciousness. This could occur through unintentional intravascular injection, generally avoided by pulling back the plunger of the syringe and injecting only if there is no blood return (discussed previously). Note that this is not entirely reliable if using small-gauge needles (30 or smaller) or if back-pressure is applied too forcefully. Systemic accumulation of anesthetics can also be an issue for patients on other interacting medications, or with hepatic or renal disease, or the rare genetic defect in serum pseudocholinesterase important for ester LA breakdown. Ensure the patient is screened beforehand for relevant potential metabolic issues, and avoid giving more medication than anticipated.

Other complications
Other adverse effects resulting from LA injection include local infection, nerve damage with later neuroma formation, hematoma (particularly in patients with a bleeding diathesis), and local injury to adjacent structures, depending on the site of injection. The patient's specific anatomic features (eg, skull defects, local infection, previous surgery) must also be identified, and avoided.

SPECIFIC NERVE BLOCKS: TECHNIQUES AND CLINICAL RESULTS IN THE LITERATURE
Greater Occipital Nerve Block

Anatomy and surgical approach
The greater occipital nerve (GON) is the primary branch of the second cervical root (C2) and innervates the scalp from the external occipital protuberance to the vertex. It crosses the semispinalis muscle traveling superiorly, and subsequently becomes subcutaneous after crossing the trapezius muscle. This latter landmark is on average about 3 cm from the midline and 2 cm below the external occipital protuberance (**Fig. 1**).[19] As a

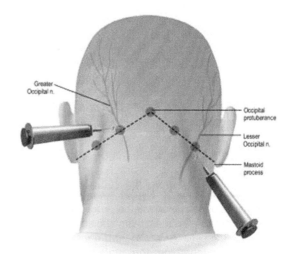

Fig. 1. Injection sites for greater and lesser occipital nerve blockade. (*From* Levin M. Nerve blocks in the treatment of headache. Neurotherapeutics 2010;7(2):199; with permission.)

practical estimate, it is located approximately two-thirds of the distance on a line from the center of the mastoid to the greater occipital protuberance. It is adjacent to the occipital artery, which is usually palpable. The nerve itself is approximately less than 2.5 mm in diameter at this point[20] and often perceptibly palpable, although many providers simply go by landmarks. Approximately 2 mL of bupivacaine or lidocaine, or a mixture of the two (commonly in 1:1 ratio), should be injected subcutaneously into this area for the desired effect.

Clinical results in the literature

The two conditions commonly treated with GON blocks are occipital neuralgia (or "neuritis") and cervicogenic headache. Refractory migraine can also sometimes respond to this technique, as can cluster headaches and other select etiologies.

Outcomes in the clinical literature for these conditions are generally good. A retrospective study of 184 patients with occipital neuralgia showed long-lasting improvement following GON steroid injections with a mean of 31 days of relief.[21] Cervicogenic headache is a somewhat controversial diagnosis with no clear diagnostic tool, but can often also be alleviated with GON blockade. In a study of 100 patients diagnosed with cervicogenic headaches all responded to repeated GON blocks.[22] This procedure was also effective in a study of 52 patients with broader headache etiologies including cervicogenic, migraine, or tension-type headaches.[23] Chronic tension-type headache may be somewhat resistant to GON block according to another study,[24] despite many patients localizing their symptoms to the occipital region.

GON block seems to be effective in many patients with migraine,[25] although controlled studies were limited until more recently. A randomized, multicenter, double-blind, placebo-controlled study[26] found that GON blockade was effective for chronic migraine, and safe and cost-effective.

GON blockade also seems to be effective in the acute, and possibly prophylactic, treatment of cluster headache.[27] A double-blind, placebo-controlled study[6] of GON block ipsilateral to the cluster headache side found that 80% of the treated group responded (none responded in the saline placebo group) with alleviated pain, lasting for several weeks.[28]

Chronic daily headache (the common denotation for headaches that occur on 15 days per month or more) encompasses a challenging subgroup of patients, particularly in specialty headache and pain clinics. Most headache specialists believe these patients actually represent a subgroup of migraine patients known as chronic migraine, with many refractory to pharmacologic and nonpharmacological approaches. A study of the benefits of GON block in a type of chronic daily headache (transformed migraine) showed positive results.[7] Further study is required, because intractable chronic daily headache is a significant health problem with little proven therapy.

GON block also has been successful in other headache types including post-lumbar puncture headache,[29] refractory trigeminal neuralgia,[30] and refractory hemicrania continua.[31]

Lesser Occipital Nerve Block

Anatomy and surgical approach

The lesser occipital nerve (LON) is derived from the cervical plexus (C2, C3) and supplies the inferior and more lateral scalp and skin of the upper neck. This nerve can be blocked by injecting one third of the way from the center of the mastoid to the greater occipital protuberance, on the same line used for GON block (see **Fig. 1**). Using actual measurements, it is usually about 6.5 cm lateral to the midline, and approximately 5.3 cm below a line drawn between the auditory canals.[32]

Clinical results in the literature

Similar to the GON, the LON has been implicated in severe occipital neuralgia and even cervicogenic headaches. When performed, LON blocks are often used in conjunction with GON blocks, particularly in those who experience headaches more laterally in the occipital region. However, there are unfortunately no studies that firmly support LON anesthetic blockade in headache disorders.

Auriculotemporal Nerve Block

Anatomy and surgical approach

The auriculotemporal nerve is a branch of the mandibular division of the trigeminal nerve, which supplies sensation over the ear and temporalis muscle. Blockade can be performed by injecting superior to the posterior portion of the zygoma just anterior to the ear (**Fig. 2**). If this block is successful, anesthesia is usually described over the temporal fossa.

Clinical results in the literature

Although blockade of the auriculotemporal nerve is not often used for headache disorders, certain patients have benefited. One report described six cases of auriculotemporal neuralgia caused by various etiologies, and blockade of this nerve resulted in complete or near-complete relief of their pain.[33] However, efficacy for other headache syndromes, such as migraines, is generally

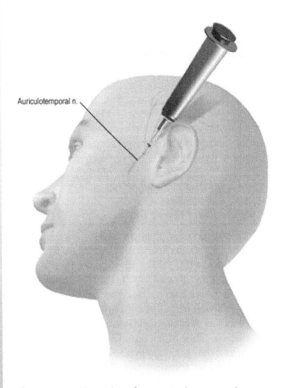

Fig. 2. Injection site for auriculotemporal nerve blockade. (*From* Levin M. Nerve blocks in the treatment of headache. Neurotherapeutics 2010;7(2):200; with permission.)

anecdotal or studied in combination with other simultaneous nerve blockades.[34]

Supraorbital and Supratrochlear Nerve Block

Anatomy and surgical approach

The supraorbital and supratrochlear nerves are branches of the ophthalmic division of the trigeminal nerve. These nerves are prone to traumatic injury because of their superficial locations (also making them easily accessible to nerve block procedures). Headaches after frontal trauma involving pain and/or tenderness localized to just above the orbital ridge should raise suspicion for this diagnosis. The supratrochlear nerve is blocked by injecting just above the eyebrow over its medial border (**Fig. 3**). To anesthetize the supraorbital nerve, the injection can be done approximately 2 cm lateral to the supratrochlear nerve, or the needle is advanced laterally through the same puncture that was used for the latter.

Clinical results in the literature

This technique seems to have efficacy in treating supraorbital neuralgia. In a study of supraorbital nerve (SON) and/or GON blockade in 29 patients with migraine, 25 patients (85%) had a favorable response. However, this report did not include

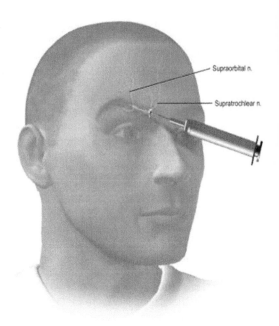

Supraorbital n.

Supratrochlear n.

Fig. 3. Injection sites for supratrochlear and supraorbital nerve blockade. (*From* Levin M. Nerve blocks in the treatment of headache. Neurotherapeutics 2010;7(2):200; with permission.)

data for SON blocks alone.[35] Blockade of both supraorbital and supratrochlear nerve was reported as efficacious for acute refractory migraine.[36] Supraorbital nerve block in particular has also been effective in a few small studies of hemicrania continua[37] and perhaps somewhat for cervicogenic headache (but less so compared with GON blockade).[23]

Infraorbital Nerve Block

Anatomy and surgical approach

The infraorbital nerve is the main branch of the maxillary nerve (V2) off the trigeminal nerve (cranial nerve V). It innervates a strip of skin between the upper lip and the lower eyelid. Blockade of this nerve is beneficial for headache featuring facial pain, but there are several anatomic variations that can pose increased risk of iatrogenic injury. An intraoral approach is often used for dental practice, but extraoral approach seems superior in attaining a wider distribution of the block (and theoretically better clinical efficacy), because of application of the anesthetic to the nerve more proximal to the infraorbital aperture. A careful landmark-based measurement approach is likely sufficient for the extraoral approach.[38] Ideally, injection between 5 and 8 mm inferior to the infraorbital margin, and about 2.5 cm lateral to the facial midline, seems most optimal (**Fig. 4**).[38] Keep in mind that the nerve itself lies deep to the ample subcutaneous tissue in that area and the

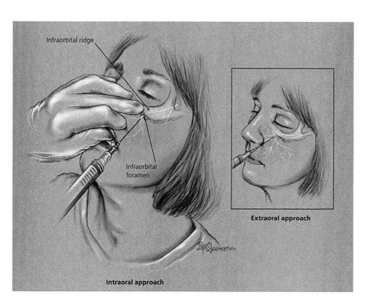

Fig. 4. Injection site for infraorbital nerve blockade. (*From* Latham JL, Martin SN. Infiltrative anesthesia in office practice. Am Fam Physician 2014;89(12):959; with permission.)

underlying quadratus labii superioris muscle. Great care should be taken to avoid patient movement or other circumstances that could risk orbital trauma or damage to nearby vessels. Never use anesthetics containing vasoconstrictors given proximity to the facial artery.

Clinical results in the literature

There are limited direct studies of infraorbital nerve block efficacy on headache syndromes. One study described 26 patients with migraine diagnoses who had a combination of bilateral infraorbital and supraorbital nerve blocks three times in 9 days, and followed them for months afterward. This open-label study showed consistently decreased migraine burden and impact on daily life (based on MIDAS scale scores) that continued through the 6 months after treatment.[39] A small double-blind placebo-controlled randomized design study of 20 trigeminal neuralgia patients (idiopathic and traumatic etiologies) found no benefit of infraorbital nerve blocks.[40]

Sphenopalatine Ganglion Block

Anatomy and surgical approach

The sphenopalatine ganglion (also referred to as the pterygopalatine ganglion) contains sensory fibers that contribute to the maxillary branch of the trigeminal nerve, and both parasympathetic and sympathetic fibers. Anesthesia of the sphenopalatine ganglion can be done via transcutaneous or intraoral injection, but a simpler and less invasive (and less risky) approach is topical application of LA to the mucosa in the lateral nasal cavity wall. This done with the patient supine, with the tip of the nose pointed vertically and the head turned

slightly to the side of the block. A long, cotton-tipped applicator should be saturated with 4% lidocaine solution and inserted into the ipsilateral nare and applied to the lateral posterior wall of the nasal cavity (**Fig. 5**), repeated until pain relief is obtained.

Clinical results in the literature

Sphenopalatine ganglion blockade initially was proposed as an acute treatment option for cluster headache, based on reported acute cluster headache response to cocaine applied to the

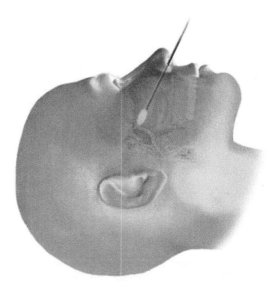

Fig. 5. Procedure for intranasal administration (sphenopalatine ganglion blockade). (*From* Levin M. Nerve blocks in the treatment of headache. Neurotherapeutics 2010;7(2):201; with permission.)

sphenopalatine ganglion intranasally.[41] Results have been generally positive using lidocaine,[42,43] although in one study of 30 male patients with cluster headache there was only marginal efficacy.[44] Still, for patients with intractable cluster headache, this seems a reasonable option. Often patients can learn to do this technique themselves, usually with good results. Sphenopalatine ganglion has also shown effectiveness in alleviating chronic migraine, including one small double-blind, placebo-controlled, randomized study.[45]

Cervical Facet and Spinal Root Block

Anatomy and surgical approach

Upper cervical facet injections are sometimes used for headache treatment, particularly of occipital localization. This headache pain can sometimes be reproduced on noxious stimulation of the atlanto-occipital joint, the lateral atlantoaxial joint, the C2-C3 zygapophysial joints, or intervertebral disk.[46] The most common facets targeted are the C2-C3 and C3-C4 joints (**Fig. 6**); more inferior facets are not commonly pursued. Potential adverse effects include local hemorrhage, infection, nerve trauma, sensory loss, weakness, or paresthesias; one must also be vigilant of nearby vascular structures including carotid and vertebral arteries. Thus, these procedures require a specialized fluoroscopic procedure room equipped with a portable imaging system ("C-arm") and a practitioner skilled with these tools for proper placement of the injection needle or catheter.

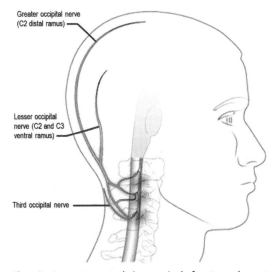

Fig. 6. Areas targeted in cervical facet and root blockade. (*Adapted from* Bhagia SM, Slipman CW, Brigham CD. Cervicogenic headache. In: Slipman CW, editor. Interventional spine: an algorithmic approach. 1st edition. Elsevier, Saunders: Philadelphia;2008. p. 737–51; with permission.)

Clinical results in the literature

There is unfortunately a lack of clear evidence of efficacy for cervical facet and root blockades and headache relief, although one open label study demonstrated significant relief in most patients after injections of LA into the lateral atlantoaxial joints.[47] The second cervical root is a target in some headache syndromes particularly when they have previously responded to GON blocks. Likewise the third cervical root has been targeted for headaches thought to be caused by "whiplash," or other cervical injury or pathology.[48]

Trigger Point Injections

Anatomy and surgical approach

Trigger points are focal areas of allodynia stemming from myofascial pain, which can add to or cause certain headache syndromes. Thought to represent a sustained muscle contraction emitting pain mediators, they are usually tender palpable in various anatomic locations, without evidence of other culpable cause (eg, cellulitis). This painful area can potentially be mitigated by local injection therapy, most commonly in the trapezius, sternocleidomastoid, and temporalis muscle areas (**Fig. 7**). Localization involves direct palpation and injection (1–2 mL of lidocaine and/or bupivacaine or mixture) into the center of the tightened muscle tissue itself (gripped between thumb and forefinger when possible). Beyond this, the preparation and postoperative care are similar to that for nerve block procedures described previously.

Clinical results in the literature

Many practitioners perform trigger point injections for a variety of headache syndromes, most commonly for chronic tension-type headache and chronic migraine.[49] Several studies have demonstrated efficacy, most notably for tension-type headaches, both episodic[50] and chronic.[51] Other smaller studies have shown some efficacy for migraine[52] and cervicogenic headache and vestibular migraine, when in combination with GON blocks.[53]

Onabotulinum Toxin Injections

Anatomy and surgical approach

Fixed-site, fixed-dose injections of onabotulinum toxin A (Botox) are a somewhat surprising addition to the headache prophylaxis repertoire in recent years, after Food and Drug Administration approval for the treatment of chronic migraine in 2010. The technique involves multisite injections (31 sites for each treatment; **Fig. 8**) of the head and neck, outlined in the original PREEMPT trial.[54,55] These sites include bilateral trapezius

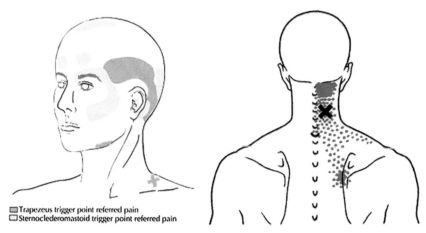

Fig. 7. Trigger point morphology and some injection sites targeted in headache disorders. (*From* Trigger Point Dry Needling (TDN). Berthoud Athletic Club. Available at: http://www.bacinfo.com/physical-therapy/. Accessed November 30, 2015.)

(three sites each), cervical paraspinal (two sites each), occipitals (three sites each), temporalis (four sites each), corrugator (one site each), frontal (one site each), and unilateral procerus (single site) muscle locations. The provider should administer 5 U of botulinum toxin in each injection site, in a manner similar to standard nerve block injection although targeting the muscle bundles instead of the nerves. However, a smaller needle size (generally 30 gauge) is used. Standard techniques described previously still hold in terms of prevention of accidental bloodstream injection of the toxin. The effects of onabotulinum toxin are not evident until approximately 24 hours afterward in terms of decreased muscle tension, and the effect on headaches may take a few days to become evident. Adverse events for this procedure most often include pain at injection sites, weakness, and issues related to weakness (eg, ptosis). The possibility of these potential outcomes should be

discussed thoroughly before the procedure during consent, and future attempts at the procedure can involve dose adjustment to balance therapeutic effects with these potential side effects.

Another issue to be aware of is the potential development of an immunogenic response, because onabotulinum toxin is an exogenous protein. As such, the use of this toxin can cause the (rare) development of immune-mediated adverse events (eg, hypersensitivity or allergic reactions), or neutralizing antibodies that result in loss of therapeutic effect over time.

Clinical results in the literature
The mechanism of action for onabotulinum toxin in chronic migraine is thought to include inhibition of calcitonin gene-related peptide and substance P release among the trigeminovascular system.[56,57] In recent years two multicenter, randomized, open-label placebo-controlled studies showed

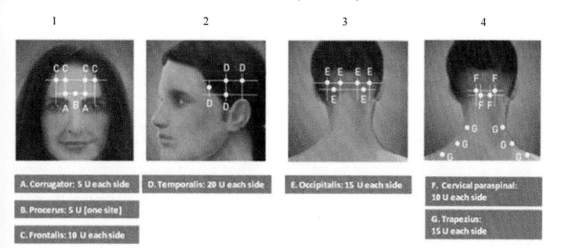

Fig. 8. Onabotulinum toxin injection. (*Courtesy of* Allergan, Inc, Irvine, CA; with permission.)

that onabotulinum toxin was highly effective in decreasing migraine headache frequency (ie, as a prophylactic therapy), decreased headache disability, and also improved quality of life.[54,55] Onabotulinum toxin for chronic migraine was also deemed safe and well-tolerated by patients when administered every 12 weeks for several treatment cycles.[58] Onabotulinum toxin is starting to be expanded for other headache types; a recent pilot study (although open-label and uncontrolled) showed sphenopalatine injection of onabotulinum toxin decreased the frequency of cluster headache.[59] However, onabotulinum toxin does not seem to be effective for episodic migraine and tension-type headaches.[60]

SUMMARY

Although there is limited evidence from properly controlled studies, peripheral nerve blocks are an increasingly viable treatment option for selected groups of patients with headache, particularly those with intractable headache or facial pain. Local tenderness overlying superficial nerves of the scalp and face might be predictive of good results with local nerve blockade but this too is not yet clear. GON block, the most widely used LA procedure in headache conditions, is particularly effective, safe, and relatively easy to perform in the office. Adverse effects are few and infrequent. These procedures can result in rapid relief of pain and allodynia, and effects may last for several weeks or months. Use of these nerve block procedures and potentially onabotulinum toxin therapy should be expanded for patients with intractable headache disorders who may benefit, although more blinded, sham-controlled studies are needed to firmly establish efficacy and ensure clinical safety.

REFERENCES

1. Levin M. Nerve blocks in the treatment of headache. Neurotherapeutics 2010;7(2):197–203.
2. de Craen AJ, Tijssen JG, de Gans J, et al. Placebo effect in the acute treatment of migraine: subcutaneous placebos are better than oral placebos. J Neurol 2000;247(3):183–8.
3. Headache Classification Committee of the International Headache Society (IHS). The international classification of headache disorders, 3rd edition (beta version). Cephalalgia 2013;33(9):629–808.
4. Strichartz GR. The inhibition of sodium currents in myelinated nerve by quaternary derivatives of lidocaine. J Gen Physiol 1973;62(1):37–57.
5. Anthony M. Cervicogenic headache: prevalence and response to local steroid therapy. Clin Exp Rheumatol 2000;18(2 Suppl 19):S59–64.
6. Ambrosini A, Vandenheede M, Rossi P, et al. Suboccipital injection with a mixture of rapid- and long-acting steroids in cluster headache: a double-blind placebo-controlled study. Pain 2005;118(1–2):92–6.
7. Ashkenazi A, Matro R, Shaw JW, et al. Greater occipital nerve block using local anaesthetics alone or with triamcinolone for transformed migraine: a randomised comparative study. J Neurol Neurosurg Psychiatry 2008;79(4):415–7.
8. Lambru G, Lagrata S, Matharu MS. Cutaneous atrophy and alopecia after greater occipital nerve injection using triamcinolone. Headache 2012;52(10): 1596–9.
9. Shields KG, Levy MJ, Goadsby PJ. Alopecia and cutaneous atrophy after greater occipital nerve infiltration with corticosteroid. Neurology 2004;63(11): 2193–4.
10. Lavin PJ, Workman R. Cushing syndrome induced by serial occipital nerve blocks containing corticosteroids. Headache 2001;41(9):902–4.
11. Campbell JN. Nerve lesions and the generation of pain. Muscle Nerve 2001;24(10):1261–73.
12. Bartsch T, Goadsby PJ. Stimulation of the greater occipital nerve induces increased central excitability of dural afferent input. Brain 2002;125(Pt 7):1496–509.
13. Bartsch T, Goadsby PJ. Increased responses in trigeminocervical nociceptive neurons to cervical input after stimulation of the dura mater. Brain 2003;126(Pt 8):1801–13.
14. Busch V, Jakob W, Juergens T, et al. Functional connectivity between trigeminal and occipital nerves revealed by occipital nerve blockade and nociceptive blink reflexes. Cephalalgia 2006;26(1):50–5.
15. Piovesan EJ, Kowacs PA, Tatsui CE, et al. Referred pain after painful stimulation of the greater occipital nerve in humans: evidence of convergence of cervical afferences on trigeminal nuclei. Cephalalgia 2001;21(2):107–9.
16. Blumenfeld A, Ashkenazi A, Napchan U, et al. Expert consensus recommendations for the performance of peripheral nerve blocks for headaches–a narrative review. Headache 2013;53(3):437–46.
17. Robbins MS, Kuruvilla D, Blumenfeld A, et al. Trigger point injections for headache disorders: expert consensus methodology and narrative review. Headache 2014;54(9):1441–59.
18. Barrington MJ, Watts SA, Gledhill SR, et al. Preliminary results of the Australasian Regional Anaesthesia Collaboration: a prospective audit of more than 7000 peripheral nerve and plexus blocks for neurologic and other complications. Reg Anesth Pain Med 2009;34(6):534–41.
19. Vital JM, Grenier F, Dautheribes M, et al. An anatomic and dynamic study of the greater occipital nerve (n. of Arnold). Applications to the treatment of Arnold's neuralgia. Surg Radiol Anat 1989; 11(3):205–10.

20. Guvencer M, Akyer P, Sayhan S, et al. The importance of the greater occipital nerve in the occipital and the suboccipital region for nerve blockade and surgical approaches: an anatomic study on cadavers. Clin Neurol Neurosurg 2011;113(4):289–94.

21. Anthony M. Headache and the greater occipital nerve. Clin Neurol Neurosurg 1992;94(4):297–301.

22. Rothbart P, Fiedler K, Gale G, et al. A descriptive study of 100 patients undergoing palliative nerve blocks for chronic intractable headache and neck ache. Pain Res Manag 2000;5:243–8.

23. Bovim G, Sand T. Cervicogenic headache, migraine without aura and tension-type headache. Diagnostic blockade of greater occipital and supra-orbital nerves. Pain 1992;51(1):43–8.

24. Leinisch-Dahlke E, Jurgens T, Bogdahn U, et al. Greater occipital nerve block is ineffective in chronic tension type headache. Cephalalgia 2005;25(9): 704–8.

25. Ashkenazi A, Young WB. The effects of greater occipital nerve block and trigger point injection on brush allodynia and pain in migraine. Headache 2005;45(4):350–4.

26. Inan LE, Inan N, Karadas O, et al. Greater occipital nerve blockade for the treatment of chronic migraine: a randomized, multicenter, double-blind, and placebo-controlled study. Acta Neurol Scand 2015;132(4):270–7.

27. Peres MF, Stiles MA, Siow HC, et al. Greater occipital nerve blockade for cluster headache. Cephalalgia 2002;22(7):520–2.

28. Afridi SK, Shields KG, Bhola R, et al. Greater occipital nerve injection in primary headache syndromes: prolonged effects from a single injection. Pain 2006; 122(1–2):126–9.

29. Matute E, Bonilla S, Girones A, et al. Bilateral greater occipital nerve block for post-dural puncture headache. Anaesthesia 2008;63(5):557–8.

30. Weatherall MW. Idiopathic trigeminal neuropathy may respond to greater occipital nerve injection. Cephalalgia 2008;28(6):664–6.

31. Rozen T. Cessation of hemiplegic migraine auras with greater occipital nerve blockade. Headache 2007;47(6):917–9.

32. Dash KS, Janis JE, Guyuron B. The lesser and third occipital nerves and migraine headaches. Plast Reconstr Surg 2005;115(6):1752–8 [discussion: 1759–60].

33. Speciali JG, Goncalves DA. Auriculotemporal neuralgia. Curr Pain Headache Rep 2005;9(4): 277–80.

34. Govindappagari S, Grossman TB, Dayal AK, et al. Peripheral nerve blocks in the treatment of migraine in pregnancy. Obstet Gynecol 2014;124(6):1169–74.

35. Caputi CA, Firetto V. Therapeutic blockade of greater occipital and supraorbital nerves in migraine patients. Headache 1997;37(3):174–9.

36. Dimitriou V, Iatrou C, Malefaki A, et al. Blockade of branches of the ophthalmic nerve in the management of acute attack of migraine. Middle East J Anaesthesiol 2002;16(5):499–504.

37. Guerrero AL, Herrero-Velazquez S, Penas ML, et al. Peripheral nerve blocks: a therapeutic alternative for hemicrania continua. Cephalalgia 2012;32(6): 505–8.

38. Aggarwal A, Kaur H, Gupta T, et al. Anatomical study of the infraorbital foramen: a basis for successful infraorbital nerve block. Clin Anat 2015; 28(6):753–60.

39. Ilhan Alp S, Alp R. Supraorbital and infraorbital nerve blockade in migraine patients: results of 6-month clinical follow-up. Eur Rev Med Pharmacol Sci 2013;17(13):1778–81.

40. Bittar GT, Graff-Radford SB. The effects of streptomycin/lidocaine block on trigeminal neuralgia: a double blind crossover placebo controlled study. Headache 1993;33(3):155–60.

41. Barre F. Cocaine as an abortive agent in cluster headache. Headache 1982;22(2):69–73.

42. Costa A, Pucci E, Antonaci F, et al. The effect of intranasal cocaine and lidocaine on nitroglycerin-induced attacks in cluster headache. Cephalalgia 2000;20(2):85–91.

43. Hardebo JE, Elner A. Nerves and vessels in the pterygopalatine fossa and symptoms of cluster headache. Headache 1987;27(10):528–32.

44. Robbins L. Intranasal lidocaine for cluster headache. Headache 1995;35(2):83–4.

45. Cady RK, Saper J, Dexter K, et al. Long-term efficacy of a double-blind, placebo-controlled, randomized study for repetitive sphenopalatine blockade with bupivacaine vs. saline with the Tx360 device for treatment of chronic migraine. Headache 2015; 55(4):529–42.

46. Mellick GA, Mellick LB. Regional head and face pain relief following lower cervical intramuscular anesthetic injection. Headache 2003;43(10): 1109–11.

47. Aprill C, Axinn MJ, Bogduk N. Occipital headaches stemming from the lateral atlanto-axial (C1-2) joint. Cephalalgia 2002;22(1):15–22.

48. Bogduk N, Marsland A. On the concept of third occipital headache. J Neurol Neurosurg Psychiatry 1986;49(7):775–80.

49. Blumenfeld A, Ashkenazi A, Grosberg B, et al. Patterns of use of peripheral nerve blocks and trigger point injections among headache practitioners in the USA: results of the American Headache Society Interventional Procedure Survey (AHS-IPS). Headache 2010;50(6):937–42.

50. Karadas O, Gul HL, Inan LE. Lidocaine injection of pericranial myofascial trigger points in the treatment of frequent episodic tension-type headache. J Headache Pain 2013;14:44.

51. Karadas O, Inan LE, Ulas U, et al. Efficacy of local lidocaine application on anxiety and depression and its curative effect on patients with chronic tension-type headache. Eur Neurol 2013;70(1–2): 95–101.

52. Garcia-Leiva JM, Hidalgo J, Rico-Villademoros F, et al. Effectiveness of ropivacaine trigger points inactivation in the prophylactic management of patients with severe migraine. Pain Med 2007;8(1): 65–70.

53. Baron EP, Cherian N, Tepper SJ. Role of greater occipital nerve blocks and trigger point injections for patients with dizziness and headache. Neurologist 2011;17(6):312–7.

54. Dodick DW, Turkel CC, DeGryse RE, et al. OnabotulinumtoxinA for treatment of chronic migraine: pooled results from the double-blind, randomized, placebo-controlled phases of the PREEMPT clinical program. Headache 2010;50(6):921–36.

55. Diener HC, Dodick DW, Aurora SK, et al. OnabotulinumtoxinA for treatment of chronic migraine: results from the double-blind, randomized, placebo-controlled phase of the PREEMPT 2 trial. Cephalalgia 2010;30(7):804–14.

56. Whitcup SM, Turkel CC, DeGryse RE, et al. Development of onabotulinumtoxinA for chronic migraine. Ann N Y Acad Sci 2014;1329:67–80.

57. Szok D, Csati A, Vecsei L, et al. Treatment of chronic migraine with onabotulinumtoxinA: mode of action, efficacy and safety. Toxins (Basel) 2015;7(7): 2659–73.

58. Diener HC, Dodick DW, Turkel CC, et al. Pooled analysis of the safety and tolerability of onabotulinumtoxinA in the treatment of chronic migraine. Eur J Neurol 2014;21(6):851–9.

59. Bratbak DF, Nordgard S, Stovner LJ, et al. Pilot study of sphenopalatine injection of onabotulinumtoxinA for the treatment of intractable chronic cluster headache. Cephalalgia 2015;36(6):503–9.

60. Jackson JL, Kuriyama A, Hayashino Y. Botulinum toxin A for prophylactic treatment of migraine and tension headaches in adults: a meta-analysis. JAMA 2012;307(16):1736–45.

Index

Note: Page numbers of article titles are in **boldface** type.

Oral Maxillofacial Surg Clin N Am 28 (2016) 435–442

http://dx.doi.org/10.1016/S1042-3699(16)30051-6

1042-3699/16/$ – see front matter

Printed and bound by CPI Group (UK) Ltd, Croydon, CR0 4YY

08/05/2025

01864686-0010